THE CITY & GUILDS TEXTBOOK

LEVEL 3 ADVANCED TECHNICAL DIPLOMA IN BEAUTY AND SPA THERAPY

HELEN BECKMANN
CLAIRE DAVIS
DEE GERRARD

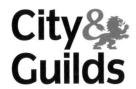

About City & Guilds

City & Guilds is the UK's leading provider of vocational qualifications, offering over 500 awards across a wide range of industries, and progressing from entry level to the highest levels of professional achievement. With over 8500 centres in 100 countries, City & Guilds is recognised by employers worldwide for providing qualifications that offer proof of the skills they need to get the job done.

Equal opportunities

City & Guilds fully supports the principle of equal opportunities and we are committed to satisfying this principle in all our activities and published material. A copy of our equal opportunities policy statement is available on the City & Guilds website.

Copyright

First edition 2016

ISBN 978 0 85193 363 4

Publisher Charlie Evans

Content Development Manager Hannah Cooper

Junior Content Project Manager Loren Bowe

Senior Production Editor Natalie Griffith

Cover design by Select Typesetters Ltd

Typeset by GreenGate Publishing Services, Tonbridge, Kent

Printed in UK by Cambrian Printers Ltd

British Library Cataloguing in Publication Data

A catalogue record is available from the British Library.

Publications

For information about or to order City & Guilds support materials, contact 0844 543 0000 or centresupport@cityandguilds.com. Calls to our 0844 numbers cost 5 pence per minute plus your telephone company's access charge. You can find more information about the materials we have available at www.cityandguilds.com/publications.

Every effort has been made to ensure that the information contained in this publication is true and correct at the time of going to press. However, City & Guilds' products and services are subject to continuous development and improvement and the right is reserved to change products and services from time to time. City & Guilds cannot accept liability for loss or damage arising from the use of information in this publication.

City & Guilds
1 Giltspur Street
London EC1A 9DD

www.cityandguilds.com
publishingfeedback@cityandguilds.com

CONTENTS

ACKNOWLEDGEMENTS

I would like to thank my family for their understanding and support – my husband Howard, my children Connor and Alexandra, and my mother Hazel.

Helen Beckmann

Thank you in particular to my wonderful family: Andy, Amy and Beth and my Mum who have supported me during the writing of this book – for their love and understanding.

Claire Davis

City & Guilds would like to sincerely thank the following:

For invaluable beauty therapy expertise

Janice Brown, Sarah Fillaudeau, Claire Davis, Anita Crosland, Emma Mackay

For taking photos

Phil Jones Photography

For supplying pictures for the front cover

Shutterstock, Phil Jones Photography

For their help with photoshoots

Loren Bowe, Janice Brown, Hannah Cutler, Tony Davis, Diana Docwra, Sarah Fillaudeau, Sasha Fillaudeau, Manjit Gill, Grace Gray, Natalie Griffith, Nicki Hobbs, Sherry-Lee Jackson, Victoria Painting, Kelly Rawlings, Emma Yeoman, Cambridge Regional College.

PICTURE CREDITS

Every effort has been made to acknowledge all copyright holders as below and the publishers will, if notified, correct any errors in future editions.

Alamy ©Peter S Noyce p67; **Andrew Buckle/Andover College** pp34, 66, 74, 75, 88, 91, 92, 111, 479; **Andrew Buckle/Bedford College** pp49, 53, 58, 68, 72, 81, 84; **Andrew Buckle/Cambridge Regional College** pp47, 104, 344, 470, 471, 479, 508, 539; **Andrew Buckle/ Canterbury College** pp77, 101, 106, 257, 262; **Andrew Buckle/ Havering College** pp4, 20, 24, 65; **Andrew Buckle/Hertford Regional College** pp83, 88, 105, 109, 158, 379; **Andrew Buckle/ Warwickshire College** pp14, 59, 84, 87, 259, 494, 495, 499, 501, 503, 504, 505, 506, 510, 552, 555; **The Carlton Spa and Beauty Group** pp321, 322, 327, 389; **Di Vapor** p511; **Elemis** p107; **Epping Forest College** p21; **FakeBake** pp477, 478; **Glow Images** ©Superstock p79; **iStock photo** ©Dušan Kosti´c p179, ©Grzegorz Kula p179, ©Scott Harms p205, ©scottjay p150, ©Simon Ivarsson p165, ©Stanislav Komogorov p158, ©Ziga Lisjak pp149, 179; **Health and Safety Executive** p183; **House of Famuir Limited** (HoF) pp 321, 322, 335, 342, 402, 404, 418; **Jessica Cosmetics** p113; **Lash FX** pp535, 536, 537, 544, 539; **London College of Beauty Therapy** pp108, 111, 327, 330, 331, 334, 345, 350, 384, 441; **Phil Jones Photography** pp 1, 2, 5, 14, 21, 22, 24, 25, 28, 29, 32, 35, 36, 37, 40, 56, 60, 75, 96, 98, 100, 102, 103, 105, 255, 266, 271, 273, 275-280, 283, 284, 287-304, 305, 306, 308, 313, 314, 315, 317, 320, 321, 323-325, 327, 329, 330, 332, 334, 337-338, 341, 351-353, 358, 359, 361, 365, 367, 375, 381-382, 388, 390-391, 392, 396-397, 399, 402, 403, 405, 417, 418, 419, 421, 422, 423, 438-440, 444, 451, 456, 463-467, 469, 471, 472, 475, 480-484, 491, 496, 513, 514, 515, 517, 518, 519, 520-523, 527, 529, 530, 538, 540-543, 545, 547, 548, 549, 551, 553, 556, 559, 561-563, 565, 567-570; **PAT** p71; **Pierre Marcar/ Kent Beauty Academy** pp81-83, 305, 393-395, 453; **Rex Features** ©CDC-Collins/Phanie p153; **Royal International** p327; **Science Photo Library** pp153, 180, ©Alexander Tsiaras p180, ©BSIP Guillaume p147, ©Dr. Chris Hale p161, ©CNRI p142, ©Cordelia Molloy p140, ©David Parker p150, ©Dr Harout Tanielian pp140, 146, ©Dr H.C.Robinson p145, ©James Stevenson p149, ©JOTI p533, ©Dr. Ken Greer/Visuals Unlimited, Inc. p148, ©Life In View p148, ©Mauro Fermariello p141, ©Dr P. Marazzin pp5, 66, 141, 143,146, 148, 149, 150, 152, 153, 154, 162, 165, 180, 181, 269, 309, 533, 534; ©Scott Camazine p318,

Disclaimer

Please note that all of the equipment and products shown in this book are examples to illustrate what you may use in your learning centre and/or salon. There are a range of different brands available and whilst City & Guilds do not promote one brand over another, we recommend that you use equipment and products from the same brand when carrying out specific treatments. In most instances, these items have been constructed and formulated specifically to work in harmony with other equipment and products of the same brand and we cannot guarantee compatibility or end results with other brands. If you are unsure as to whether certain equipment or a product of one brand can be used in conjunction with another, please consult your supervisor or contact the brand's company directly for further advice.

CITY & GUILDS' NATIONAL ADVISORY COMMITTEE FOR BEAUTY

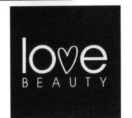
MAC

City & Guilds

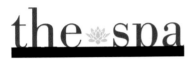
the spa

BABTAC MEMBER

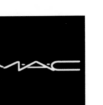
HALE
COUNTRY CLUB & SPA

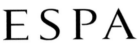
ESPA

susancressy spa & beauty therapy in practice

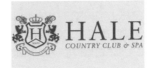
love
BEAUTY

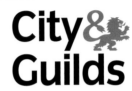
Sb
Sanctum Beauty

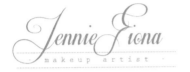
Jennie Fiona
makeup artist

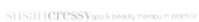
CR citrusrooms

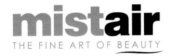
mistair
THE FINE ART OF BEAUTY

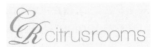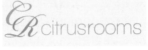
essie
USA's nail salon expert. Since 1981.
PROFESSIONAL APPLICATION

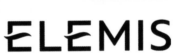
ELEMIS

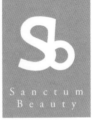
CheshireSkinClinic

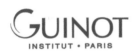
GUINOT
INSTITUT · PARIS

HOUSE OF FAMUIR
COSMETIC, HEALTH & BEAUTY

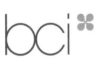
bci
beauty concepts international

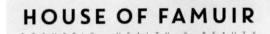
STEREX
ELECTROLYSIS INTERNATIONAL LIMITED

TAMARIND

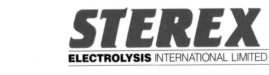
L'ORÉAL
PARIS

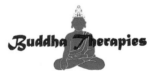
Buddha Therapies

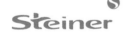
Steiner

CNHC
Complementary & Natural
Healthcare Council

benefit
SAN FRANCISCO

"Award Winning"
Holistic Health Spa and Clinic
www.buddhatherapies.com
http://www.buddhatherapiesnutrition.co.uk/

CARLTON
Professional

19 25

DECLÉOR
PARIS

JESSICA

dermalogica

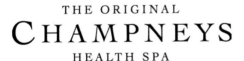
THE ORIGINAL
CHAMPNEYS
HEALTH SPA

Gemini
beauty

g GERRARD
INTERNATIONAL

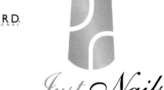
Just Nails
& a little beauty

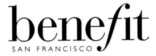
LAVASHELLS®

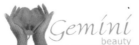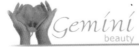
JO MALONE
LONDON

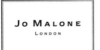
FHT
Federation
of Holistic
Therapists

accredited
voluntary
register

ABOUT THE AUTHORS

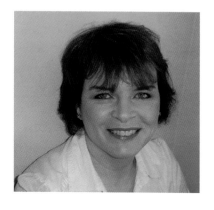

Helen Beckmann

Helen has worked in aspects related to the beauty therapy industry since she completed her qualifications 30 years ago. During this time she has worked for several salons, taught in further and higher education, been a national and international examiner, External Quality Assurer, and a consultant for City & Guilds for the past 14 years. She has owned her own beauty and holistic therapies salon where she managed three therapists, continuing to practise up until two years ago. She has a keen interest in updating her skills and continuing her professional development. She is at present in her final year of study for her second degree.

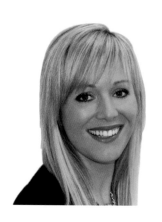

Claire Davis

Claire has worked in the beauty industry for 23 years, after studying fashion, interior design, and beauty therapy to Level 4 standard. She ran her own beauty salons for 10 years and set up a training academy 15 years ago. She expanded into the world of digital virtual learning and developed Virtual Beauty training resources. From here, she has been working with City & Guilds, project managing the Level 3 video e-learning and SmartScreen resources. She is a firm believer that working with determination is all you need to achieve your goals in life.

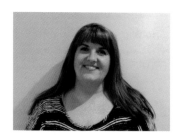

Dee Gerrard

After training as a beauty and holistic therapist, Dee has worked in salons, freelance, in her own salon and then in education. She loves working with people and even after 20 years says she still gets a buzz from learning new treatments and techniques. Dee became a college lecturer as she needed a new challenge; she feels that it has been a very rewarding career and she has been lucky enough to work with some great teams and people especially at the Manchester College. Her aim has always been to improve the standards and professionalism of therapists joining our industry today and she feels that she is very fortunate to have a career where she can do that.

ABOUT THE CONTRIBUTORS

Anna Allington

Provide electrical epilation

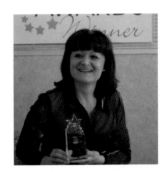

Anna has been a qualified beauty/holistic therapist for over 25 years, with a portfolio that includes teaching in further education, coordinating training for a European health spa, examining internationally, consultancy work through international seminars and practical workshops to improve and update skills in all areas of the beauty therapy industry. Anna currently owns Academia International – Beauty Therapy Training Ltd, which is based in Oxfordshire and has an active role in training students to Levels 2, 3 and 4 Beauty Therapy. Her ethos for success is commitment, quality, hard work and a passion for beauty therapy, which encourages all of her students to establish fulfilling careers within the health and beauty industry.

Penny Hallworth

Promote and sell products and services to clients

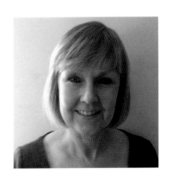

Penny has over 30 years' experience in the beauty industry. Her career has covered salon therapy, teaching in further education and various roles in the cruise ship spa sector, from therapist to supervisor overseeing spa standards and business and latterly becoming Head of Training at the Steiner Training Academy. Penny loves to use her experience in beauty to teach and inspire others to deliver the best customer experience and develop great business skills. She is currently teaching and training at various establishments in the education and business sectors.

Andrea Plimmer

Monitor and maintain the client's spa journey and provide dry spa treatments

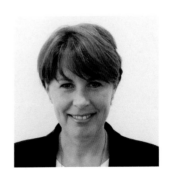

Andrea Plimmer is Director of Vocational Education at Trafford College, having previously managed hairdressing, beauty therapy, spa, hospitality, travel and tourism at the college. She has extensive knowledge and experience of the beauty and spa industry over the past 20 years including working in the UK, overseas and on cruise ships. She currently teaches on a foundation degree in spa management and is the co-author of several beauty resource packs and a Level 2 and 3 spa book. She has combined her passion for the spa industry and travel into inspiring students through education and training.

FOREWORD

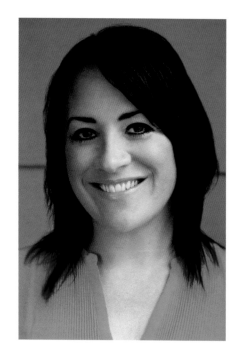

I have been working in the beauty and spa therapy industry for over 20 years and have absolutely loved every second. My initial training equipped me with the skills, knowledge and confidence to enable me to have a successful and varied career. This industry has presented exciting opportunities for me, such as working in salons and health spas, presenting on television and moving into Further Education, to both teach and manage a beauty therapy department. I also worked as a consultant for City & Guilds producing and developing qualification content and assessment material for the UK and international markets. I now work as the Hair and Beauty Portfolio Manager within City & Guilds and look after all of the national and international qualifications for beauty and spa therapy, nail technology, media, theatrical and special effects make-up, complementary therapies, hairdressing and barbering.

In response to the changing educational landscape and the desire to re-shape our portfolio offer in line with employer needs, City & Guilds have produced this fantastic textbook to help support you with your chosen qualification. A career in beauty or spa therapy will provide you with an incredible industry to work in and a City & Guilds qualification is recognised across the world. This textbook has a number of inspirational features and will give you a broad insight into the practical and underpinning knowledge required to complete your qualification. It's also a great reference tool once you are qualified. The images, step-by-step guides and end-of-unit 'Test your knowledge' questions all work really well together to give you a comprehensive support resource. The authors and contributors have fantastic breadth and depth of knowledge between them and are well thought of in the education sector and beauty industry, so you are learning from the best!

Beauty and spa therapies are diverse and exciting – whether you choose to work in salons, spas, hotels or cruise ships, you career will be inspirational and challenging. It's a wonderful and global industry to work in. I would like to take this opportunity to wish all who are studying the City & Guilds Level 3 Advanced Technical Diploma in Beauty & Spa Therapy the very best of luck throughout their chosen careers.

Emma Mackay

Hair and Beauty Portfolio Manager
City & Guilds

HOW TO USE THIS TEXTBOOK

The chapters in this textbook are numbered to match the units in your City & Guilds Level 3 Advanced Technical Diploma in Beauty and Spa Therapy qualification. Each chapter covers everything you will need to understand in order to complete your end assessment.

Each unit in the qualification makes reference to values and behaviours, and health and safety. This textbook has two separate chapters dedicated to these areas, so you can refer to the chapters directly for in-depth information whenever you see the values and behaviours or health and safety boxes in the margins.

Throughout this textbook you will see the following features:

HANDY HINT

Spas with an ice room encourage clients to rub ice all over their bodies to cool down and get an invigorating sensation.

HANDY HINTS are particularly useful tips that can assist you in your revision or help you remember something important.

Iontophoresis

The introduction of water-soluble substances into the skin.

KEY WORDS in bold in the text are explained in the margin to aid your understanding.

INDUSTRY TIP

The left kidney sits slightly higher than the right.

INDUSTRY TIPS are useful tips that will help you in the workplace.

WHY DON'T YOU...
Look at your bare foot. Can you make out any of the bones of the tarsals?

WHY DON'T YOU ... boxes suggest ideas to help you practise and learn.

Activity

Research endometriosis. Present your findings in an interesting way.

ACTIVITIES help to test your understanding and learn from your colleagues' experiences.

VALUES & BEHAVIOURS

Identifying the client's expectations

Communicating with clients

VALUES AND BEHAVIOURS boxes link to the sections in the Values and behaviours chapter for you to recap learning.

Watch a video of body analysis on SmartScreen (unit 305).

SmartScreen icons indicate where there is an accompanying video of a consultation or treatment routine available.

HEALTH AND SAFETY boxes link to sections in the health and safety chapter for you to recap learning.

The green IMPROVE YOUR MATHS badge identifies items that combine improving your understanding of beauty and spa therapy with practising or improving your maths skills.

The purple IMPROVE YOUR ENGLISH badge identifies items that combine improving your understanding of beauty and spa therapy with practising or improving your English skills.

At the end of each chapter are some 'Test your knowledge' questions. These are multiple-choice questions, designed to prepare you for assessment and to identify any areas where you might need further training or revision.

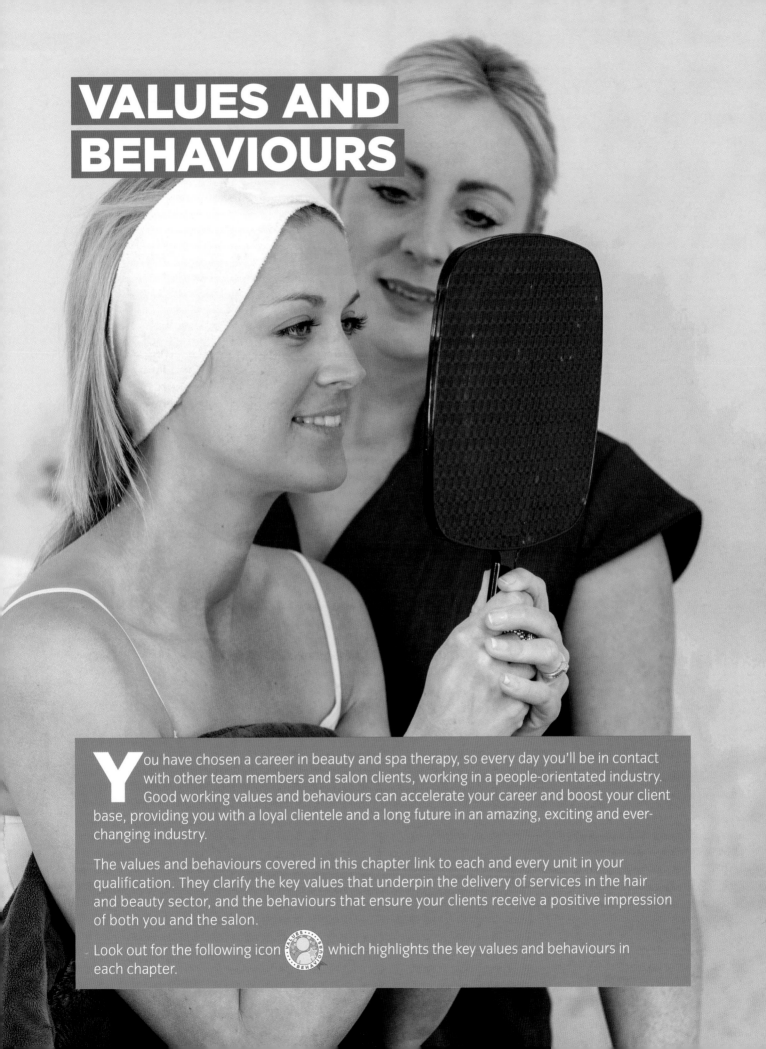

VALUES AND BEHAVIOURS

You have chosen a career in beauty and spa therapy, so every day you'll be in contact with other team members and salon clients, working in a people-orientated industry. Good working values and behaviours can accelerate your career and boost your client base, providing you with a loyal clientele and a long future in an amazing, exciting and ever-changing industry.

The values and behaviours covered in this chapter link to each and every unit in your qualification. They clarify the key values that underpin the delivery of services in the hair and beauty sector, and the behaviours that ensure your clients receive a positive impression of both you and the salon.

Look out for the following icon which highlights the key values and behaviours in each chapter.

Values

Values are our working ethics, the moral code we work to, and our principles and beliefs. Every person is unique and his or her personal views will vary, but when working in the beauty sector we need to standardise our ideals, and follow and promote the expected industry values set out in this chapter.

Willingness to learn

When working in the beauty therapy industry, you must be prepared to work hard. Being on your feet all day, working with the general public and learning new skills all require a strong disposition. You'll need motivation and enthusiasm for this kind of work, and a keenness and eagerness to learn new skills.

You'll need to be ready and prepared for every eventuality, such as:

- clients arriving without appointments
- clients and therapists running behind appointment times
- changes to appointments and services booked
- absent team members
- the ever-changing fashions and skills required to maintain your career.

Being a willing participator in the spa/salon and focusing on the high standards required from your spa/salon will help you to improve your performance and develop your career.

Complete services in a commercially viable time

Working to a commercially viable time when carrying out services in the salon or spa is important. Clients are allocated a time when they book their beauty appointment and they expect that appointment to run to time. There are times when appointments will run late: this may be because clients are late for appointments or occasionally services overrun, but you will be expected to complete most of your services in the timeframes allocated to ensure the spa/salon operates as smoothly as possible.

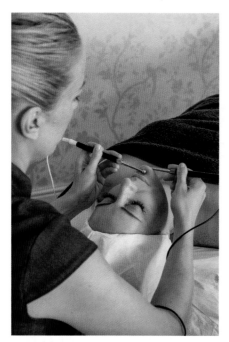
Complete the service in a viable time

VALUES & BEHAVIOURS

You will carry out services on a variety of people: some will have different values from you, and some will have different backgrounds, upbringing, cultures, religion and beliefs and may behave unexpectedly. You will need to learn to adapt to these differences and respect other people's values, beliefs and points of view, even if you do not share them.

Activity

If you failed to work to commercially viable times or clients were regularly later to appointments, the spa/salon would run behind schedule. If you have eight clients booked in your appointment column today and run 12 minutes late with every client, how late will you be leaving?

THE CITY & GUILDS TEXTBOOK

Organisational and industry standards of appearance

Within the beauty therapy industry, personal appearance and the spa/salon's dress code can vary immensely. Some spa salons have a uniform such as a tunic and trousers or a dress and a colour preference such as all black. Always ensure you prepare your work clothes in advance with a clean, ironed uniform.

Your appearance

Along with the receptionist, every member of the team should look presentable and represent the industry and their salon. Ensure you allow enough time before work to prepare yourself for your working day.

The following diagram shows areas of appearance that are important.

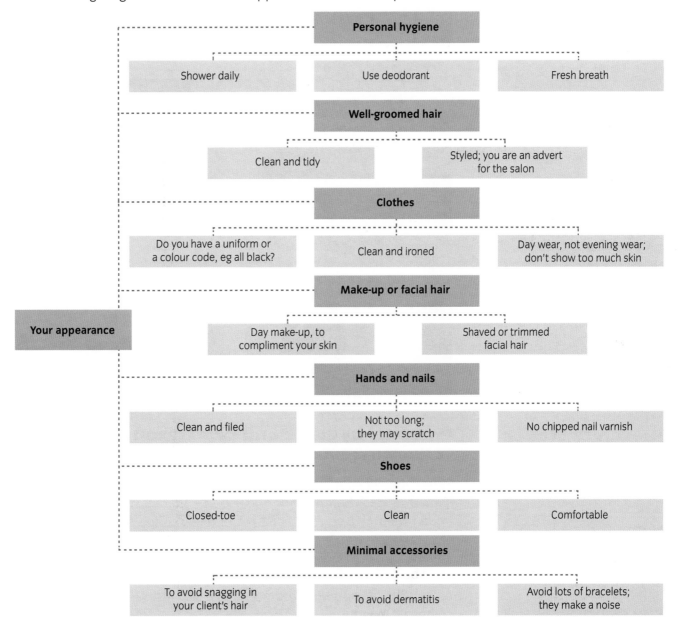

Activity

Which of these photos give positive impressions of the therapist and which give negative impressions?

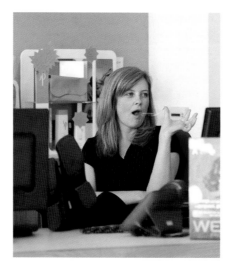 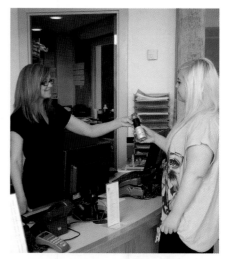

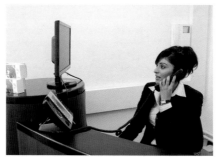 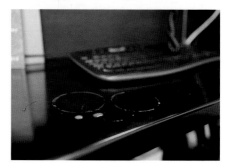

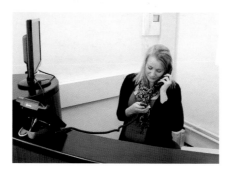 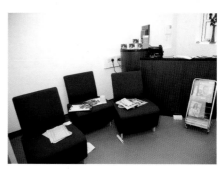

Personal hygiene and protection requirements

Start your day after a good night's rest, ensuring you brush your teeth, shower or wash before work, and use a deodorant. Wear a clean, ironed uniform. If you are a smoker, or enjoy coffee or spicy foods, always ensure you have mints or similar handy to freshen your breath. Your hair should always represent the industry you are in and look clean and tidy and off your face. You may choose to wear a little make-up to help you look well groomed, and nails must be clean and not chipped if painted.

Maintain personal hygiene

Staff should ensure that their own personal hygiene is maintained; this is how:

- Shower before work.
- Wear clean clothes.
- Wear deodorant.
- Brush your teeth every morning.
- Ensure your hair is clean and tied back off your face.
- Keep breath fresh throughout the day.
- Do not attend work with infectious conditions.

For safety reasons, wear closed-toed flat shoes. Never wear open-toed shoes, as you may injure yourself if you drop any sharp objects such as tweezers on them. Avoid wearing jewellery so that you don't catch your client's skin.

Activity

Identify infectious conditions that may keep you away from work.

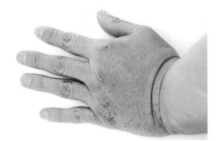
Dermatitis

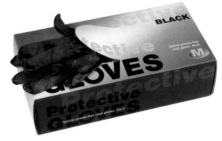
Wear non-latex disposable gloves

Protect your hands and clothes

It is important to protect your hands to avoid occupational dermatitis. Dermatitis can occur when your skin comes into contact with substances that can irritate the skin and cause allergies. Dermatitis is not contagious to others but it can spread around your own skin. Although most commonly found on the hands, it can appear on the face, lips, arms and cause irritation to the eyes. The good news is that it can be avoided. Follow these five simple steps to healthy hands:

1 Wear non-latex disposable gloves.
2 Dry your hands thoroughly after wetting.
3 Moisturise your hands regularly.
4 Use new gloves for every client.
5 Check your hands regularly for signs of contact dermatitis.

INDUSTRY TIP

Remember: poor standards of health and hygiene can cause offence to your clients, spread germs and allow cross-contamination.

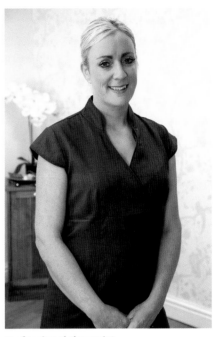
Professional therapist

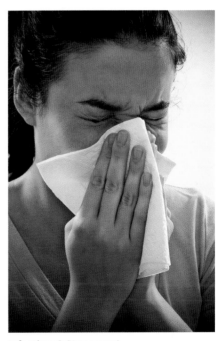
Infectious? Stay away!

Dermatitis can be recognised by the skin's:

- dryness
- itchiness
- redness
- cracking
- bleeding and swelling
- blistering.

PPE (personal protective equipment) for the therapist and the assistant includes:

- gloves to protect your hands from products
- an apron to protect your clothes from product damage.

If you suffer from asthma or allergies, wear a mask, particularly when spray tanning or using any products that may be particularly strong-smelling or give off fumes, eg nail products.

Flexible working attitudes

Where possible, have an adaptable approach to your daily work and always expect the unexpected. Be willing to change your working pattern to suit the needs of the business, and try to be flexible during your working day to meet client demands, without affecting other client services. Be respectful to all staff, visitors and clients and understand that everyone has differences: this includes values and beliefs, religion and culture, and personal views.

You need to be able to adapt to different situations, such as working under pressure or dealing with a regular client.

Would you treat a regular client differently if the spa salon were busy or quiet? How would you react if you were short of staff in the spa salon, or had to deal with a power failure?

> **VALUES & BEHAVIOURS**
>
> Treat everyone equally, ensuring that you do not make any unsuitable comments regarding age, gender, disability, sexual orientation, race, religion, marital status, and so on.

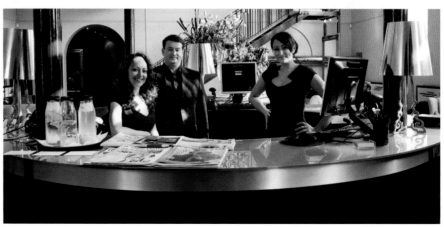

Teamwork makes a great salon

How to adapt to different situations

A routine service	A busy salon	A quiet salon	Staff shortages	Power failure
You should already have built a good rapport with your regular clients, but this doesn't mean you don't need to try. Treat all clients like it's their first visit and impress them every time.	Make sure you give every client the attention they deserve, no matter how busy you are. Apologise if you're running a little late with the service and explain that the salon is busy. Reassure your client that you have plenty of time for their service. Don't panic and don't rush the service.	If you're not busy, don't assume your client isn't. Don't slow down the service. Use the extra time you have to discuss and promote products and services to the client and give extra advice.	If you have staff absences to cope with, always explain the situation to your clients. If they understand the situation they are more likely to sympathise and not get upset if services run late. If a therapist is absent, check whether anyone else can look after the client and work together as a team to manage the workload together. Remain calm, work methodically and do not rush your services.	Your salon should have a **contingency plan** for emergencies such as a power failure. Try to contact all clients in advance to warn them of the power failure and offer an alternative appointment time. Ask if they would prefer an alternative treatment if you are unable to use the equipment that requires power. If the power fails in the middle of a service your manager will tell you what the salon procedure is. Remain calm, reassure your client that the treatment will be completed or you will offer her an alternative treatment. Remain professional. Remember – you can cope!

Activity

Consider your strengths and areas to develop. List the tasks and roles where you need to develop further and how you are going to do this.

Contingency plan

Back-up or secondary plan.

In a team meeting, allow 15 minutes for each staff member to create a mission statement that creates focus on the business. Discuss as a team your statements and why you chose them.

(Materials needed: pens, paper.)

The entire team now choose a single statement or vision that represents the business. At the end of this activity, make sure that all spellings, grammar and punctuation are accurate and decide on the mission statement you are going to use for the business.

Teamwork and assisting others

A salon operates effectively when everyone works as a team, and with one common goal – the client experience being the main focus.

Maintain customer care

Client care is paramount in establishing effective relationships, so ensure you always treat clients well.

This is how to treat your clients:

- Respect them.
- Look after their belongings.
- Protect their clothes.
- Show an interest.
- Listen to them.
- Offer advice.
- Discuss their outcome of the treatment.

Respect diversity of clients

If your client has mobility problems, discuss with them the best way you can adapt the treatment so they are comfortable and can enjoy it.

If your client arrives wearing a head scarf or burka, ask them if this is for religious purposes. If so, ask how you can carry out their treatment while respecting their religion. Can you ensure there aren't any males around if a Muslim lady has her hair on show? Maybe you could offer them a later appointment when the salon is quieter or before or after opening hours?

If you have a client who is transgender, you may be unsure of how your client would like to be referred to – male or female. It is okay to ask your client how they would like to be referred to, and this will prevent you from offending them. Build a relationship with your client so that they feel they can discuss things with you and they feel comfortable with the choices they have made.

Communicate with your client

The first impressions of the salon will start at reception so ensure that the reception area is neat and tidy. A selection of up-to-date magazines for clients to read while they wait for their appointment may keep them happy if the service is running late. Always communicate with clients, advise them if the therapist is running a little late and offer them a drink to make them feel at ease.

Salon staff should always:

- speak politely
- introduce themselves
- welcome and greet the client by their name
- generally refer to the client by name
- offer refreshments
- give advice about products and services available in the salon.

Salon staff should not:

- chew gum
- leave the reception unattended
- let the phone ring more than three times
- make a client wait to be attended to
- take personal calls
- use jargon or technical terms.

When questioning and talking with clients, you are using your communication skills. Remember that how you communicate can make a positive or negative impression on your client of you and your salon.

Activity

Which of the following comments are good and which are poor? From the poor sentences you identify, how would you rephrase them to make them better?

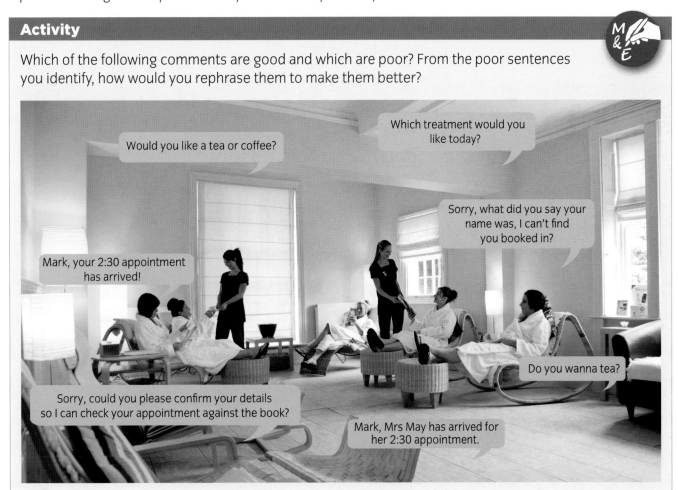

Positive attitudes

You spend many hours at work, so working relationships are important. Be helpful and friendly to your co-workers; smile, avoid sarcasm, control your reactions, be appreciative, and be happy with other people's success. Offer encouragement and give genuine compliments to others, such as: 'congratulations on your promotion', 'your client's nails looked lovely', 'you look nice' and so on.

Statistics show that people working in the beauty industry are some of the happiest people at work. Enjoy your job and have fun while working; look your best, remain optimistic and upbeat and get back up, even after a fall. Set yourself goals and go after them, and don't complain if things don't go your way – just try again next time.

Professional behaviour

It is important to be professional at all times, both in the salon environment and outside of the salon. It is important when wearing your uniform outside of the salon that you remain professional as people may recognise where you work or you may be seen by clients. The way in which a person behaves reflects on the image of the salon.

Acting in a professional way gives out the message that you are a dependable and responsible person. It also gives people confidence in your ability to do your job well.

Professional behaviour includes:

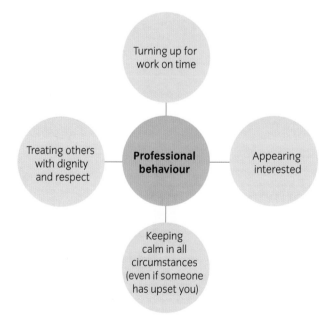

Turning up for work on time

Appearing interested

Keeping calm in all circumstances (even if someone has upset you)

Treating others with dignity and respect

Professional behaviour

Following the standards of your profession/industry codes of conduct means:

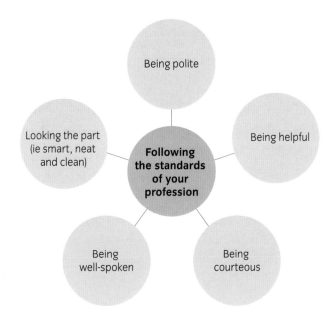

Negative behaviour

If you don't act in a professional way, it can lead to friction and upset within the workplace. Negative behaviour will often have an impact on everyone within the working environment.

Negative behaviour will have an impact on everyone you work with, including both internal and external colleagues. Negativity is stressful for everyone. It can create a poor working environment and can lead to conflict within the team.

> **HANDY HINT**
>
> If someone has upset you, discuss it with them face to face. Always be constructive, communicate clearly and in a friendly manner, and don't talk about them behind their back.

> **HANDY HINT**
>
> Remember that everyone is different and value everyone's opinion even if you do not agree with them. Treat people fairly and professionally.

Personal and professional ethics

Your personal ethics and your salon's professional ethics are often very similar, because they are about right and wrong. Although professional ethics are more formal than our personal ethics they both generally involve treating people correctly, being honest and fair.

Personal ethics

Personal ethics are very subjective and individual. Our beliefs are formed by our everyday life experiences and our background, and can vary from person to person. Personal opinions, those of family and friends, our communities, culture or religion may form our views on what is morally right or wrong. Our personal beliefs are reflected in how we interact, respect and treat people, how honest and fair we are and even how loyal we are to our employers.

> **HANDY HINT**
>
> If you make a mistake at work, admit to it. Problems are far easier to rectify if the salon is aware of the problem and the situation can be resolved quickly. Therefore it is less likely to affect the salon services. Your honesty and open apology are more likely to earn you respect from your colleagues, rather than disdain as a result of the error itself.

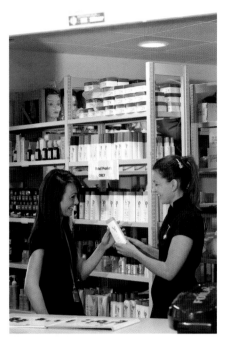

Help your colleagues

HANDY HINT

It is important to remain objective and follow your salon's professional ethics, even if this means reporting a colleague for doing something wrong, as this may affect the running of the business.

Activity

Discuss with a colleague what you would do if you encountered the following scenarios:

- You realise after a client has left the salon that you accidentally charged them too much for their beauty treatment.

- You accidentally spill a product on your client's trousers.

- A colleague has confided in you that they have taken some beauty products from the retail stand for personal use.

- A colleague has taken a client's phone number from their record card for personal use.

When you and your colleague have discussed how you would deal with the above scenarios, present your answers to other colleagues. Clearly explain why and how you came to your conclusions.

Professional ethics

Professional ethics are more about company rules and regulations, what we must adhere to when working with clients and co-workers. It includes the salon code of conduct and may include client confidentiality, respecting the diversity of clients and co-workers, reporting concerns that may affect the salon business and following legal requirements. It should also include how the company and others treat you.

Self-management

Being a self-manager is important in work; it helps you organise yourself, take ownership of your own responsibilities, and take the initiative with change. Self-management is about taking charge of your own future, working towards goals, taking and managing risks, dealing with pressure and managing your emotions. It's your contribution to your work – being organised, responding positively to change, planning and managing your time effectively. If you can't self-manage, you may struggle to progress through life and advance with your career. Failing to manage yourself could lead to unhappiness and potentially unemployment.

Take the initiative, set yourself clear goals and targets to work towards, self-appraise and reflect on your own strengths and weaknesses and monitor your own progress. Ask for feedback from peers and your employer and take on board their criticism.

Self-management skills

A good self-manager:

- manages and adapts to change, takes risks and seeks advice
- has a flexible and adaptable approach to work and learning
- manages emotion, anger, conflict and stress
- thinks outside the box – problem-solving
- works towards goals, showing initiative, commitment and perseverance
- deals with competing pressures and builds self-confidence.

Activity

Write a career progression plan about where you want to be in six months' time, one year and where you would like to be in five years' time. Add achievable personal SMARTER targets to work towards.

SMARTER targets:

- Specific – what exactly do you need to do/achieve?
- Measurable – how will you know you have achieved the target?
- Agreed – do both you and your manager agree on and understand what the target is that has been set?
- Realistic – are you realistically likely to be able to achieve the target and is it relevant to your role and ability?
- Time-bound – when do you need to achieve the target by?
- Evaluated – what is the date that has been set to evaluate progress so far?
- Reviewed – what is the date that has been set to review the outcomes?

At the end of the activity, check your spellings, punctuation and grammar. Make sure it reads well and, if need be, ask someone else to check it for you too.

Creativity

If you think of a great idea, but don't do anything with it, you are imaginative, not creative. Creativity is about thinking of something and then acting on it. You can bring your creative thinking into your workplace to create new treatments, for example.

Being creative, using your imagination and producing ideas and having the commitment to drive these forward are skills that employers are calling out for. It can take courage to express your ideas though – fear

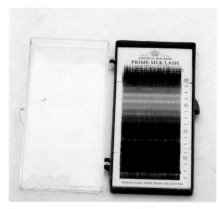

You can bring your creativity to the workplace

of ridicule or lack of interest can sometimes prevent us from speaking out loud and expressing our ideas. So be brave and rather than think 'I can't', think 'why not?'

When thinking creatively you need to generate and explore your ideas and those of others. Sometimes you need to work alone but at times you need to know when to work together. You'll need to explore ideas, experiment and practise, learn from mistakes and make adaptations to the original concept, ask questions and maybe observe others at work. Try keeping an ideas book, noting your visions and writing down what inspires you, as this may prevent great ideas being forgotten about.

Communication techniques

In the salon, spa or nail studio, the majority of communication with people is face to face. However, there is a growing trend towards the use of technology (eg email, text messaging and social media sites such as Facebook and Twitter). It is important to be aware of the effect that distance can have on communication.

During conversation only 7% of what we communicate comes from the words we use, 38% comes from the tone of voice we use to say the words and 55% comes from our body language or non-verbal communication. You can therefore see how important it is to pay attention to your tone of voice when communicating over the phone. The tone of your voice will say far more than the words you use.

The way we communicate can be divided into three categories:

- verbal communication
- non-verbal communication
- listening skills.

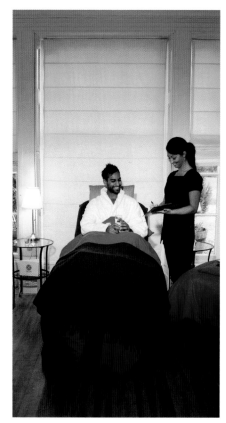

A therapist talking to her client

Verbal communication

Verbal communication is any communication that is spoken and includes sounds such as laughing or any noises we may make to agree with something or confirm a decision (eg uh-huh). When speaking to people you need to be aware of how you are speaking to them. You must make sure you:

- are not aggressive
- speak clearly and calmly
- do not use technical jargon unless it is necessary.

In order to establish and manage a client's expectations, it is necessary to ask them questions. There are two types of questions:

- open questions
- closed questions.

HANDY HINT

When addressing your colleagues and clients you will not speak to them in the same way as you do to your friends. You need to speak to colleagues and clients in a more formal and professional manner.

Open questions

Open questions are used to start a conversation and find out information. They allow you to find out information as they give the client a chance to give you a more detailed response. Open questions often begin with what, why, when and how. During a consultation, a therapist is likely to ask the following types of open questions:

- What causes your stress?
- Which treatments have you had before?
- How does your skin feel normally?

Closed questions

Closed questions are used to:

- confirm information (eg Can I confirm that your appointment is for an Indian head massage?)
- get a short response – yes or no (eg Is that pressure firm enough?)

close a conversation or shorten it if the client is talkative (eg Is there anything else I can help you with today?).

Tone of voice

You will need to adapt your tone of voice to the treatment that you are doing. During a quiet treatment such as a body massage you would speak clearly in a soft, friendly tone, but while working on someone's nails, you would chat at a normal tone and be able to express yourself more freely through your voice. Smile when you speak because it softens how you sound and look. When emphasising a point or asking a question, raise your voice a little at the end of the sentence. Always remain courteous and never talk to colleagues loudly in a salon/spa. If you need some help from a therapist, ask politely and respectfully. Never display any animosity that may be present in the team or engage in idle chat with a colleague when you should be focused on your client.

Telephone manners

When you answer the telephone, smile, as it shows in your voice; speak clearly and say good morning/afternoon to the caller. Always state your name, to let the caller know who they are speaking to.

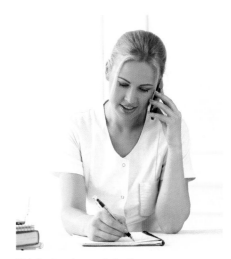

Think about your telephone manners

Activity

In groups, discuss examples of poor telephone manners and think about your own experiences.

Activity

From the following list, which is the best way to answer the phone and why?

- Hello, Indulgence. Can I help you?
- Good afternoon, Indulgence Beauty Salon. Sarah speaking. How may I help you?
- Good morning, Sarah speaking. How can I help?
- Hello, Sarah at Indulgence speaking. Can I help you?

Non-verbal communication

When communicating with clients, it is very important that you listen. Always give your clients enough time to express their wishes, and smile and nod to acknowledge you understand. Maintain eye contact and show an interest in what is being said.

Body language

When you communicate you do so verbally and non-verbally. Body language is a method of non-verbal communication and can be positive as well as negative. It can give away secrets about whether you are telling the truth, listening to your client and interested in what your client is saying.

Non-verbal communication and body language include:

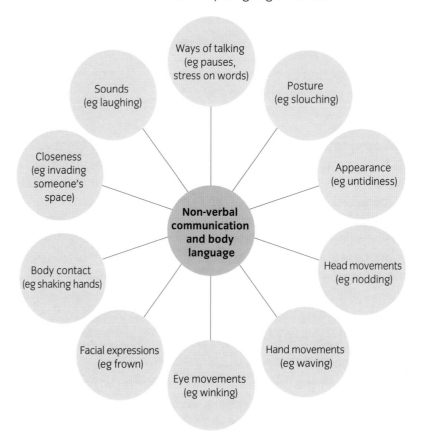

Engage in positive body language by:

- smiling – you are happy and approachable
- maintaining eye contact – you are listening
- having a good open body posture – you are alert and ready for work
- keeping a little distance – respect for personal space
- showing open palms – openness and honesty.

Watch out for negative body language, which includes:

- crossed arms, closed-in body posture – defensive behaviour and a closed mind

- talking with your hand in front of your mouth – you are not being honest or truthful

- scratching behind the ear or rubbing the back of the neck – the listener is uncertain

- poor posture – unprofessional and indicates tiredness.

Written communication

Written communication is anything that includes written words, not just letters. Some types of written communication include:

- websites
- posters
- email
- price lists
- blogs
- Twitter
- text messages
- Facebook (social media)
- aftercare leaflets
- client record cards
- leaflets.

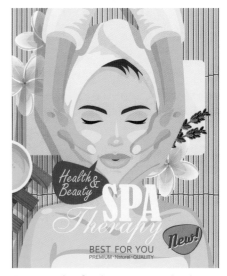

An example of written communication

Any written information relating to the salon or spa should be clear and **concise**. You should proofread, spell check and check the grammar in any material before it is issued as it is a representation of your salon or spa because it reflects on your professional image.

Concise

Short.

Email and text messaging

If your salon asks you to contact a client via text message or email, you should avoid using text abbreviations. Always write words in full and check the spelling. Text messaging and emails are still quite new methods of communicating with clients and some text messages can seem impersonal and blunt. Remember, your client can't see your smiling face or hear the friendly tone in your voice when reading an email or texts, so re-read the message to ensure it is friendly and professional, and not too abrupt or direct.

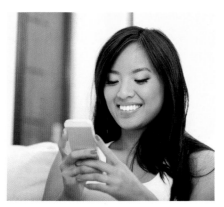

Make sure your email and text messages are professional in tone

Activity

A client emails the salon asking for a beauty treatment next Tuesday at 3pm and you respond with the following email:

> Hi Jan
>
> No worries, we can def fit u in on Tues. Who does your treatment for you? Gems free, will she do? Wot you want doing? Can U let me no? See you l8r.
>
> Millie.

Discuss with a colleague what is wrong with this email, listing all the problems and spelling errors. Re-write the replying email professionally.

Activity

Use the internet to search for salon websites.

Discuss with your colleagues whether you think these salon websites would be useful to clients.

Identify salon websites you like and explain why.

Identify salon websites that you would improve and explain your reasons.

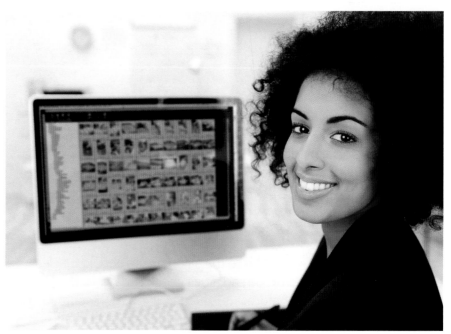

Research on the internet

Listening skills

When someone else is talking to you, you should make sure you listen. During a client consultation you should always listen more than you talk. By listening rather than talking, you will gather valuable information. This will assist you when you are deciding which recommendations you are going to make. It also shows the client that you are interested in what they have to say and that it is important.

At the end of the consultation, it is a good idea to repeat back the important points of the conversation to make sure that you have fully understood the information and that you haven't made any assumptions. This technique is known as summarising and confirming.

Visual aids

Visual aids are a fabulous tool for use when explaining treatments. For example, it is really useful if you have access to before and after photos to show clients the results that a treatment can achieve. If a client has never used a particular product or had a particular treatment before, show them the equipment and products that you are going to use during their treatment and explain the treatment.

Adapt your methods of communication to suit the client's needs

An important part of good communication is being able to adapt your methods of communication to different situations. For example, if a client has a hearing problem, is blind or partially sighted or has a learning disability, you may need to adapt your communication in the following ways.

WHY DON'T YOU…
In pairs, practise a consultation using a visual aid (eg a product). Ask your partner for feedback. Did it help with the consultation? Was it useful to be able to demonstrate/show something? How was it useful? What improvements could you make?

Communication difficulty	How to adapt your communication
Learning disabilities	Speak clearly. Be patient. Avoid technical jargon. Repeat information and check client's understanding.
Deaf or partial hearing	Face the client. Use eye contact. Speak normally but clearly. Do not shout at the client. If possible, use visual aids (eg pictures of the treatment). Try to discuss the client's needs in a quiet area without other sounds and distractions. Be patient.
Blind or partially sighted	Speak normally and clearly. Try to discuss the client's needs in a quiet area without other sounds and distractions. Be patient. Guide your client through the salon – offer your client your shoulder as assistance and walk in front them. Mention any steps and potential dangers as you go.

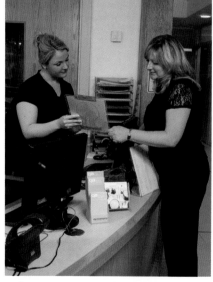

A therapist using product boxes as visual aids with a client

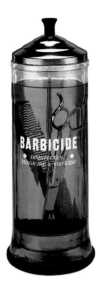

Barbicide

Effective, hygienic and safe working methods

It is essential that salon cleanliness be maintained throughout the day. This will ensure that a professional image is given to your clients. Always use towels and couch roll for each client and ensure that the salon floors are kept free of product left over from a treatment. At the start of a service you must ensure that products and equipment are ready for use, and when you have finished, tidy your trolley and return any products you are not using to the product area and dispose of any used consumables. After every service you must ensure that your products and equipment have been cleaned and sterilised, ready for the next client and to prevent cross-contamination.

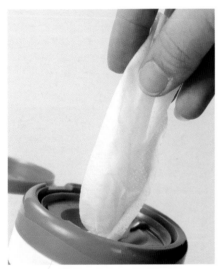

Chemical wipes

Sterilise tools and equipment

Tools and equipment must be sterilised in an appropriate manner. Salon sterilisers consist of disinfectants, an autoclave and an ultraviolet (UV) light.

There are three methods of sterilisation used in beauty salons:

- chemicals
- moist heat
- ultraviolet.

Chemicals

This method is often used in beauty salons. The chemicals are placed in a jar or container after they have been washed and cleaned to remove dirt. The chemical mixture must completely cover the tools. It is an effective method if used correctly. Chemical sprays are also available for tools that cannot be immersed in liquid.

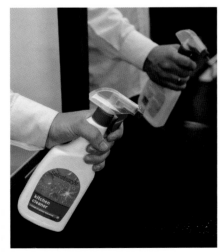

Chemical sprays

A common liquid disinfectant is Barbicide, but some salons may use sanitising sprays. Items suitable for a liquid disinfectant are placed in the solution for about 20 minutes; some chemicals will sterilise and destroy all micro-organisms, while others will disinfect or sanitise by destroying most micro-organisms. Remember to mix neat Barbicide with water.

Moist heat

This method is created by the use of an autoclave, which heats water up to a very high temperature (higher than boiling water). It will kill most common bacteria found in beauty salons.

Autoclaves are the most effective method of sterilising. They use heat to steam clean and sterilise equipment, which usually takes about 20 minutes.

Ultraviolet

Ultraviolet light rays are used to kill bacteria. Tools are cleaned first, then placed in a sterilising cabinet. This method is not used as much today, as you need to keep turning the tools around in the cabinet for the light rays to cover all sides of the tools to work.

Sanitising using UV lights takes longer as the equipment needs to be placed in the cabinet for about 20–30 minutes and then turned over and treated for a further 20–30 minutes. This method is effective only if used with cleaned sterile equipment and the equipment is turned properly.

Always wash metal tools with warm soapy water before sterilising them. Have a duplicate of tools so you can leave the used tools to thoroughly sterilise in the autoclave.

Comfort for you and the client

Therapists work long days and spend many hours standing, particularly when massaging. It is very important that you stand correctly to minimise fatigue and reduce the risk of injury caused by a bad posture. Poor posture can cause back problems and long-term illness, so always remember your stance when massaging and posture throughout other treatments, not only when you are standing but also when you are sitting.

> **HANDY HINT**
>
> As a rule when cleaning, disinfecting and sterilising equipment and tools, clean with detergent and water, sterilise in an autoclave and disinfect with a chemical liquid or a UV light.

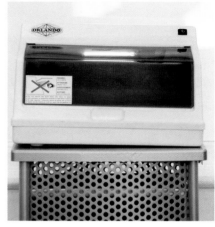

UV light cabinet

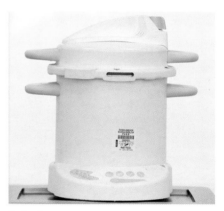

Autoclave

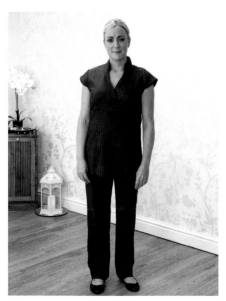

Correct posture

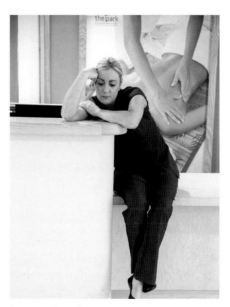

Incorrect posture

Client comfort is very important, especially as some treatments can take longer than others. To maintain your client's comfort, ensure you provide a cushion for the bottom of their back if they are sitting for long periods of time or a bolster or pillow to put under their knees if they are lying down. You will need to know how to adapt the treatment accordingly for your client's needs based on their consultation.

Always ensure that you position your equipment and trolley within easy reach for your comfort and make sure you have everything on the trolley prior to inviting your client in to the treatment room. This will also enable you to work efficiently and save time, maintaining a professional image at all times.

HANDY HINT

If you are right-handed, keep your trolley on the right-hand side, and the opposite if you are left-handed.

Safe use of electrical equipment

Always check that electrical equipment is maintained and checked regularly and that all employees receive training in the use of the equipment, following manufacturer's instructions.

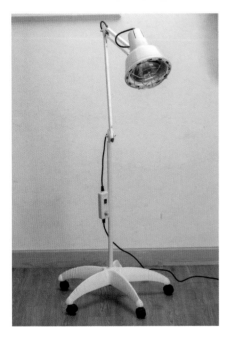

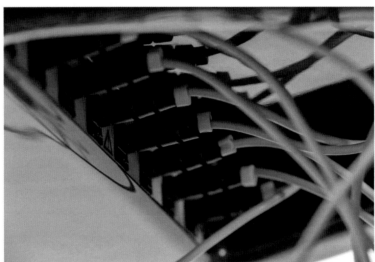

Always check and maintain electrical equipment

Make sure you:

- understand the instructions before using any electrical equipment: if you don't, ask
- always switch off at the mains before connecting or disconnecting any electrical appliance
- dry hands thoroughly before using electrical equipment
- check equipment looks clean and in good repair before using
- report any damaged electrical tools or equipment, including cables and plugs and remove from use.

For more information, refer to the Electricity at Work Regulations.

Adhere to instructions

To ensure the smooth running of the spa salon and to follow good health and safety practice, it is of vital importance that you follow your workplace policies and any instructions of suppliers and manufacturers.

Workplace policies are important to follow as it helps maintain a safe and healthy working environment. Within a salon environment the key policies and procedures cover the following:

- maintenance of the salon and the equipment in the salon
- ventilation of the salon, temperature and lighting
- salon hygiene, cleanliness and the disposal of waste material
- workspace in the salon (workstation and seating)
- condition of floor and traffic route through the salon
- drinking water supply
- area for rest, eating and changing (if required), storage of clothing
- sanitary conveniences
- areas of glazing in the salon (windows, doors and partitions).

Activity

List as many of your workplace policies as you can.

Suppliers' and manufacturers' instructions

Your salon's representative or supplier may provide you with products, tools, equipment, salon fixtures and fittings and retail items to use within the salon and during the treatment. When you are using tools and equipment it is important that you read any manufacturers' instructions (MFIs) and follow the advice given by your supplier. Also follow the MFIs for advice on storing, handling, using and disposing of products.

Following instructions properly ensures that you use equipment correctly, which not only prolongs the life of the item, but also ensures the safety of yourself and others. Always follow the MFIs for equipment specific to the treatment.

Behaviours

Behaviours are the way we conduct ourselves and perform in the workplace; they are the way we look after people and demonstrate our manners, they are the deeds we do, and how we carry out our activities on a day-to-day basis. The industry's expected behaviours are covered in this section of the chapter.

Meet your salon's standards of behaviour

Your personal presentation and behaviour must protect the health and safety of both you and others. It must also meet with legal requirements and follow your workplace policy.

Your personal image reflects on your salon's professional image. Always ensure you are fit for work and follow good standards of personal hygiene. Seek guidance from your manager before going to work if you have a potentially infectious condition, for example a cold, 'flu, eye infection or stomach bug.

Your behaviour should reflect the standard expected of you in the salon and reduce the risk of harm to yourself and others. You are representing your salon, and the image you give of yourself has an impact on the whole business. Always act professionally, speak politely to visitors and clients, and promote equality and diversity for all.

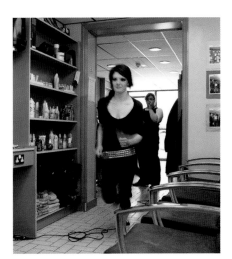
Never run in the salon!

Greet the client respectfully and in a friendly manner

When greeting clients, always ensure you are friendly, courteous and respectful. Check whether the client has booked the appointment under their first name or surname and, if unsure, you should refer to them using their title and surname, until your client advises otherwise. Always be helpful and assist them with their coat; make them feel welcome and valued. Clients are visiting the salon for treatments, so the experience should be a treat.

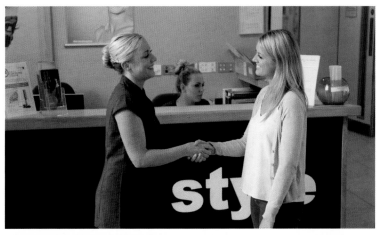
Be friendly and respectful

Activity

At some point all of us have entered a store and been poorly greeted by an uninterested staff member. Discuss with your colleagues how that made you feel, what was wrong with the service and whether you have since returned to that store.

THE CITY & GUILDS TEXTBOOK

Communicate with clients

Spas and salons are in a very fortunate position. More and more people are shopping online and customer service in many industries is therefore deteriorating. Your potential clients cannot get their beauty treatments via the internet, so you have the potential for a long-lasting client base if you serve them well. Happy clients will want to return to you and not your competitor. All it takes is great customer service and a great result.

Establish an effective rapport with clients

It is perfectly natural if you don't get on with everyone you meet. Personal beliefs and individual interests make people unique, but when it comes to working in the spa salon, you must work harmoniously with your colleagues and clients, and maintain a professional working relationship at all times.

As soon as a client walks through the door, you must make them feel valued and special. Conversations with your clients should be targeted around them, their interests and activities, making them feel that you are interested in what they do. Always try to engage your client in a neutral, friendly conversation, avoiding views on politics, religion and controversial subjects. Always show respect towards your client's views but minimise expressing your own opinions and try to avoid talking about what you have been doing: this is a time for them.

The small talk and personal details discussed with your client individualise the treatment you offer. Remembering small details of conversations from previous visits goes a long way to building a good **rapport** with your client.

Identify and confirm the client's expectations

It is your responsibility to identify and confirm your client's requirements and expectations, and to decide whether they're achievable. Your clients may have certain medical conditions that may restrict or prevent a treatment so it is important to be realistic about what is possible and either adapt the treatment accordingly or offer them an alternative treatment.

Be confident in what you have learnt and remember the power of internet search engines. If you are unsure about anything, ask your manager or colleagues and, if they are also unsure, check on the internet. You will find a lot of information there about medical conditions and other information that will assist you in making the right decision for your client.

Be courteous and helpful

It is important that you are always polite and courteous to your clients. Ask after their well-being, make them the focus of your conversation and be as helpful as possible. You could also make a note of some

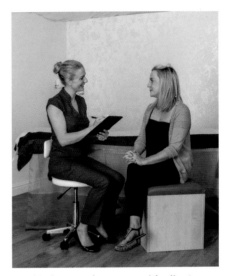

Establish a good rapport with clients

VALUES & BEHAVIOURS

Avoid discussing topics that involve politics or religion as some people have very strong views and opinions, and these topics could lead to a heated debate.

Rapport

A personal link or understanding between people.

INDUSTRY TIP

A good way of encouraging clients to purchase products that you have recommended is to let them try them. Give your client the product and let them try it on their skin.

personal details on their record card so you can refer to them and ask how they are on their next visit. You must always provide them with advice, explain your findings of the treatments, and make any recommendations of aftercare and future services.

Always offer a future appointment to your client and advise on costs of the services and how long the service will take.

Disability Discrimination Act 2005

The Disability Discrimination Acts of 1995 and 2005, which have now been superseded by the Equality Act 2010, aim to ensure that disabled people are treated in a fair and equal way. The Acts place duties on providers of goods, facilities and services and make it unlawful for a service provider to discriminate against a disabled person.

Respond to sensitive reactions

During the treatment, always keep an eye on your client and be aware of sensitive reactions. If you are treating a particular area in body massage, for example, keep an eye on areas that may cause the client pain or discomfort and check that they are okay and adapt the treatment as necessary. It is equally important to be sensitive to the client's feelings during consultation and aftercare discussions.

Type of client	Potential problem	How to deal with it
Confident and bubbly	Asking for services in a way that indicates they know more than they do. Might not be open to listening to your ideas.	Express your advice clearly with detailed explanations of why you recommend certain services. Use open questions to clarify their requirements.
Shy and nervous	May not explain their requirements clearly.	Make your recommendations suitable for the client needs. Use open questions to clarify their requirements.
Early arrival	The salon may not be able to carry out the service before the allocated appointment.	Check whether the therapist can accommodate an early client. See if another therapist is available. Explain the outcome to the client and offer refreshments if the client chooses to wait.
Late arrival	There might not be time to carry out the service and the client may need to rebook.	Ask the therapist if they can accommodate the late client. Check whether another therapist can accommodate the client. Offer an alternative service that suits the time allocations. Offer to rebook the client.
Angry	The client may raise their voice and upset you. They may cause a scene in the salon and other clients may overhear.	Remain calm and polite. Don't get defensive but stay objective. Don't raise your voice. Move the client to a discreet area if possible. Refer the complaint to your manager and explain clearly to the client what you are doing and why.

Type of client	Potential problem	How to deal with it
Confused	There is potential for the service requirements not to be met if the client is confused. Client cannot give meaningful consent to treatment if they are confused.	Look at your client's body language and use open and closed questions to identify which areas need further discussion or advice.
Limited mobility or mobility impaired	Access to all salon areas may be difficult. A client may be offended if you treat them unfairly.	Always follow the Equality Act 2010/**Disability Discrimination Act 2005** and treat clients fairly. Don't patronise disabled clients. Don't assume someone needs help but ask if they require any.
Hearing impaired	Clients may struggle to understand or hear you clearly over background noise. Potential for misunderstandings.	Ensure you speak face to face to aid lip-reading. Use visual aids to clarify understanding. Reduce background noise where possible. Speak clearly but don't shout.
Vision impaired	The client may not see potential hazards in the salon.	Offer guidance to the client when moving around the salon. Make them aware of any steps or hazards ahead and move obstacles where possible. Speak clearly to guide them to your voice and where you are.
Non-fluent English speakers	Misunderstandings	Speak clearly, using non-technical terms. Keep your language simple. Use images, visual aids or write down what you are suggesting.

Activity

Some religions and faiths prevent women from having their head or hair uncovered in front of men. With a colleague, research faiths and religions, and identify any that may affect hairdressing services. Why is it useful for you to have a basic understanding of faiths and religions?

How would you adapt the treatment accordingly?

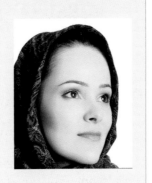

Activity

How would you deal with a client who asks why their appointment is running late?

WHY DON'T YOU...
Describe the signs of an angry client and those of a confused client.

HANDY HINT
Remember to treat all clients equally and respect the diversity of clients in your salon.

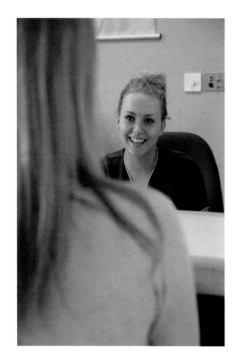

Promptly assisting a client

You will need to respond to your clients' needs in a variety of situations, such as at reception when booking appointments, during a consultation and throughout the service. Clients will also seek advice on aftercare and recommendations on retail products for maintaining the style between visits. Always ensure you work within the limits of your own authority and refer to a senior staff member or your manager for guidance when needed.

Behave professionally

It is important to be professional at all times, both in the salon environment and outside of the salon.

It is important when wearing your uniform outside of the salon that you remain professional because people might recognise where you work or you might be seen by clients. Within the salon it is important to behave in an appropriate and respectful manner towards your colleagues and clients at all times. The way in which a person behaves reflects the image of the salon.

Being professional also includes following safe and hygienic working practices in line with salon requirements and legislation. These are covered in more detail in the chapter on Health and safety legislation.

Personal space

Personal space refers to the area around us that we consider to be private. If you invade someone's personal space and get too close for comfort, they may feel uneasy. Personal space varies from person to person and situation to situation. You will need to enter a client's personal space during some treatments so make sure you are aware of it and how clients may feel.

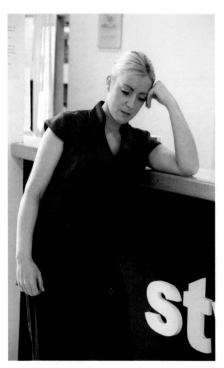

Negative behaviour, such as appearing bored, will leave a poor impression on a client

Use effective consultation techniques to identify treatment objectives

The consultation process is an essential part of any beauty or spa treatment. It will allow you to get to know your client and find out their hopes, fears and expectations (ie their objectives for the treatment).

Having a knowledge of the client's needs will allow you to select the most suitable treatment and products and even to start to think about products that will benefit them after the treatment has been completed.

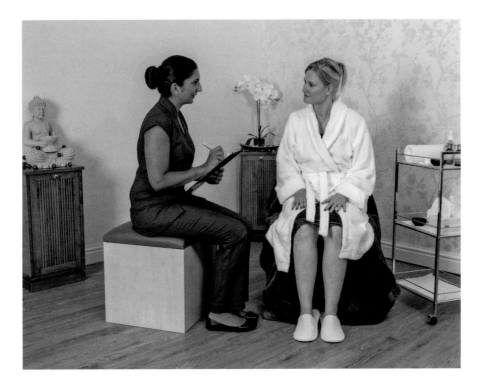

During the consultation you should:

- record important or key information
- assess whether a treatment is suitable for the client
- find out and record what the client hopes and needs to achieve from the treatment (ie their expectations)
- decide on which product or treatment will meet the client's needs
- explain the **features**, **actions**, **benefits** of the treatment and any **special points** in relation to the particular treatment
- provide an opportunity for the client to discuss the treatment and ask questions
- establish a rapport with the client and build confidence
- agree on the treatment objectives so the correct products and treatment can be used and any adaptations to the treatment can be made to suit the client's needs
- take details of the client's medical history so you can adapt the treatment if there are any **contra-indications** and provide the most suitable treatment
- take details of any previous treatments so that you can use this information when deciding which procedure to use
- carry out, if needed, an analysis of the client's posture and/or a skin sensitivity or patch test
- add the results of a skin sensitivity test to the consultation form or client's record card
- check for contra-indications.

Features

A description (of the treatment).

Actions

What will take place (during the treatment).

Benefits

Effects (that the treatment is likely to have).

Special points

Any particular information to be aware of (about the treatment).

Contra-indication

A reason why a treatment cannot be carried out or needs to be adapted.

Review

Assessing or examining something again.

The very first consultation that you have with a new client will always be more in-depth than later consultations. When the client returns for future treatments, a shorter **review** consultation should still be performed and the treatment plan amended according to the client's needs.

A consultation should not only be performed at the start of every treatment but also when the client makes their booking. If the receptionist is not a trained therapist, they must seek advice from senior therapists or managers about the questions they need to ask and the advice they need to give. When the client books their appointment always ask them if they have had the treatment before. For example, if they have never had a body massage before they may not be aware that they will need to undress. By finding out whether the client has had a treatment before, you will be able to provide them with the correct advice so that they come prepared for the treatment.

Activity

For Level 3 treatments, write a list of questions that the receptionist needs to ask clients when they are booking.
Put together an information pack to help any new starters, including descriptions of the treatments, approximate timings and the questions the receptionist needs to ask when taking a booking.

INDUSTRY TIP

Skin sensitivity or patch tests usually need to be carried out at least 24 hours before an appointment.

INDUSTRY TIP

During the consultation process it is essential that you find out about and record details of clients' medical histories in case there are any conditions (contra-indications) that might restrict or prevent the treatment.

Contra-indications

A contra-indication is a reason why a treatment cannot be carried out. A contra-indication might prevent the client from being treated at all, or it might require the treatment to be restricted or modified. Checking for contra-indications must be done prior to any treatment. Ask the client whether they have any conditions that might be relevant to the treatment. The client should then sign and date the consultation form to confirm that the information is accurate.

In some cases contra-indications will just restrict treatments. For example, a bruise or an area of broken skin will need to be avoided. If you need to adapt your treatment, you should always explain to the client how and why and get their agreement before you start. In some cases, it might be more advisable for the client to rebook the treatment for another time when they can more fully benefit from the experience.

The following contra-indications will either prevent or restrict treatment so you need to make sure you are familiar with them. For further information on each of the contra-indications listed, refer to chapter 302, Anatomy and physiology.

> **INDUSTRY TIP**
>
> Sometimes professional advice for treatment can be obtained from a pharmacist, eg for skin infections or allergies.

Contra-indications that prevent treatment

Contra-indication	Action	Contra-indication	Action
Fungal infection	Seek medical advice for treatment. Wait until infection has got better or skin conditions have improved.	Chemotherapy	Seek medical advice prior to treatment.
Bacterial infection		Radiotherapy	
Infestation		Deep vein thrombosis	
Viral infection		Disorder of the nervous system (eg epilepsy, multiple sclerosis, etc)*	
Severe skin condition (eg eczema or psoriasis)			
Eye infection			

* Disorders of the nervous system can prevent or restrict a procedure depending on the treatment that the client is receiving. Please check each chapter for further details of nervous system contra-indications.

> **INDUSTRY TIP**
>
> If there is a reason why you cannot carry out a treatment you must explain tactfully to the client why the treatment cannot go ahead.

Contra-indications that restrict treatment

Contra-indication	Action	Contra-indication	Action
Broken bone	Treatments may need to be modified or an alternative treatment offered. A note from the client's GP may be required.	Allergy	Treatments may need to be modified or an alternative treatment offered.
Recent scar tissue		Varicose veins	
Hyperkeratosis		Undiagnosed lump	
Skin allergy		Recent fracture or sprain	
Cuts and abrasions		Respiratory condition	
Epilepsy		Circulatory condition (eg phlebitis)	
Diabetes		Pregnancy	
Heart disease		Obesity	
High or low blood pressure		Nail condition	
Skin disorder			
Piercings			

INDUSTRY TIP

Remember, to avoid breaching client confidentiality, it is important not to discuss personal information about a client with anyone else in the salon.

Seek medical advice

If you think that the client should seek medical advice, then suggest this. Remember that you are not qualified to make a medical diagnosis and so it is important that the client sees a medical professional.

If the client speaks to their medical practitioner and they have agreed that the treatment can go ahead, you should record this. Make notes on the client's record card and get the client to sign to confirm the information and agree to the treatment going ahead. This is known as a disclaimer.

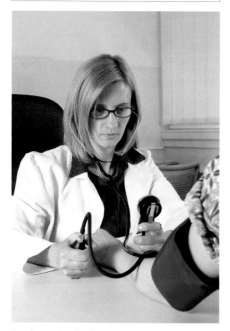

Seek medical advice

Manage client expectations

It is important that you explain what is realistically achievable with a treatment. Be truthful at all times. The client will be more disappointed if you give them an unrealistic expectation than if you are honest and explain that a single treatment will not have the same result as a course of treatments. For example, if a female client wants a toned body after one electrical muscle simulation (body faradic) session, it may not be possible. You will need to explain to the client how the treatment works and why they will see better results over a course of treatments. If the client will never achieve a toned body, even with a course of treatments, be honest and tactful and suggest other more suitable treatments.

Once you have agreed the treatment objectives with the client and decided what the treatment will include, you should write down the information in the client's treatment plan. You should make a note of any changes to the treatment that need to be made. Ask the client to sign the consultation form. Their signature indicates that they are happy to have the treatment you have recommended as recorded on their record card. Make sure the treatment plan and record card are accurate and filed away securely and in line with the Data Protection Act (see pages 82–83). This will help to maintain client confidentiality.

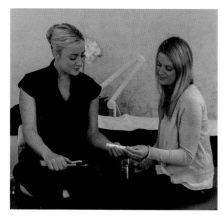

A therapist providing treatment advice to a client

Make product and treatment recommendations to meet client requirements

When you make product recommendations or sell treatments or products, it is important to:

- know all the treatments that the salon provides so you can advise and make recommendations
- have a thorough knowledge of the particular product or treatment you are recommending (ie, its features and benefits)

- make sure that the products you are offering the client are appropriate to the treatment that has been performed
- record the information on the client's record card.

For more information on selling products, please see chapter 301, Promote and sell products and services to clients.

Evaluate client feedback

It is important to gain feedback from the client. Feedback helps you to:

- evaluate the effectiveness of a treatment
- understand how you can improve a treatment
- learn from your experiences.

When you have completed a treatment you should seek confirmation from the client that they are satisfied with the result of the treatment. If the client previously purchased a product, check they were happy with it.

Activity

Gaining client feedback is one method of finding out how you can improve your skills as a therapist. Can you think of any other ways of finding out how to improve the way you work?

Methods of gaining feedback

Ideally, you should use a range of methods to gather feedback as different information can be gained from each method:

- verbal questions
- observation – was the client's body language relaxed during the treatment? Did they appear to enjoy their treatment?
- written questionnaires.

It is essential to gain feedback from clients as it is one way in which you can improve the service that both you and the salon provide. Do not be nervous about asking clients about their treatment. Ask open questions rather than ones that will just get a one-word (yes or no) answer. You want their feedback to be constructive to help you improve. If the client is happy with their service, hopefully they will come back and ask for you specifically. Always thank the client for their feedback whether it is negative or positive.

INDUSTRY TIP

If you want honest feedback from a client, get a colleague to ask the client for the feedback. Clients might be more likely to give honest feedback to someone else.

INDUSTRY TIP

One way of evaluating your customer care and quality of service is to review how many of your clients come back as repeat business – especially for regular treatments. Repeat business is usually a positive sign. However, there is always room for improvement no matter how good you think you are.

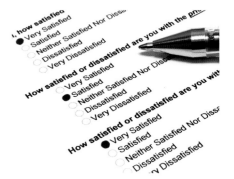

Written questionnaire

HANDY HINT

It is necessary to distinguish clients who have a genuine complaint, which needs to be taken seriously from those clients who are complaining because they want money off their treatment or a complimentary treatment. This comes with experience.

INDUSTRY TIP

You should make every effort to rectify a problem. Check the treatment schedule to make sure there is enough time to address it there and then. If not, book the client in again for a complimentary treatment after checking this with your manager.

INDUSTRY TIP

Offering the client top-quality customer service when dealing with their complaint will help to keep them as a client. It is in the salon's interest to keep clients as trying to attract new clients costs the salon money (eg marketing and advertising costs).

Resolve client complaints

If a client is unhappy with a product or treatment then it is vital that their complaint is dealt with immediately in a professional manner by:

- listening to their complaint without interrupting
- identifying exactly what the problem is
- involving the correct people (eg your manager) to deal with the client
- following relevant workplace policies for dealing with complaints
- being patient and understanding
- displaying positive body language – don't become defensive or aggressive towards the client
- offering to **rectify** the problem immediately
- offering a complimentary treatment or products (if you are authorised to do so)
- moving the client to a more private area of the salon if they are becoming loud and aggressive.

The salon should have a procedure for dealing with complaints. Depending on the nature of the complaint, you might be able to **resolve** the problem yourself. For example, the receptionist should be able to deal with complaints about bookings or retail products. If you are unable to resolve the problem you might need to refer the complaint to someone else (eg your manager) so that it is dealt with promptly and effectively.

Rectify

Put right.

Resolve

To find a solution or answer.

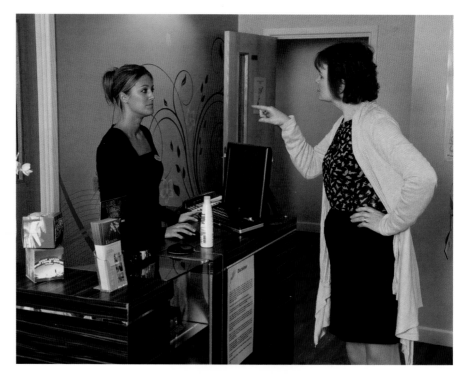

Client complaints should be dealt with calmly and efficiently

Check the client's expectations

You must check that your client fully understands the treatment process so that they feel at ease and that you have understood your client's requirements.

Use open and closed questions to check each other's understanding. Open questions usually start with what, why, how and when and give you the detail required. Closed questions are answered with a yes or no and can help to confirm what is being requested.

Always read your client's body language and look for signs of uncertainty. If your client is rubbing their neck or behind their ears, it is a sign that they are unsure and further advice/discussion is required.

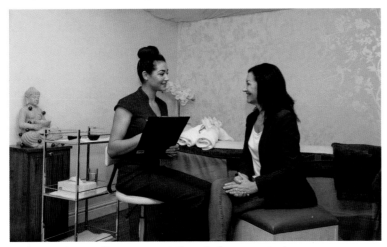

Understand your client's expectations before you start

Promptly and positively respond to questions and comments

It is important that you respond to your client's questions and comments promptly, positively and professionally to ensure your customer service is of a high standard.

Your client may have questions about the service being carried out, future services or products; ensure you answer these questions honestly and in a positive manner.

It is always easy to respond to positive feedback from a client but some comments may not be positive. A client may be unhappy for several reasons such as:

■ the time he or she had to wait for their appointment

■ the time the service took

■ the end result of the treatment

■ the cost of the service

■ the behaviour of the therapist or other staff.

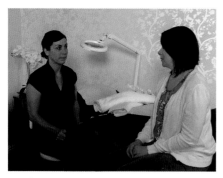

Let the client respond

When you have to deal with negative comments, you must respond in a professional manner at all times. Try to resolve the issue promptly, apologise where necessary and make any necessary arrangements to rectify the issue as soon as you can. Any comments that become complaints should be reported to your manager.

Allow the client time to respond

Before you commence with any service, ensure your client has been given the time to consider their responses and clarify their needs. Always allow additional time if your client is still unsure and offer further information if required. You must never talk over your client and should use jargon-free language when discussing services and products to help your client understand what is being suggested to them. Listen to your client and nod or repeat what is being said so they are clear you have understood.

If your client is thinking of having an alternative treatment in the future or has expressed an interest in purchasing some products, allow them time during the service to consider the benefits. Towards the end of the service, revisit the conversation, show them the products used and repeat the benefits to the client.

HANDY HINT

Always give appropriate and accurate information to your clients.

Quickly locate information

You must always ensure that the salon information systems are easily accessible. Clients require effective responses to their questions and you must be able to locate this information quickly.

If your client requires information regarding appointment times and availability, ensure the reception is tidy and the appointment book and appointment cards are available.

A price list for services and retail products should be available to clients.

Deal with any clients' complaints politely and swiftly. If your manager needs to contact the client, ensure you have all the relevant contact details and have taken notes about the nature of the complaint. Whatever the complaint, the quicker it is dealt with the quicker it is forgotten by the client.

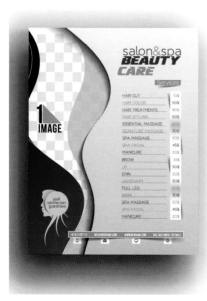

Have treatment lists to hand

Provide information about services and product

It is important that you are aware of all the services and products your salon offers. One client may see another client receiving a service or buying a product and enquire what it is. It is part of your job role and your client will expect that you can provide them with information and advice about the relevant product or service.

WHY DON'T YOU...

Identify any services that you have limited knowledge of, and ask your salon managers or peers to explain them to you.

You should keep a price list to hand, as this lists the services your salon offers and the prices charged. You should also attend any salon training regarding new products and services to ensure you are well informed and can advise your clients effectively.

Activity

Identify two or three products that you have not used for a while. Read the manufacturers' instructions on how to use each product and research the features and benefits to the client for using these products.

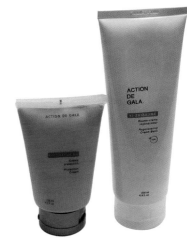

Products for a client to use at home

Recognise complicated information and check understanding

Check your client understands what has been decided by using open and closed questions to clarify what has been discussed and agreed. If the information is complicated, ensure you use non-technical language that is jargon-free.

Information that your clients require needs to be communicated quickly and effectively. Complicated information should be checked for a clear understanding and the reasons why client expectations can't be met must be explained.

HANDY HINT

Open questions require a client to give more in-depth answers and may start with why or how. Closed questions help to confirm and define details as they are answered with one-word responses like yes or no.

Activity

You have used the explanation below to describe a process to your client and she looks confused. Reword the explanation into client-friendly words that she will understand.

'Okay, Hannah. You are very tight around the deltoid and across the trapezius so I am going to relax the muscles for you by working into them with petrissage movements which will also help remove any toxins.'

Explain why client expectations cannot be met

Sadly, some clients attend the salon expecting a treatment to be carried out, but a consultation and relevant tests prove that the required service cannot be carried out. For example, a client may want a body massage but may be undergoing treatment by a medical professional that would prevent a treatment from going ahead. It is essential that you explain to your client why a service can't be carried out and you should suggest an alternative treatment. Speak clearly, be polite and give the appropriate detail. Remain professional and objective as to why the client's expectations can't be met.

Activity

List some examples of services that clients might expect but which can't be carried out due to the results of tests or the consultation. How would you explain this to your client?

Answers at the back of the book.

1 What does the term values mean?

a Morals and ethics

b Ethnicity and religion

c Culture and age groups

d Possessions and money

2 Which one of the following is the best way to deal with a client with different values?

a Avoid talking to them so that they don't get upset

b Ask detailed questions to try to understand them

c Debate with them and try to change their minds

d Respect them and adapt to their needs

3 Why is it important to have commercially viable timescales for working?

a To make sure the salon operates smoothly

b To make sure the salon closes on time

c To make sure all clients are satisfied

d To make sure no clients turn up late

4 Why is it important to wear no jewellery when working as a therapist?

a It can be uncomfortable to wear for long periods

b It can catch the client's skin

c It looks unprofessional

d It causes allergies

5 Read the following statements:

Statement one

It is recommended that layers of clothing are worn at work to regulate heat and minimise body odour.

Statement two

Shoes should be comfortable and have open toes to keep feet cool.

Which one of the following is correct for the above statements?

a True True

b True False

c False True

d False False

6 Which one of the following is the best way for a therapist to avoid contact dermatitis?

a Keeping nails short and neat

b Rinsing hands after each client

c Wearing gloves for the necessary treatments

d Applying hand cream every night

7 Why is it important to have a flexible working attitude?

a To secure a pay rise

b To keep the salon busy

c To work under pressure

d To meet changing demands

8 Which one of the following is the best action to take when a therapist is running late?

a Explain the situation to the client that is waiting

b Tell the next client to come back when it is not so busy

c Get the next client to complete their own record card to encourage them to stay

d Expect that the client can see what is happening and will understand

9 Read the following statements:

1 Being the first in the salon every day

2 Taking ownership of responsibilities

3 Being flexible

4 Working quickly

Which two of these best describe the term self-manager?

a 1 and 2

b 2 and 3

c 3 and 4

d 4 and 1

10 Which one of the following describes creativity?

a Working well with others and using their ideas

b Having good ideas and acting upon them

c Being imaginative

d Asking questions

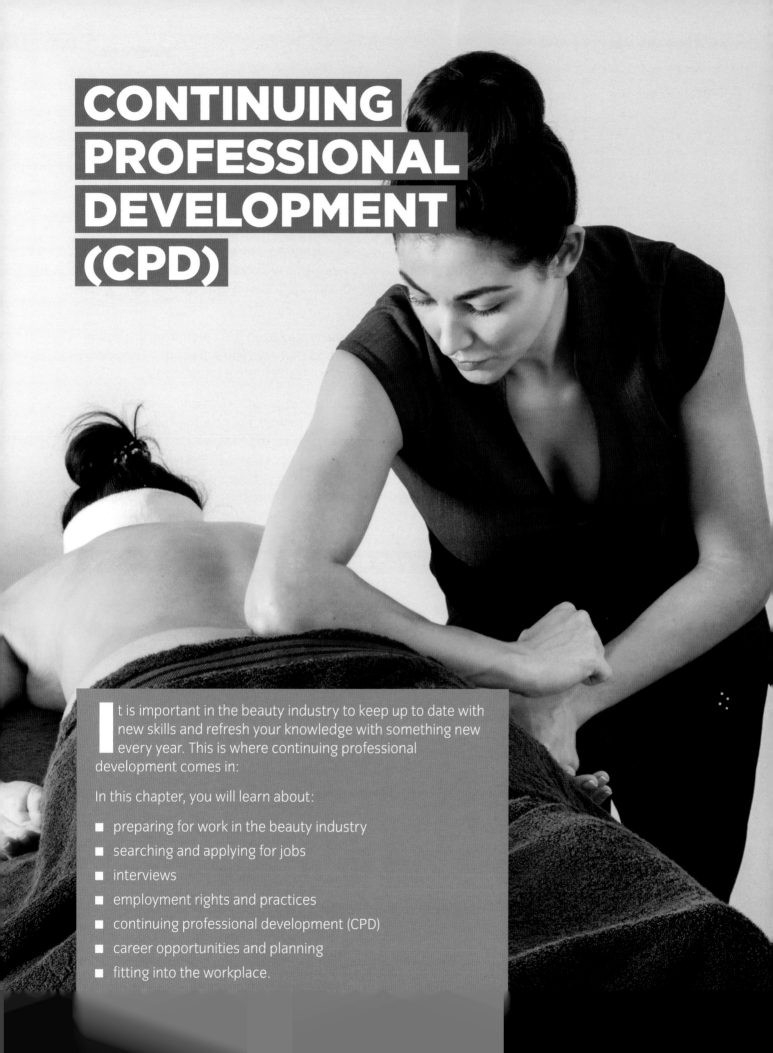

CONTINUING PROFESSIONAL DEVELOPMENT (CPD)

I t is important in the beauty industry to keep up to date with new skills and refresh your knowledge with something new every year. This is where continuing professional development comes in:

In this chapter, you will learn about:

- preparing for work in the beauty industry
- searching and applying for jobs
- interviews
- employment rights and practices
- continuing professional development (CPD)
- career opportunities and planning
- fitting into the workplace.

Prepare for work in the beauty industry

What is CPD?

CPD is an acronym for continuing professional development. The beauty industry changes all the time, with new products on the market, equipment and exciting new resources available for you to refresh your skills. As well as the practical skills, theory-based learning is also important to keep up to date with current knowledge. By attending workshops, seminars and courses you will continue learning all the new exciting things coming into our industry so you can include them in your current work.

Preparing for work involves many stages. In this chapter we are going to look at some of the stages and elements you will need to consider as you make the transition from a learner into a professional.

Every employer is different and will operate in different ways. As a new employee, part of the challenge is to work out how the knowledge and skills that you have learned can be adapted to fit with the spa or salon's practices and ethos. What is really important is to learn how to integrate into an established team and to develop the skills to fit in easily and to be confident in what you know.

Search for and apply for jobs

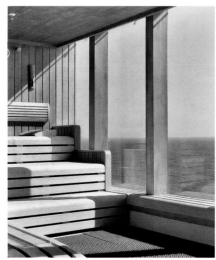
Sauna on a cruise ship

Before you start looking for a job, it is worth considering what options are available to you. There are several things you need to think about:

1 The type of spa or salon you want to work in and why. You could work in:

- a department store salon
- a beauty salon
- a spa resort
- a hotel spa
- a cruise ship.

Why do you want to work there?

What is it that appeals to you?

What skill sets do you have that make this salon a natural fit for you?

Does the salon offer additional product training or additional courses?

2 Location. Are you willing to travel for work? Is commuting an option (cost, travel time)? Is moving closer an option?

3 The benefits to your career. There will be pros and cons to every opportunity or job role. Some examples follow:

- Some spas are overnight retreats and building up regular, repeat business is difficult. You might also carry out the same treatments on a regular basis (eg massage).

- A larger organisation may have a more defined structure, making it easier to progress up the ladder if becoming a supervisor is part of your long-term career plan.

- In larger beauty salons, spas and cruise ships, it is often possible to work in a specific role to use the skills that you enjoy and excel at (eg if you are confident and have excelled at massage treatments and body treatments, there might be a specialist body therapist role).

Do your research

Once you have established the type of salon or spa that you would like to work in, you need to do your homework. Find out as much as you can about salons or spas that you are interested in working for. Use the internet to find out about them as most salons have a website. The website will allow you to get a feel for:

- the salon's clientele
- the services, treatments and products it offers
- the type of work it does
- how many staff it has.

Where to find vacancies

Job vacancies are mainly found on the internet, with a small proportion published in print media. Below you can find examples of where you can look for the right job for you:

- further education colleges (they often advertise local vacancies on their noticeboards and websites)
- local job centres
- trade publications
- industry-specific recruitment websites
- salon/spa shop windows.

Apply for jobs

Many companies also have recruitment or careers sections on their websites so you can see whether they have any vacancies and apply online.

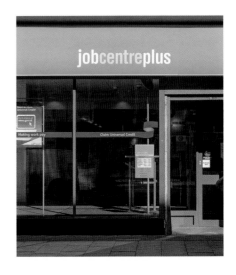

INDUSTRY TIP

If the salon/spa you are interested in working for is close by, drop by in person to see if they have any vacancies or to deliver your **CV** by hand. It makes more of an impression and meeting them face to face will help them remember you.

CV (curriculum vitae)

A short summary of your education, qualifications, previous jobs, and sometimes also your personal interests, that you send to an employer when you are trying to get a job.

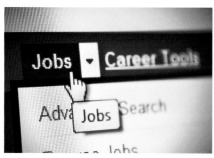

Job search online

Even if there aren't any positions available, it is still worth emailing or posting your CV to employers you are interested in working for. Good employers will keep these on file and look at them even if they aren't actively recruiting.

When sending your CV be sure to include:

- a recent, appropriate picture of yourself
- up-to-date contact details
- a brief one- to two-page summary (including dates) of your qualifications and training.

Interviews

Being a good interviewee is a skill you develop over time. However, even the most inexperienced interviewees can follow some basic rules.

Punctuality

- Be on time or early – it's never acceptable to be late.
- If you know you are going to be unable to make the interview, phone the company that is interviewing you first thing on the day of the interview and apologise for any inconvenience. Ask if you can rearrange the interview.

Look the part

Dressing smartly gives the right first impression. Make sure that:

- your hair is clean and styled
- your make-up has been applied professionally and appropriately
- your hands look moisturised, your nails are filed and a suitable length, with no chipped varnish
- your clothes are ironed
- you look clean and professional
- your shoes are clean and appropriate
- you have high standards of personal hygiene.

Don't be scruffy. Being well-presented is vital in the hair and beauty industry – a potential employer won't have much confidence that you can promote and sell treatments if you aren't well groomed yourself.

Be prepared

Most salons will require a **trade test**, otherwise known as a skills test, so be prepared. This may be part of the first interview, or you may be called back to carry out a trade test separately. Make sure you ask about this as you will need to take a clean, pressed uniform, have your hair secured appropriately, remove all jewellery and have short, varnish-free nails.

- Make sure you've done your research and can answer basic questions that the interviewer may have (eg 'What do you know about our salon/company?').

- Take anything with you that might help your application (eg portfolios, certificates, photographic work, marketing or media work you have been involved with).

- Take another copy of your CV with you to leave with the interviewer (even if you have already emailed it) and which you can refer to during the interview.

Create a positive impression

Interview questions

- Use positive body language (eg nodding, smiling, eye contact) and use a firm handshake when meeting the interviewer and at the end of the interview.

- Sit forward (avoid slouching) and make sure you are giving the interviewer your full attention.

- Take notes and don't be afraid to ask questions.

- Look enthusiastic, interested and keen.

- Don't make negative comments about former employers or salons where you have worked. It won't look good in the eyes of a potential employer.

- Provide explanations for leaving and changing jobs.

- Be prepared for some random questions – if you're not sure how to answer them, jot the questions down and come back to them.

- The interviewer is likely to ask you open questions (who, what, why, when, how, tell me) that you cannot answer yes or no to.

Finish the interview

Ask any necessary questions once the interview has finished.

Trade test

A test, often carried out after a first interview, to demonstrate your practical skills and techniques to a potential employer.

WHY DON'T YOU...
Practise answering open questions with a friend and do some role-plays of interviews.

Interview

INDUSTRY TIP

Remember you have only one opportunity to sell yourself. You won't get a second chance to make a first impression.

Employment rights and practices

Every business has a responsibility to ensure it follows the relevant rules and regulations.

As an employee, you should also be aware of your own responsibilities, as well as what your rights are and what your employer should be doing with regard to, for example, pay, contracts, time off and working hours.

Terms and conditions of employment (contract of employment)

Within two months of starting work, all employees must be given a written document outlining their terms and conditions of employment. You may initially receive a letter detailing your basic terms (salary, hours of work, number of days' holiday, supervisor/manager, etc) but the terms and conditions of employment/a contract is the main document given to all employees.

Terms and conditions of employment contracts

Every member of staff requires an employment contract. The list below shows the detail that is required to fulfil a legal contract:

- employee's name
- employer's name
- place of work
- date employment is to begin
- date employment is to end (if a temporary contract)
- employee's hours of work
- how often an employee is paid
- rate of pay
- amount of holiday an employee is entitled to
- sick pay entitlement
- details of any disciplinary and grievance procedures
- notice periods (for both employer and employee)
- an outline of the employee's responsibilities
- any specific terms and conditions relating to the business.

Grievance and disciplinary procedures

These will give details about the company's procedures for dealing with a grievance or disciplinary matters. They will outline the process for raising a grievance and the procedures (eg verbal and written warnings) for taking disciplinary action against an employee. They will also contain details of how an employee can appeal against any action.

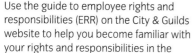

HANDY HINT

Use the guide to employee rights and responsibilities (ERR) on the City & Guilds website to help you become familiar with your rights and responsibilities in the workplace.

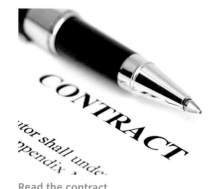

Read the contract

Employee handbook/rules and regulations

Some salons will have their own employee handbook. An employee handbook should include information on rules and regulations (eg appearance, sickness, reporting procedures, reporting absences from work, booking holidays). If a salon doesn't have a handbook, the same information that is included in the handbook (ie rules and regulations) might be issued verbally or put on the staff noticeboard. Other relevant information (eg on reporting lines and management or supervisory structure) may be given verbally.

Job description

It's important to know exactly what is expected of you. A job description should provide a short summary of the job role you are undertaking and outline the requirements of the job from the company's perspective.

Just having knowledge isn't enough to succeed in this job: you've also got to have the right personality. Technical skills are important but alone they won't make you a good beauty therapist.

As well as having an outgoing, friendly and talkative personality, beauty therapists should also be:

- self-motivated
- professional
- keenly aware of health and safety issues
- able to create a calm environment where clients can relax
- a good listener
- able to treat client information with confidentiality.

Appraisal and review system

As part of your development and training, you are likely to have an appraisal to review your performance and plan for future development. You will have opportunities to discuss progression with your manager during your appraisal and review.

Training agreements

Training can be quite costly for employers. On starting a job, it may be necessary to sign an agreement to repay any training costs should you leave the company within a certain time period (normally six months to a year) after starting the job.

Health and safety procedures

Employees should be made aware of any health and safety procedures and should be given appropriate training. Any health and safety

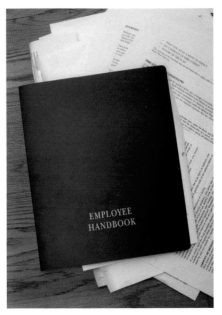

Employee handbook

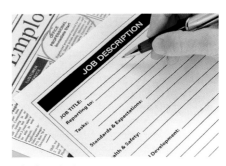

Job description

> **INDUSTRY TIP**
>
> Appraisals are a two-way discussion. They should be an opportunity to look at your professional development as well as discussing your performance and sales targets.

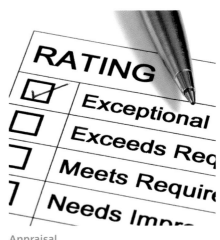

Appraisal

WHY DON'T YOU...
Find out how the appraisal and review system works for the salon you will be employed in. Ensure that you fully understand the appraisal system and how it will work.

Interpersonal skills

Communication skills.

INDUSTRY TIP

Make sure you take control of your own ongoing development and training. It will be beneficial to you in the long term to make sure your skills are kept up to date and developed. See it as an investment in your future as well as a commitment to your development from the company you work for. Ensure you are positive about and participate fully and willingly in any future training plans.

HANDY HINT

Any time you have away from the salon floor has a direct impact on costs to the salon, so if you are allowed to attend off-the-job training make sure you are grateful to your employer for allowing you to participate.

Subsidised

Where part of something has been paid (eg by an employer) to keep the price low.

training should be held during an employee's normal working hours. The training should not only cover safe working practices in the salon but also products used in the salon.

Continuing professional development

Wherever you choose to work, make sure they have a programme of ongoing development. This is vital for your professional development and motivation. You need to be able to undertake training and education on a long-term basis to strengthen and develop your skills and improve your weaker areas. As a newly qualified therapist, you will still be working out what are your strengths and weaknesses (both in terms of your technical and **interpersonal skills**). As you gain more experience you will become aware of areas that you could improve on. It is therefore important to develop a healthy attitude towards professional development and learning from the start.

Depending on the type of salon you start off in, it may be necessary to undergo some further on-the-job training straight away. Some salons will want to refine your skills so you can deliver services to their required level. Any further training needs may be established during the skills test or trade test after a successful first interview or it may come to light during a performance review or appraisal.

On-the-job training might involve further training in-house during working hours from colleagues who specialise in the areas that you need to develop. Alternatively, it may be necessary to attend off-the-job training with specific manufacturers and suppliers whose products you are using within the salon. Off-the-job training isn't always **subsidised** or paid for by your employer.

Areas for improvement

From a salon owner's perspective, there are traditionally some areas where college leavers' skills need attention and further development when it comes to working in a productive, commercial salon. Aside from the technical skills which need further development over time to become perfect, professional and speedy, interpersonal skills usually need further improvement. Learning how to manage relationships with clients successfully comes with time and experience.

As a newly qualified therapist it is often consultation and customer service skills that need further development. Learning to interpret body language and non-verbal communication signals and using open questions (to probe) and closed questions (to clarify) to establish clients' expectations will help you develop good relationships with clients and create a meaningful treatment plan for future bookings. It is always good for you to look up to a team leader/manager during your initial stages of employment and for them to guide you through.

Carrying out a detailed consultation is essential to understanding and confirming the client's expectations. It will be your job to establish, meet and exceed these expectations and a repeat booking will only be guaranteed if you are able to do this.

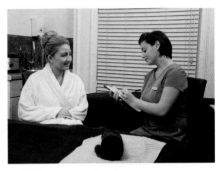

Address any weak areas

Career opportunities and planning

The hair and beauty industries are broad and provide a diverse range of career opportunities. The sector continues to grow and now employs 1.5% of the UK's working population. The variety of opportunities and experiences available to you will depend on the type of salon you work in. Most salons in the UK will carry out day-to-day treatments rather than undertaking treatments for celebrities or being involved in media work. However, some salons may be involved in seminars, shows and photographic work. There are opportunities to work all over the world if you are in the right place at the right time or take the right career path for you.

INDUSTRY TIP

Watch and learn how more experienced colleagues carry out consultations and develop good relationships with clients. Get your supervisor or manager to help you reach the required levels by using role-plays and real-life scenarios to help you practise your interpersonal skills.

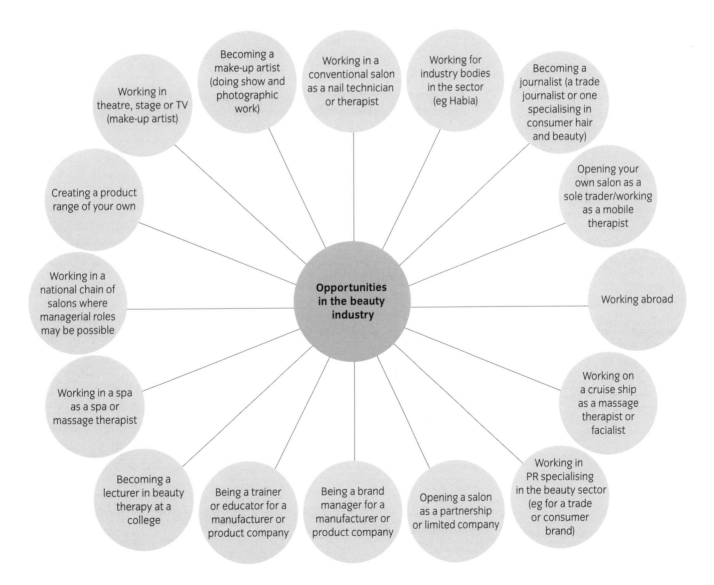

Opportunities in the beauty industry:

- Working in theatre, stage or TV (make-up artist)
- Becoming a make-up artist (doing show and photographic work)
- Working in a conventional salon as a nail technician or therapist
- Working for industry bodies in the sector (eg Habia)
- Becoming a journalist (a trade journalist or one specialising in consumer hair and beauty)
- Creating a product range of your own
- Opening your own salon as a sole trader/working as a mobile therapist
- Working in a national chain of salons where managerial roles may be possible
- Working abroad
- Working in a spa as a spa or massage therapist
- Working on a cruise ship as a massage therapist or facialist
- Becoming a lecturer in beauty therapy at a college
- Being a trainer or educator for a manufacturer or product company
- Being a brand manager for a manufacturer or product company
- Opening a salon as a partnership or limited company
- Working in PR specialising in the beauty sector (eg for a trade or consumer brand)

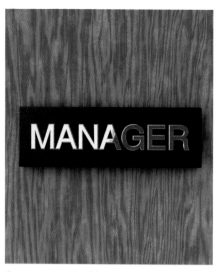

Career opportunities

Proactive

Taking control of a situation.

Mentor

A more experienced person who trains and supports new employees.

VALUES & BEHAVIOURS

It is important to be able to adapt to new situations, have flexible working attitudes and a willingness to learn.

What next?

Many stylists or therapists at the highest level take a **proactive** approach to ensuring they are fully up to speed with new innovations and that they keep up to date with new techniques and treatments. It is important as a newly qualified therapist to:

- watch and learn from colleagues who are at a more senior level – make sure you benefit from their knowledge and expertise

- attend any out-of-hours training that you can and any sessions where other members of the team share knowledge and skills that they have gained from training

- attend update sessions, seminars and courses run by product companies and manufacturers

- take an active role in your own professional development and training by attending workshops or seminars relevant to your interests

- go to trade exhibitions and shows where you can see industry names in action, watch practical demonstrations and keep in touch with industry developments and innovations.

Fit into the workplace

Working in a salon is all about teamwork so demonstrating that you are a good team player is vital. As the saying goes, 'there's no I in team'.

Make sure you buddy up with an existing team member who can help show you the ropes. Having a good **mentor** to follow is an essential part of learning. Knowing the ins and outs of the salon's working practice and salon etiquette will help you understand the unwritten rules of the salon.

Dos and don'ts of fitting into the salon team

Dos

- Follow the examples of other team members, even if it isn't what you are used to. Every salon operates differently, so for example if people in your workplace clear up after each other, follow their lead.

- Make a real effort to fit in. Take up any social invitations and try to get to know your new colleagues.

- Be sure to take part in any further education opportunities the salon is offering. Think of yourself as a sponge soaking up information about your new workplace.

- Keep up with the pace and speed of the team. Get used to the timings of treatments.

- Fit in with the way the team works. Observe and follow the way they work and their conduct in the salon.

- Show a willingness to put yourself out by staying late and coming in early if required – it is all about building respect and relationships.

Don'ts

- Don't alienate yourself by sticking to old routines and regimes. Make sure you are open-minded about new ways of working and understand what is and isn't appropriate salon etiquette.

- Don't expect to fit in straight away. Give yourself time to integrate into the team.

- Don't show off or talk yourself up. Your new team members will be impressed by your standard of work and behaviour so you should let your work speak for itself.

- Don't knock salon procedures that you are unfamiliar with. They may not be a familiar way of working but if they are how your new workplace operates, get used to them.

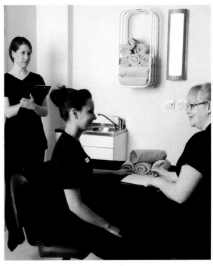

Be prepared to observe and learn from others

Summary

Fitting into a salon team is not easy and will certainly take time but by ensuring you follow the dos and don'ts you can make the transition smoother. Following the examples of other team members will certainly make the process more painless and will help you feel comfortable with your new colleagues.

Being a successful therapist in the commercial world means not only becoming technically, creatively and artistically proficient but also skilled at building good relationships with your clients based on trust and mutual understanding. Therefore developing your interpersonal skills is vital; having good communication skills is equally as important as delivering skilful and competent treatments.

As with any service industry, being on good form (ie delivering good conversation, making people feel at ease and ensuring they are comfortable and looked after) is as important as performing the treatment well. An experienced therapist knows when to talk and when to let a client relax so watch and learn from those who have already developed this skill to learn how to recreate the same ambience yourself.

> **HANDY HINT**
>
> Always bear in mind that you are a business within a business. Each and every client you meet has the potential to become one of your regulars and help expand your client base through personal recommendation and word of mouth.

Case study: Gina Charalambous

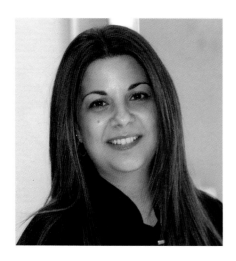

Beauty Director, Metrospa

The majority of junior therapists I have met have come through the conventional route of going to college to gain their Level 1, 2 and 3 qualifications. Although you have passed your exams, transferring your skill base into a spa or beauty salon will often prove scary. For any newly qualified therapist there are five main areas you need to consider when working in a salon.

Personal appearance

Many therapists seem to forget that they are the biggest advertisement for their own skills. It is only too obvious when visiting spas and other beauty salons how poor personal appearance can let a therapist down. If you want a client to have confidence in the treatments you are offering, their first point of reference is how you look. Being well groomed, having clean hair and nails, simple, classic and carefully applied make-up and a properly ironed uniform are a must for any therapist.

Technique

College will have provided you with the basic techniques for carrying out beauty treatments. However, a newly qualified therapist must always remember that their skills provide a base from which they need to move on and develop further with training. You must adapt your basic knowledge to the beauty brand/salon you are representing.

Client satisfaction

The clients you will now be looking after may prove much more demanding than the models you have practised on at college. Watch how the other therapists in your workplace deal with their clientele. Ask if a more senior therapist can be your mentor and shadow them when they are doing treatments to watch and learn. This will prove invaluable and will give you an insight into the speed you will need to be working at and how to develop good interpersonal relationships with clients.

Time-keeping

Be aware of your treatment list (or **column**) and your time-keeping. You may well be part of a larger team and in order to work well and efficiently in a busy salon you will need to finish your treatments on time so that the salon continues to run smoothly. If you are not busy, use your time constructively. If appropriate, practise on other team members and be proactive in asking more senior members of staff if there are any jobs

Column

A column of appointments (ie the day's appointment schedule).

that need doing. In helping out around the workplace, you will demonstrate you are a team player and develop an awareness of all the elements needed in the smooth running of the business.

Attention to detail

Finally, the biggest area for improvement in newly qualified therapists is attention to detail. Clients will expect the highest standards, so how you finish a manicure (ie how well you apply the polish), for instance, may make all the difference between a client having faith in you to do other treatments or not. Learn to accept nothing less than expert standards. If you have areas of weakness, practise, practise, practise!

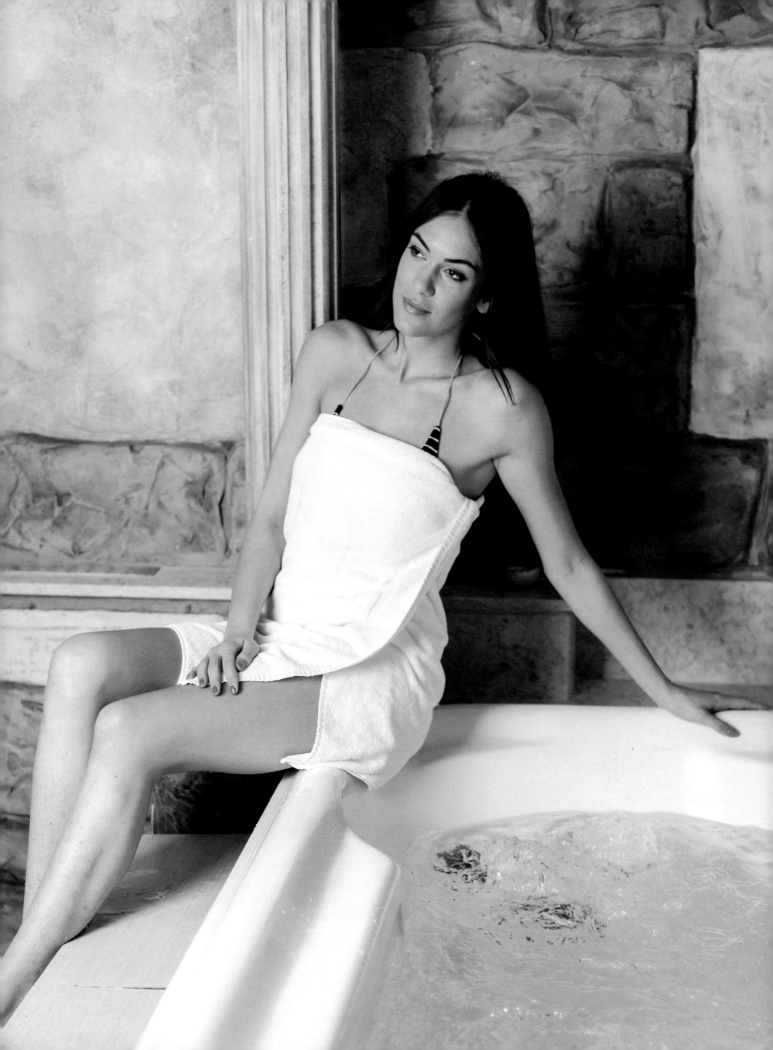

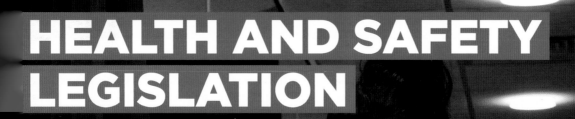

HEALTH AND SAFETY LEGISLATION

Health and safety is an essential part of your job role: you have a duty of care to work colleagues, clients and visitors to the salon.

This chapter will help you expand on your health and safety knowledge you learnt at Level 2 and learn about the different legislation you have to abide by when working in a beauty salon or spa.

In this chapter, you will learn how to:

- carry out a risk assessment
- monitor health and safety in the salon
- laws relating to health and safety
- laws relating to **consumer** protection
- other relevant legislation.

You will need to use this chapter together with all the other chapters and refer back to it.

Legislation

Consumer

Someone who pays for goods or a service.

Legislation

Laws that are made or passed by Parliament.

Acts

Laws.

Regulations

The rules under each Act.

By-law

A local council rule.

In order to make sure you are following health and safety regulations, you need to be familiar with all the **legislation** that is relevant to the workplace.

Acts or **regulations** that are set and passed by the government consist of sets of rules or guidelines that must be followed by law. While they apply to all businesses, we will be looking at how these Acts and regulations are important to the beauty and spa industries. Failure to meet legal requirements can result in a fine and, in very serious cases, the loss of the business and possibly imprisonment. Legal requirements vary between local authorities so it is essential that businesses find out about the local **by-laws** to show they are acting professionally and follow the expected industry standards.

Laws relating to health and safety

HANDY HINT

Don't worry about the year that an Act is given; it is the content that is important.

In this part of the chapter you will learn about the:

- Control of Substances Hazardous to Health (COSHH) Regulations
- Electricity at Work Regulations (EAWR)
- Environmental Protection Act
- The Cosmetic Products (Safety) (Amendment) Regulations 2012
- Health and Safety (Display Screen Equipment) Regulations
- Health and Safety (First-Aid) Regulations
- Health and Safety at Work Act (HASAWA)
- Local Government Miscellaneous Provisions Act
- Manual Handling Operations Regulations
- Personal Protective Equipment (PPE) at Work Regulations
- Provision and Use of Work Equipment Regulations (PUWER)
- Reporting of Injuries, Diseases and Dangerous Occurrences Regulations (RIDDOR)
- The Regulatory Reform (Fire Safety) Order (RRO)
- Workplace (Health, Safety and Welfare) Regulations.

HANDY HINT

Trading Standards is a local authority service that enforces a range of legislation. Approximately 100 Acts and 600 sets of regulations are enforced by Trading Standards officers.

Health and Safety at Work Act

The Health and Safety at Work Act (HASAWA) imposes duties on employers to ensure that they provide a safe place of work for everybody affected by their activities. This Act also imposes a duty on employees to ensure that they comply with the employers' safety arrangements and do not behave in a way that endangers others. The Act applies to people who are self-employed too.

The HASAWA is an enabling Act that allows the government to make further laws, known as regulations, with approved codes of practices (ACOP) that detail how employers must comply with them. The various health and safety regulations include guidelines on:

■ health and safety policies

■ risk assessments

■ hygiene, cleanliness and disposal of waste

■ heating, lighting and ventilation

■ work facilities and maintaining a safe and healthy work environment

■ safe use of chemicals

■ personal protective equipment (PPE)

■ fire safety

■ safe use and maintenance of work equipment

■ manual handling (lifting and carrying).

HANDY HINT

Acts are dated when they are passed, but as they are reviewed and have changes called amendments made, they get a revised date. Many Acts are reviewed and amended regularly as laws change.

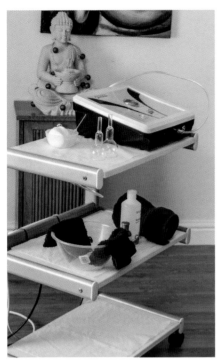

Work areas must be clean and tidy

The Health and Safety at Work Act is the main Act, known as an umbrella Act, which means it contains a number of other Acts, each covering specific aspects of health and safety within it.

Employer's responsibilities

Under the HASAWA and other regulations, an employer is not just responsible for the health and safety of their clients but also the staff, clients/customers and any visitors (such as product representatives, area managers and tradespeople). Your employer must:

- maintain the workplace and make sure it is safe to work in
- give staff appropriate training and supervision
- keep access and exit points clear and free from hazards at all times
- provide a suitable working environment and facilities that comply with the HASAWA
- make sure the salon's health and safety systems are reviewed and updated.

Employee's responsibilities

The employee's responsibilities under the HASAWA are to themselves, their colleagues and clients. You must:

- maintain the health and safety of yourself and others who might be affected by your actions
- work together and communicate with your employer about health and safety issues, so that your employer can keep within the law.

Who is the person responsible for reporting health and safety matters? **You are.** If you see a health and safety problem, you must deal with it or report it. Everyone is responsible for maintaining a safe place of work.

Carry out a risk assessment

Hazard

Something that can cause harm.

Risk

The likelihood of a hazard causing harm.

A **hazard** is something that can cause harm, eg electricity, chemicals, working up a ladder, noise, a keyboard, a bully at work, stress, etc. A **risk** is the chance, high or low, that any hazard will actually cause somebody harm.

A risk assessment is a process carried out within the salon to review and report any potential risks. A risk assessment helps you protect your work colleagues, clients and visitors to the salon. Remember, a hazard has the potential to cause harm. You are not expected to remove all risks from the salon but you are expected to protect people as far as is reasonably practical. People entering the salon have a right to be protected from harm. Failure to follow procedures can result in legal action and loss of business. If your salon employs five or more people you are required under the Health and Safety at Work Act (HASAWA) to record the findings of a risk assessment.

There are five steps to a risk assessment:

1 Identify the hazards.

2 Identify the risks by deciding who might be harmed and how.

3 Evaluate the risks and decide on precautions.

4 Record your findings and identify who should implement them.

5 Review your assessment and update if necessary.

Level of risk

A hazard may not necessarily become a risk. You need to assess a risk based on the likelihood of it occurring. This will allow you to decide on the level of risk. The level of risk is worked out using the following calculation, assigning the numbers from the lists below:

Risk level = consequence of exposure × likelihood of occurrence

Consequence

1 – no injury

2 – minor injury

3 – moderate injury

4 – major injury

5 – injury resulting in death

Likelihood

1 – very unlikely

2 – unlikely

3 – possible

4 – likely

5 – almost certain

Risk level

1–3 = low risk

4–6 = medium risk

8–12 = high risk

15–25 = extremely high risk

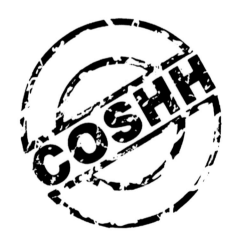

INDUSTRY TIP

Any item blocking a fire exit is a high-level risk.

INDUSTRY TIP

In winter months it is often dark while we are at work so lights bulbs should be tested regularly to ensure that they are working and available when needed to make sure that any risk is reduced.

The result of this calculation will allow you to evaluate the level of risk and make suitable decisions about how to manage it.

The following table gives some examples of low-level risks and high-level risks:

Hazard	Low-level risk	High-level risk
Trailing wires	At the back of the treatment area out of the way.	Trailing across the treatment area.
Blown bulb	If good natural light. During daytime.	In a dark stairway – a risk of tripping and falling.
Stock delivery	Left in the corner of the stock room.	In the middle of a walkway – a risk of tripping over it and injury.
Chemical hazards	Stored and handled correctly using the manufacturers' instructions.	Stored in incorrect conditions (eg products may be flammable). Used incorrectly without referring to manufacturers' instructions.

Why and when a risk assessment should be carried out

A risk assessment should be carried out to ensure safety in the salon. Almost anything in the salon can be a hazard and become a risk. It is therefore your responsibility, along with your employer, to prevent these hazards from becoming risks for the safety of yourself and others.

A risk assessment must be carried out as a result of:

- a change to the salon environment
- the introduction of new treatments or products
- a change in personal circumstances.

A change to the salon environment

A change to the salon environment could mean a total salon refit or something small, such as the installation of a ramp for disabled access. Whatever the change within the salon, the impact on the staff and people visiting the salon must be considered. Even a new shelving system in the stock cupboard or dispensary may need a risk assessment to work out the safest place to store certain items.

> ### Activity
>
> Think of the way products and equipment are stored in your salon. List where you would put the following items so that they were stored safely and correctly:
>
> - talc
> - massage oil
> - lash glue
> - eye make-up remover
> - epilation needles
> - water testing kit.

The introduction of new treatments or products

It is always exciting to get brand-new products and offer your clients a new treatment. Before you start to use new products or introduce new treatments you must understand the risk they could pose to the client and the therapist carrying out the treatment. For example, if your salon was introducing a new skincare range and you were to put the products on clients' skin without reading the manufacturer's instructions, what could happen?

> **INDUSTRY TIP**
>
> Products containing chemicals are widely used in beauty and spa therapy. You must always read and follow the manufacturers' instructions. Products should be stored safely and in line with the manufacturers' instructions. The stock storage area of the salon should be accessible only to authorised members of staff.

> **HANDY HINT**
>
> If you do not have steps or a ladder, you must not place anything on high shelves if the result is that you have to stand on tiptoe or overreach to get it.

> **INDUSTRY TIP**
>
> Failure to carry out a risk assessment could put colleagues and visitors to the salon in danger.

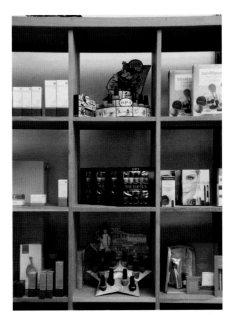

A risk assessment may need to be carried out for a new shelving system in the salon

> **HANDY HINT**
>
> If your salon is going to offer a new treatment, such as body electrotherapy, you will need to check with your insurance company to make sure you are insured to offer this treatment.

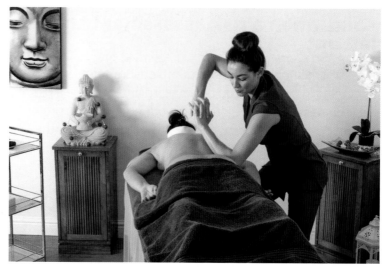

A new treatment

A change in personal circumstances

Therapists' circumstances may change during the time that they are employed at a salon. For example, a work colleague may become pregnant. A risk assessment would therefore need to be carried out to identify any areas of her work she might no longer be able to participate in. The salon may also take on a new member of staff who is too tall or too short to use the salon's couches. A risk assessment would need to be carried out to prevent injury or long-term damage to them from poor posture.

Activity

If you or a work colleague becomes pregnant, you will have to carry out a risk assessment. Look on the Health and Safety Executive's (HSE's) website, www.hse.gov.uk/mothers/index.htm, for more information. List five main points you need to consider when carrying out a risk assessment for a pregnant colleague.

Necessary actions

The salon has many potential hazards. If you notice a hazard, it is your responsibility to report it and carry out a risk assessment before it becomes a risk and an injury occurs. When you have carried out a risk assessment and identified the possibility of a risk, you must decide on the necessary actions to take. You will need to:

- record the risk assessment
- report the risk to the salon manager or owner.

Once you have completed the risk assessment you will need to make an action plan. Your action plan will need to include:

- long-term actions to ensure that the risks are dealt with and continue to be managed (eg routinely checking a piece of fixed equipment to make sure the same fault does not happen again)
- training for employees (eg a health and safety course and relevant information for staff to read)
- regular checks that will need to take place to make sure that the hazards and risks identified by the risk assessment are controlled
- staff responsibilities for maintaining and preventing the hazards and risks that you identified
- updated risk assessment information.

> **HANDY HINT**
>
> Focus on more significant risks rather than smaller, less severe risks.

Record the risk assessment

A risk assessment can be recorded in a number of different ways:

- a checklist
- a report
- a form or table.

Once you have decided the way in which you are going to report your risk assessment, you need to think about the information that needs to be included:

- What are the hazards?
- Who might be harmed?
- What is the level of the risk?
- What steps are already in place to manage the risk?
- What additional or follow-up action needs to be taken and by whom?
- How will follow-up actions be put into place?
- What is the target date for putting into place follow-up action?
- What is the completion date for follow-up action?

An example of a risk assessment is shown in the table on pages 62–63.

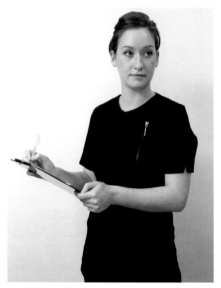

A therapist using a checklist to carry out a risk assessment

> **PAT**
>
> Portable appliance test. Appliances need to be checked by a qualified electrician at least once a year.

Report the risk assessment

It is important that you report the findings of a risk assessment to your manager or the salon owner. They need to be informed of your findings to be able to make the necessary improvements or changes.

> **HANDY HINT**
>
> Do not speak to staff about risk assessment actions when they are working. Organise a staff meeting before work when they aren't busy. Put a list of your risk assessment actions on the wall in the staffroom and tick them off once they are completed.

Hazard (details of equipment or activity)	Who might be harmed?	What additional action needs to be taken?	How will additional actions be put into place?	Level of risk	Likelihood of risk	Target date	Completion date
Sharps (such as epilation needles): ■ cross-infection ■ needle-stick injuries. 	Staff Clients	Clients: To sit or lie correctly on a treatment couch. Staff: Dispose of sharps in sharps box to avoid needle-stick injuries, cross-contamination of blood.	Check all clients are positioned correctly prior to treatment that involves sharps (eg electrolysis). Demonstrate correct posture for sitting at staff meetings. Sterilise equipment. Nominate a member of staff to be responsible for the sharps bin. First-aid training.			22/4/17	26/5/17
Water: ■ skin irritations from contact with water. 	Staff	Wear PPE as needed. Dry and moisturise hands correctly.	Check hands daily for signs of dermatitis. Inform staff of risk of dermatitis and signs of dermatitis at regular meetings and new staff induction. Get information leaflets from the HSE. Monitor PPE.			16/5/17	3/6/17
Products and chemicals: ■ incorrect usage ■ client skin sensitivities. 	Staff Clients	Clients: Always carry out a skin test on clients when using products (eg self-tan) with active ingredients. Staff: Read and follow manufacturers' instructions. Follow COSHH.	Staff must always use previous record cards to check for skin sensitivities and carry out patch tests. Update all record cards.			27/5/17	1/6/17

Hazard (details of equipment or activity)	Who might be harmed?	What additional action needs to be taken?	How will additional actions be put into place?	Level of risk	Likelihood of risk	Target date	Completion date
Electricity: ▪ faulty equipment ▪ dangerous positioning and storage of equipment ▪ incorrect usage. 	Staff	Visually check all equipment prior to use. Clean all equipment. Store equipment away from water. Follow EAWR	Make sure equipment is **PAT** tested and working correctly. Staff must follow manufacturers' instructions.			12/4/17	31/5/17
Posture: ▪ musculoskeletal injuries (eg neck and back pain) from standing for long periods. 	Staff	Staff should make sure they stand at the correct height. Staff to take regular breaks.	Employer to provide suitable stools and couches. Employer to make sure staff wear sensible footwear.			25/5/17	1/6/17

HANDY HINT

Make sure that you recap your knowledge of health and safety requirements and issues you covered at Level 2.

HANDY HINT

If you have new information regarding health and safety, it is your responsibility to pass it on.

HANDY HINT

It is always beneficial to revise the regulations that relate to your work environment and keep up to date with changes. In your working day your activities are covered by more health and safety regulations than you realise!

HANDY HINT

Health and safety laws are always changing and being updated to help protect you. Always check the HSE's website (www.hse.gov.uk) for the most up-to-date information.

Informing staff

Once you have completed a risk assessment, it is important that everyone working on the premises or anyone entering the premises is informed of any changes to procedures or policies as quickly as possible. Staff can be notified of any changes at staff meetings. For clients and visitors to the salon you can put a notice up or advise them verbally (eg 'We now have a ramp to make it easier if you find the steps to the treatment rooms difficult'). Whichever way you decide is best to communicate this information, make sure everyone is aware and informed.

Update risk assessment information

It is important to keep up to date with health and safety and update any risk assessments.

When you work in a busy salon, you don't always have time for formal talks to discuss health and safety. However, it is vitally important that staff are aware of health and safety at all times and that information and updates are passed on to them.

Health and safety support

Even when you have worked in the salon for a long time, you must not take health and safety for granted. Just because there has never been an injury before, doesn't mean there never will be.

As well as being aware of new health and safety requirements, you must make sure you are familiar with existing requirements and the latest information about products, chemicals or work-related diseases (eg dermatitis). It is also important to remember the basic industry requirements for health and safety.

In this part of the chapter you will learn about:

- the health and safety support that should be provided to staff
- procedures for dealing with different types of security breaches
- the need for insurance.

At Level 3, you will be expanding your role to monitor health and safety in the workplace and you will be supporting others to ensure all health and safety requirements are met. This will include regular monitoring and reviewing of the following key hazards and risks, so that they can be controlled and managed:

- sterilisation and disinfection
- work-related diseases (eg dermatitis)
- slips, trips and falls.

Sterilisation and disinfection

Sterilisation and **disinfection** are key areas where you can control risks to prevent harm to yourself and others. The consequences of not carrying out sterilisation and disinfection could be:

- loss of business

- creating an unprofessional image (eg because of a dirty, unhygienic couch or broken and dirty equipment)

- legal action from clients or colleagues (eg because of cross-infection or cross-contamination from unclean equipment and tools).

To prevent this you must:

- make sure you are fully trained and understand how the equipment for sterilisation and disinfection works

- always follow the manufacturers' instructions to give you the maximum level of sterilisation or disinfection.

Methods of sterilisation and disinfection

The following diagram shows the equipment used for the methods of sterilisation and disinfection.

Sterilisation

The total removal or destruction of all living micro-organisms, including their spores.

Disinfection

The destruction of micro-organisms but not their spores. Disinfection is less effective than sterilisation.

HANDY HINT

Disinfecting spray or wipes can be used on certain tools and equipment.

HANDY HINT

UV cabinets are good for storing sterilised instruments to keep them sterile.

Methods of sterilisation and disinfection

Autoclave:
- Only for sterilising metal and glass.
- Uses steam to sterilise.
- Heats water under pressure to 120°C.
- Only method of sterilisation in the salon.
- Kills organisms within 20 minutes.

Ultraviolet (UV) cabinet:
- Objects are exposed to ultraviolet rays.
- Only disinfects tools.
- Not suitable for tools with unexposed surfaces.
- Takes at least 15 minutes.

Chemicals (eg Barbicide):
- Only disinfects tools.
- Tools must be fully immersed.
- Tools need to be left in solution for recommended time.

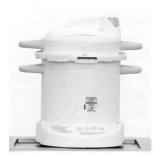

Autoclave

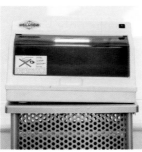

UV cabinet

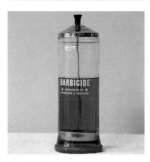

Barbicide

HANDY HINT

Chemical solutions lose their effectiveness over time so they need to be changed regularly.

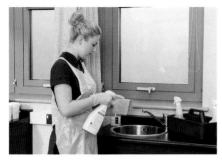

A therapist disinfecting a sink

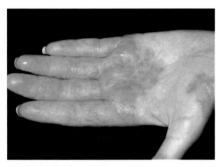

Dermatitis

INDUSTRY TIP

Objects need to be turned over in a UV cabinet to make sure that all surfaces are exposed to the rays and are disinfected.

WHY DON'T YOU...
Find out more information about dermatitis by looking at the HSE's Bad Hand Day campaign (www.hse.gov.uk).

INDUSTRY TIP

Your employer should provide disposable powder-free and latex-free gloves as part of your personal protective equipment (PPE).

HANDY HINT

Follow these four simple steps to avoid dermatitis:

1 Wear non-latex, powder-free gloves when dealing with chemicals and products or when required.

2 Dry your hands thoroughly after washing them.

3 Moisturise your hands regularly.

4 Check your hands regularly for signs of contact dermatitis. If you notice any signs of dermatitis, let your salon manager know and seek further advice from a pharmacist.

Dermatitis

It is important to protect your hands with gloves to avoid dermatitis. Dermatitis is a skin condition affecting the epidermis and dermis. It happens when the skin comes into contact with substances that can irritate it and cause allergies. The skin becomes sore, dry, red and cracked with blisters. Dermatitis is not contagious but can spread on your own skin. Beauty therapists and hairdressers are more likely to get dermatitis because of the need to wash their hands regularly and because of exposure to products that may become irritants.

Common workplace injuries

Slips, trips and falls

Slips and trips are the most common cause of injury in the workplace. You must stay alert to the dangers of slips, trips and falls. They can cause serious injury and may end in legal action. You need to be alert to the causes of slips, trips and falls and try to prevent them.

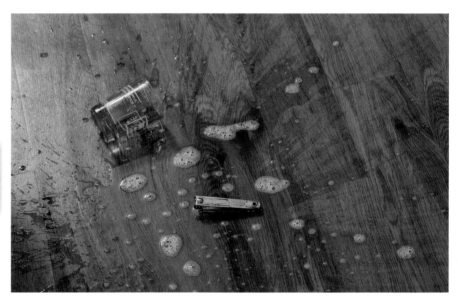

Liquids spilt on the floor are a slip hazard

The following list shows hazards that can be caused in a salon if a health and safety/risk assessment is not carried out.

- uneven flooring
- spillages that haven't been cleaned up
- incorrect/unsuitable footwear
- trailing cables and leads
- obstructions to walkways
- running in the salon
- poor lighting
- no health and safety policy in place.

Workplace (Health, Safety and Welfare) Regulations

The Workplace (Health, Safety and Welfare) Regulations require everyone in the workplace to help maintain a safe and healthy working environment. You and your employer should follow **environmentally friendly** working practices.

Employer's responsibilities

Your employer's responsibilities under the regulations are to:

- maintain equipment and the workplace
- regulate temperatures
- make sure working conditions and the size and shape of the room suit the number of staff employed
- make sure there is sufficient lighting and ventilation
- make sure all walkways are clear of hazards
- provide toilets and washing facilities
- provide drinking water and facilities for staff to rest, eat meals and change clothing
- provide secure areas or lockers for employees' clothing and property
- make sure all lights above the stairways and at fire exits are working.

Employee's responsibilities

Your responsibilities under the regulations are to:

- make sure all doors, fire exits and stairways are kept free of **obstructions** and hazards
- make sure you know the fire **evacuation** procedure
- prevent infection and **contamination** by keeping the salon's workstations, mirrors, floors, gowns, towels, equipment and tools clean
- keep the salon tidy to prevent accidents, such as tripping over trailing electrical wires
- clean up spillages immediately to prevent slippery surfaces
- report any problems that you are unable to deal with to your employer.

Environmentally friendly

Safe for or good for the environment.

HANDY HINT

The number of toilet and washing facilities must be sufficient for the number of employees and customers using the premises.

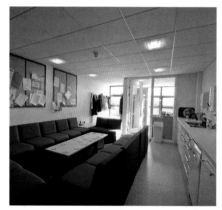

A clean and tidy staffroom

Obstruction

Something that blocks a path.

Evacuation

Leaving an area, eg in an emergency.

Contamination

The presence of something unwanted that might be harmful.

Provision and Use of Work Equipment Regulations

The Provision and Use of Work Equipment Regulations (PUWER) require that all the equipment in the salon (both new and second-hand) must be used for its intended purpose only and kept in good working condition.

Employer's responsibilities

Your employer's responsibilities under the regulations are:

- to provide you with training to use the equipment as it is intended
- to make sure that the equipment is properly built and fit for use
- to ensure all work equipment is properly maintained including equipment supplied by employees.

Employee's responsibilities

Your responsibilities under the regulations are:

- to make sure you know how to use the equipment in the salon properly and safely
- to use equipment only for its intended purpose (eg do not use a warm wax heater for heating paraffin wax).

Greenhouse gas emissions

The release of gases into the atmosphere that absorb infrared radiation. These gases contribute to the greenhouse effect and global warming.

Therapist instructing a colleague

Local Government Miscellaneous Provisions Act

The Local Government Miscellaneous Provisions Act requires all businesses to be registered with the local authority, first so that the government knows they exist and second so that they can be **monitored** and regulated. Your employer must make sure they take the relevant steps to register for the services they are offering.

A business must show that its standards meet the rules and regulations set out in the local council's by-laws. By-laws are a set of local laws that deal with local issues and tell a business how it must act with regards to health and safety, hygiene and cleanliness. Specific by-laws relate to specific business practices (eg ear piercing and electrolysis). You may have to obtain a licence to practice so always check with your local council. Some councils have downloadable copies of their by-laws on their websites.

This Act also gives local authorities the power to inspect business premises and to act if something falls below the required standard.

Monitored

Kept an eye on.

Control of Substances Hazardous to Health Regulations

Various chemicals are seen as hazardous (eg cleaning substances and bleach). The Control of Substances Hazardous to Health Regulations, otherwise referred to in the industry as COSHH, identify dangerous chemicals. Hazardous substances can enter the body through **ingestion**, **absorption** or **inhalation**. A hazardous substance in the workplace can put a person's health at risk and cause disease or injury, such as asthma, cancer or dermatitis.

Hazardous substances must be **identified** by specific symbols that you should be able to recognise. All suppliers must legally provide guidelines on how their materials should be stored and used. All products identified as hazardous must, by law, be listed and a COSHH risk assessment must be **accessible**. Be aware that substances that seem to be harmless can be hazardous if used or stored incorrectly. A risk assessment should be carried out for each substance used in the salon. Low-risk products should be used instead of high-risk products wherever there is an **alternative**.

Ingestion

Taking into the mouth and digestive system (ie eating).

Absorption

The process whereby chemicals or nutrients enter the bloodstream via the stomach or intestines.

Inhalation

Breathing in.

Identified

Recognised or pointed out.

Accessible

Easy to get to.

Alternative

A different possible choice or outcome.

Under COSHH you must make sure that any hazardous substances are stored, handled, used and disposed of correctly and safely. The best way of remembering this is by following **SHUD**:

- **S**torage: keep in a locked cupboard at room temperature when not in use; ideally this cupboard should also be **fire retardant**.
- **H**andling: wear appropriate personal protective equipment (PPE) such as gloves, mask and apron.
- **U**sage: use according to the manufacturer's instructions or workplace guidelines.
- **D**isposal: make sure you dispose of all hazardous waste in a hazardous waste bag; the local authority or a private company will collect the waste and **incinerate** it. Hazardous waste usually consists of tissues, cotton wool and wax strips that have been in contact with bodily fluids (eg blood).

The manufacturer's instructions will explain how to store, handle, use and dispose of chemicals or substances. The local by-laws will tell you how to dispose of them. Be considerate to the **environment** and follow the local authority's guidelines on waste and refuse. Your salon's policy will explain where to store and mix the chemicals and where to dispose of them in the workplace.

Employer's responsibilities

Your employer's responsibilities under the regulations are:

- to make sure COSHH health and safety information sheets are available for substances and chemicals in the workplace
- to make sure chemicals are disposed of according to local by-laws and with respect to the environment
- to ensure that a COSHH risk assessment is undertaken.

Employee's responsibilities

Your responsibilities under the regulations are:

- to follow SHUD
- to read and follow the manufacturer's instructions, local by-laws and your salon's policy
- to know where to find the COSHH information sheets.

Because the following substances have their own specific regulations, COSHH does **not** cover:

- lead
- asbestos
- radioactive substances.

Fire retardant

Made of material that slows down the spread of fire.

Incinerate

To burn something to ashes.

Environment

This can mean both the natural world around you as well as the things around you, which often have an effect on you.

WHY DON'T YOU...
Make a list of all the items in your salon that would come under COSHH – everything from washing powder to peroxide. Ask your tutor or manager to check your list.

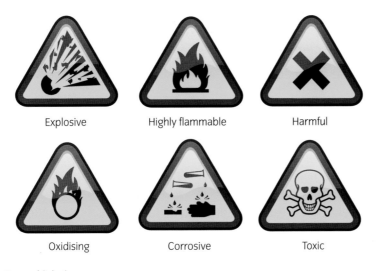

Explosive Highly flammable Harmful

Oxidising Corrosive Toxic

Hazard labels

Electricity at Work Regulations

The Electricity at Work Regulations (EAWR) requires all electrical **appliances** to be used with caution and handled correctly. Electrical equipment must be maintained in a condition suitable for use, checked and tested on a routine basis.

Appliance

A device or piece of equipment made to perform a specific task.

Employer's responsibilities

Your employer's responsibilities under the regulations are to make sure that all electrical equipment:

- is in a safe working condition
- is portable appliance tested (PAT) by a qualified electrician at least once a year (some appliances might need checking more frequently)
- is visually checked by salon employees routinely and frequently.

PAT requires anything that has a cable and a plug to be tested. A record must be kept. Insurance companies require all electrical equipment to be routinely tested. Each appliance must have a sticker on the plug to show the last date tested and when it is next due.

Employee's responsibilities

Your responsibilities under the regulations are to:

- not use electrical appliances unless you have been trained
- use appliances correctly and to switch them off after use
- carry out routine daily visual checks

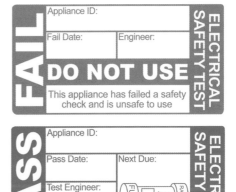

PAT testing

- not overload plug sockets
- report any faults immediately to your supervisor or manager and label the item as faulty
- not use faulty equipment.

Routine checks could be done in the morning when equipment is switched on or at the end of the day when equipment is switched off. You must check any electrical appliance you use for faults or problems (eg frayed or loose cables or flexes, broken plugs or damage to the external casing).

Equipment that has been identified as faulty must have a clear and secure label applied to it. Write down what the problem or fault is and include the date. Remove the equipment from the working area if possible until it can be repaired or disposed of.

Activity

Can you see evidence of PAT testing having taken place in your salon? What date did it take place? When is the next test due?

The Regulatory Reform (Fire Safety) Order

Emergency exit route

The safest route by which staff, clients and visitors can escape from a building

The Regulatory Reform (Fire Safety) Order (RRO) requires all premises to have basic standards of fire prevention and control and an **emergency exit route**.

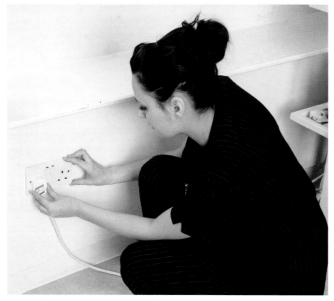

Therapist checking a plug

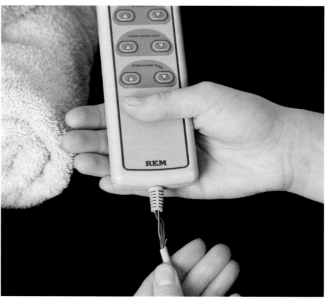

Faulty wiring

General fire safety hazards

Fires need three things to start – a source of ignition (heat), a source of fuel (something that burns) and oxygen:

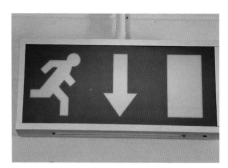

Fire exit sign

- Sources of ignition include heaters, lighting, naked flames, electrical equipment, smokers' materials (cigarettes, matches, etc), and anything else that can get very hot or cause sparks.

- Sources of fuel include wood, paper, plastic, rubber or foam, loose packaging materials, waste rubbish and furniture.

- Sources of oxygen include the air around us.

Every business/building owner must carry out a fire safety risk assessment which should be reviewed annually or following any changes. It assesses how to prevent a fire and in the event of a fire how to control it.

A fire safety risk assessment must:

- identify fire hazards
- identify people at risk
- evaluate, remove or reduce risks and protect staff, clients and visitors from risk
- record, plan, inform, instruct and train staff
- be reviewed.

Employer's responsibilities

Your employer's responsibilities under the order are to:

- keep sources of ignition and flammable substances apart
- avoid accidental fires, eg make sure heaters cannot be knocked over
- ensure good housekeeping at all times, eg avoid build-up of rubbish that could burn
- consider how to detect fires and how to warn people quickly if they start, eg installing smoke alarms and fire alarms or bells
- have the correct fire-fighting equipment for putting out a fire quickly
- keep fire exits and escape routes clearly marked and unobstructed at all times
- ensure that workers receive appropriate training on procedures they need to follow, including fire drills
- review and update the risk assessment regularly.

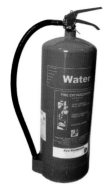

Water extinguisher

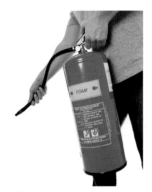

Foam extinguisher

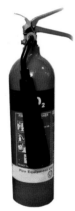

Carbon dioxide

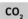

Carbon dioxide.

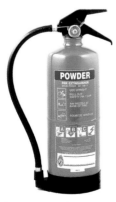

Dry powder extinguisher

Employee's responsibilities

Your responsibilities under the Act and the order are to:

■ know where the fire extinguishers and fire blankets are located in the salon

■ know which fire extinguishers can be used on different fires

■ know the evacuation procedure and where the safe meeting point is for salon staff and clients

■ ensure you receive adequate training in fire safety procedures including fire drills and make sure you know your evacuation point.

Fire safety procedures

Under the Regulatory Reform (Fire Safety) Order, new staff must be informed of fire safety procedures:

■ what to do if the fire alarm sounds

■ how to raise the alarm

■ safe evacuation procedures

■ fire assembly points.

All staff need to know where the fire extinguishers and blankets are located and which fire extinguishers can be used on different fires. The following table shows the different classes of fire and which extinguisher should be used in each case.

Class of fire	Uses	Type of extinguisher
A	Wood, paper, hair or textiles	Water extinguisher, foam extinguisher, dry powder extinguisher, wet chemical extinguisher
B	Flammable liquids	Foam extinguisher, dry powder extinguisher, CO_2 extinguisher
C	Flammable gases	Dry powder extinguisher, CO_2 extinguisher
D	Flammable metals	Specially formulated dry powder extinguisher
E	Electrical fires	CO_2, dry powder extinguisher
F	Oils	Wet chemical extinguisher, fire blanket

Personal Protective Equipment (PPE) at Work Regulations

Gloves, aprons, masks and eye protection for salon employees as well as your uniform and shoes all come under the Personal Protective Equipment (PPE) at Work Regulations. Protective equipment used for the client is not covered by these regulations. It is important that you wear the appropriate PPE to protect yourself from harm when you are working with chemicals and to minimise cross-infection. PPE Equipment that should be worn by a person at work to protect them against a health or safety risk. PPE within the beauty industry includes:

- gloves
- eye protection
- aprons.

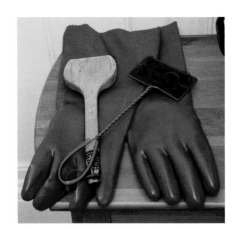

Thermal gloves for handling hot stones during massage

Employer's responsibilities

Your employer's responsibilities under the regulations are to:

- supply free of charge any PPE required for you to carry out your job
- maintain supplies of PPE so that they are always accessible
- train staff how to use PPE appropriately
- carry out risk assessments
- recommend when to use PPE.

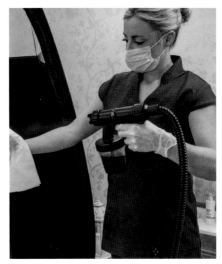

Therapist wearing a disposable protective mask

Employee's responsibilities

Your responsibilities under the regulations are to:

- wear PPE when you are mixing, handling and using chemicals or substances
- report any shortages of PPE to the relevant person so that additional stock can be ordered.

What items are PPE in the beauty industry?

- aprons – waxing/tanning
- gloves – waxing/eye treatments
- masks – tanning.

Manual Handling Operations Regulations

You are sometimes required to move equipment and stock around the salon. This is called manual handling. Always follow the Manual Handling Operations Regulations. There are correct ways to lift objects so you do not injure yourself.

According to the Health and Safety Executive (HSE), more than a third of all injuries resulting in over three days' absence from work are caused by manual handling. A recent survey showed that over 12.3 million working days are lost each year due to work-related **musculoskeletal disorders** that have been caused or made worse by poor manual handling.

Musculoskeletal disorders

Muscle and bone disorders.

Activity

Write a list of problems or disorders that might affect a therapist's muscles and/or bones if they do not follow manual handling guidelines.

Employer's responsibilities

Your employer's responsibility under the regulations is to carry out risk assessments on all employees for manual lifting to make sure they are able to lift boxes and other heavy objects without causing injury.

Employee's responsibilities

Your responsibility under the regulations is to always ask yourself: 'Can I lift this?' If the answer is no, then don't! Ask for help. If the answer is yes, remember to bend your knees and keep your back straight. Lift the weight with your thigh muscles, not your back, and keep the item you are lifting close to your body. Even if a box is light, you should ask for help if it obscures your view.

Steps to take when lifting a box:

1 Place your feet slightly apart (in line with your shoulders) with the leading leg forward.

2 Bend your knees, keeping your back straight when picking up the box.

3 Using both hands, get a firm grip of the box from underneath.

4 Lift up the box and hold it close to your body (don't twist your body).

Remember: back problems can cause a lot of pain, and can last a lifetime. You should not try to lift/move anything that is too heavy or too bulky for you to manage safely.

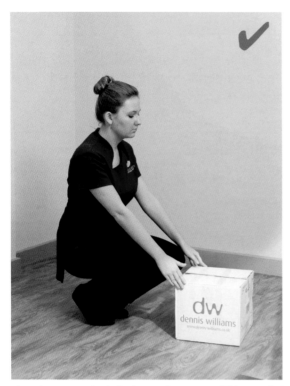
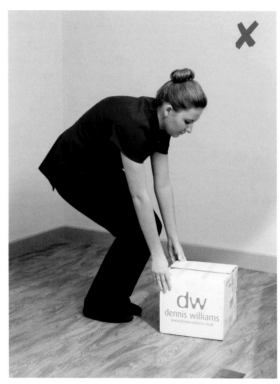

The picture on the left shows the correct lifting technique; the lifting technique on the right is incorrect. The technique on the right will put pressure on the spine and could lead to injury

Reporting of Injuries, Diseases and Dangerous Occurrences Regulations

The Reporting of Injuries, Diseases and Dangerous Occurrences Regulations (RIDDOR) require the following **occurrences** to be reported to the HSE immediately by telephone and then in writing within ten days of the incident:

- injuries resulting in over seven days' loss of work (including non-working days)

- injuries (eg falls) sustained by you, your colleagues, clients or visitors in the workplace that result in three or more days off work

- major injuries, such as amputation, dislocation, fractures (not fingers or toes), loss of sight and any other eye injuries

- any work-related incident where a person has had to spend more than 24 hours in hospital

- accidents and injuries sustained from violence in the workplace

- death in the workplace

- diseases, such as **occupational** dermatitis or work-related asthma

- dangerous occurrences (eg a gas leak) even if they occur outside working hours and no one is injured.

Occurrence

Something that happens.

Occupational

Relating to a job.

Employer's responsibilities

Your employer's responsibility under the regulations is to report any of the above occurrences and make sure that information about the occurrence has been recorded.

Employee's responsibilities

Your responsibilities under the regulations are to:

- report any work-related diseases to the person responsible for health and safety
- prevent any work-related diseases by wearing PPE
- report any accidents or injuries that happen to you at work
- prevent accidents or injuries by following safe working guidelines and maintaining a tidy environment.

Activity

Which work-related diseases might you be exposed to? Make a list. Discuss your list with your manager and colleagues.

Health and Safety (First-Aid) Regulations

Advisable

Suggested that you should.

HANDY HINT

Make sure you know where the business keeps its health and safety policies as these should be accessible.

HANDY HINT

Know where your first-aid box is kept just in case you need to access it.

Hypoallergenic

Products that do not contain any or many of the known allergens.

The Health and Safety (First-Aid) Regulations apply to all workplaces in Great Britain – including those with fewer than five employees and those with self-employed staff. The regulations require the protection of everyone in the workplace by making sure risk assessments are carried out to prevent accidents and injuries at work. It is **advisable** that at least one person has undertaken first-aid training.

A basic first-aid box or container should include:

- a leaflet giving general guidance on first aid (eg HSE's leaflet 'Basic advice on first aid at work')
- 20 individually wrapped sterile plasters (assorted sizes), appropriate to the type of work (**hypoallergenic** plasters can be provided, if necessary)
- two sterile eye pads
- four individually wrapped triangular bandages, preferably sterile
- six safety pins
- two large sterile individually wrapped unmedicated wound dressings

- six medium-sized individually wrapped unmedicated wound dressings
- a pair of disposable gloves
- eyewash kits, because of the chemicals used in salons.

The appointed person should check the contents of the first-aid container frequently and make sure it is restocked if anything is used. They should ensure the safe disposal of items when they reach their expiry date.

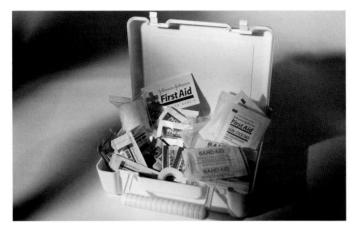

First-aid box

Employer's responsibilities

Your employer's responsibilities under the regulations are to:

- take immediate action if employees are injured or taken ill at work
- consider providing a first aider
- choose an appointed person to be responsible for first-aid arrangements
- provide a well-stocked first-aid container
- make sure all staff know who the appointed first aider is (if appropriate).

Employee's responsibilities

Your responsibilities under the regulations are to:

- avoid taking any unnecessary risks that might put you or others in danger
- report to your appointed person any first-aid supply shortages
- record any accidents in an accident book.

To record an accident in the accident book, make a note of who had the accident, the date and time of the accident and what action was taken. Record the name of any witnesses and who else was present at the time of the accident. The accident book should be kept in a central location in the salon.

> **HANDY HINT**
>
> Make sure you know where the accident record book is kept.

Health and Safety (Display Screen Equipment) Regulations

Periodic

Occurring at regular intervals.

The Health and Safety (Display Screen Equipment) Regulations protect the health of people who work with display screen equipment (DSE). This includes computer workstations or visual display units (VDU) (ie computer screens). It applies to people, such as salon receptionists, who use display screen equipment for long periods at a time as part of their job. It does not apply to occasional use, such as making appointments. Long-term use is often associated with neck, shoulder, back or arm pain, fatigue and eyestrain. Display screen equipment work is not risky but users need to follow good practice, such as setting up their workstations well and taking **periodic** breaks.

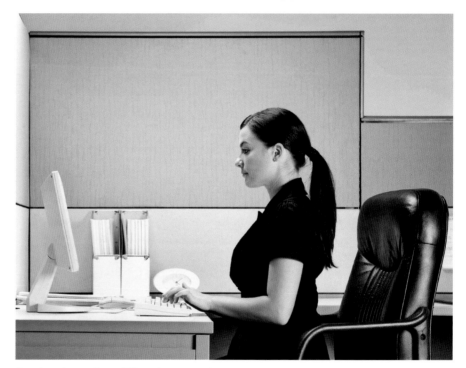

Good posture when sitting at a computer

Employer's responsibilities

Your employer's responsibilities under the regulations are to:

- carry out risk assessments on new workstations or make changes to current workstations
- re-assess workstations if staff suffer from any discomfort
- train employees in good practice for working with display screen equipment
- plan scheduling of work, regular breaks and changes of activity
- pay for employees to have eyesight tests if required.

Employee's responsibilities

Your responsibilities under the regulations are to:

- make sure you maintain good posture:

  - keep your back straight when you work and do not slouch
  - keep your feet flat on the floor when sitting

- take regular breaks if you are using display screen equipment for long periods of time and to change activity (eg if you are a receptionist change to a different task, such as filing)
- organise your desk space effectively
- keep your mouse arm straight and rest it lightly on the mouse
- use a wrist support
- keep your keyboard close to your body and do not over-stretch
- adjust the screen or lighting position where possible to suit your personal needs.

Environmental Protection Act

Any waste products from the salon must be disposed of correctly so you do not pollute the environment or harm others. You must always dispose of products by following the MFIs and local by-laws. All staff must be trained and be made aware of how to dispose of waste in a safe way.

Certain consumables need to be disposed of in a clinical yellow waste disposal bag. Check with your local by-laws to see what they require.

Laws relating to consumer protection

In this part of the chapter you will learn about the:

- Data Protection Act
- Consumer Protection Act
- Consumer Protection (Distance Selling) Regulations
- Supply of Goods and Services Act
- Sale of Goods Act
- Sale and Supply of Goods Act
- Trade Descriptions Acts
- Prices Act.

> **HANDY HINT**
>
> The Health and Safety (Display Screen Equipment) Regulations state that certain kinds of workers are entitled to have an appropriate eye test paid for by their employer. If any of your work is reliant on good eyesight you can ask your employer to pay for your eye test.

> **HANDY HINT**
>
> Further information on good posture can be found in chapter 303, Provide body massage.

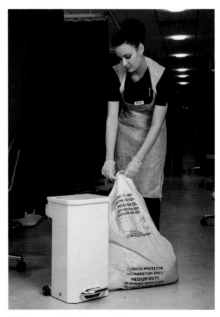

Yellow waste disposal bag

Data Protection Act

The Data Protection Act controls how personal information is used by organisations, businesses and the government.

Clients give you their personal information, such as their addresses and phone numbers, because they trust you and the salon to use it correctly. Clients' information must be protected and you must always follow the Data Protection Act. Everyone responsible for using data has to follow strict rules called data protection principles.

The Information Commissioner's Office (ICO) is the UK's independent authority set up to uphold information rights in the public's interest. It sets the rules for the Data Protection Act, which protects people's rights to confidentiality and privacy. When completing client record cards and taking contact details at reception, you must make sure you follow the requirements of the Data Protection Act. Under the Data Protection Act, businesses must register if they keep client data on a computer.

The following list shows you how personal data must be used:

- Personal information must be processed fairly and lawfully.
- Personal data should only be used for specified purposes and should not be used for anything other than the stated purposes.
- Personal information should be **accurate** and kept up to date as far as possible.
- Information should not be kept once it is no longer required for the purpose it was held for.
- Personal data should be processed **in accordance with** the Data Protection Act.
- No unauthorised person should have access to the information and the business should protect against accidental loss, destruction or damage to personal data.
- Personal information should not be **transferred** to any other country unless protection and rights are maintained during the processing of the information.

Employer's responsibilities

Your employer's responsibilities under the Act are to:

- keep only information that is needed for the business
- keep records as accurate as possible and up to date
- dispose of information carefully (eg shred paper documents) when it is no longer required
- never pass on any information to a **third party**
- limit access to records to only those employees who need it for their work.

Accurate

Correct and true.

In accordance with

Consistent with.

Transferred

Sent to or shared with.

HANDY HINT

Make sure you are familiar with how the law affects you, as you do not want your reputation as well as that of the business to be affected.

Third party

Another person or organisation that is not directly involved but may have connections with the business.

Employee's responsibilities

The Data Protection Act protects you and all the data stored about you, whether it is held on paper or on a computer. This could include medical and dental records, bank records and employment and college records. You have a right to access this information if and when you want to and you should expect it to be kept confidential. Remember this and be professional with any information you record regarding any individual.

You must keep records as accurately as you can and keep information confidential. You must not pass on any information about your clients to a third party, whether that is personal details, services that they have had or products that they have bought.

Failing to keep client confidentiality could mean losing clients and gaining a poor reputation. A client could sue the business, in which case the guilty employee could be given a warning or lose their job for **gross misconduct**.

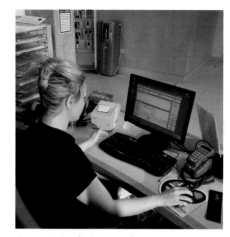

A computer being used to manage clients' records

Gross misconduct

Very bad, unacceptable behaviour.

Consumer Protection Act

In the salon, we are exposed daily to different products and we have a right to expect those products to be as safe as possible. The Consumer Protection Act safeguards staff and clients from products that do not reach a reasonable level of safety.

It is now possible to sue a supplier even without proof of the supplier being **negligent** under the Sale of Goods Act. A therapist using the product in the salon can sue the supplier if a product is faulty (even though your employer purchased it).

The Consumer Protection Act also covers:

- misleading prices, services or facilities
- price comparisons
- inaccurate conditions attached to the price.

HANDY HINT

Never give clients personal information, such as your address or phone number. It is unethical and might put you at risk. Your contract of employment might also forbid this – for example, to prevent staff from encouraging clients to have their treatments done privately in their homes.

Negligent

Failing to take proper care.

HANDY HINT

Do you know where to find the product price lists if there is a price query?

Employer's responsibilities

The employer's responsibilities under this Act are to:

- display clear prices for products and services: the client should be able to tell exactly how much something will cost
- not make false claims about a product or service nor mislead a client
- not attach conditions of sale for either a product or service that are inaccurate or misleading.

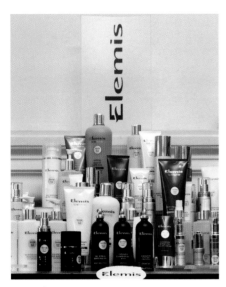

A product range

Employee's responsibilities

Your responsibilities under the Act are to:

- give clients clear prices for products and services
- be honest when you are promoting or selling a product or treatment: do not say a product or treatment does something if it does not.

Consumer Protection (Distance Selling) Regulations

The Consumer Protection (Distance Selling) Regulations make sure that when goods are purchased over the phone, from the internet or by mail order the consumer has the right to receive a refund. If there was a delivery charge this must also be refunded. However, costs incurred by the client to return the item are not included.

If you need to return something you must check the contract information, which will include the name and address of the supplier, a description and details of the goods or services and the price paid.

Employer's responsibilities

The employer's responsibilities under the regulations are:

- to give clients a refund if they are unhappy with a product but not to cover the cost of the postage to return the item
- to display **contractual** information on the website with clear terms and conditions of sale.

Employee's responsibilities

Your responsibility under the regulations is to offer and process a refund if a client wants to return a product.

Contractual

Agreed in a contract.

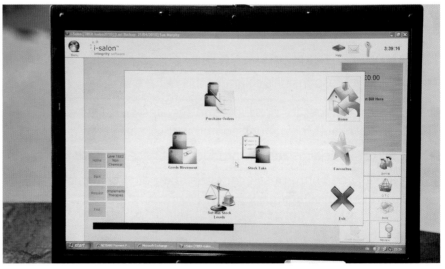

Controlling stock electronically

Supply of Goods and Services Act

Services, goods and materials provided with those services or treatments are covered within the Supply of Goods and Services Act. The Act makes sure that:

- a treatment is carried out with skill and reasonable care
- a treatment is carried out within a reasonable amount of time
- a treatment meets what it claims to do
- the charge for the service is reasonable
- any goods supplied in the course of the treatments are of a satisfactory quality and fit for purpose
- a consumer has the right to have goods replaced, repaired or compensated if they are of poor quality or are not fit for the purpose for which they have been supplied.

Employer's responsibilities

The employer's responsibilities under the Act are to:

- make sure staff are **adequately** trained
- make sure employees are aware of their responsibilities and what is expected of them during their working hours
- charge a reasonable price for a treatment service
- have clear treatment/service times and make sure therapists know and work to the treatment/service times
- state exactly what a treatment does
- make sure that the goods that the business supplies are of a good quality and fit for the purpose for which they are sold
- replace products which are faulty or not fit for the purpose for which they were sold
- **compensate** a client if a service is of a poor quality.

Adequately

To a suitable or acceptable standard.

Compensate

Give someone their money back, or to pay someone as a result of illness or injury.

Employee's responsibilities

Your responsibilities under the Act are to:

- carry out services professionally with skill and care and to offer only those treatments for which you are trained
- charge a reasonable price for services
- know and work to the service times of the salon
- state only what a treatment does (do not make up information)
- retail only products of a good quality and fit for the purpose for which they are being sold
- refer any complaint regarding faulty goods or services to a manager to action a refund or compensation.

HANDY HINT

Always check that the products you are using are in date. If they are out of date let your manager know so that they can be replaced.

Sale of Goods Act and Sale and Supply of Goods Act

The Sale of Goods Act and the Sale and Supply of Goods Act cover consumer rights including:

- goods being of satisfactory quality
- the conditions under which goods might be returned after purchase
- whether the goods are fit for their intended purpose
- goods being free from faults or defects.

If these are not followed, the consumer has the right to a replacement or refund.

Employer's responsibilities

The employer's responsibilities under the Acts are to:

- check that goods being ordered are of a satisfactory condition and free from faults
- have a clear conditions of sale policy that states when products can be returned.

Employee's responsibilities

Your responsibilities under the Acts are to:

- check stock being delivered for damage or faults and to make sure it meets **expectations**
- check stock before retailing to make sure it is in good condition and has not passed its shelf life
- accept returns within the return period and to offer a replacement or refund.

Expectation

A belief that something will happen.

Trade Descriptions Act

The Trade Descriptions Act prevents manufacturers, retailers or service industry providers from misleading consumers as to what they are spending their money on.

This Act prevents:

- services or products being falsely described or false claims being made
- giving false information, including on quality, price or purpose
- services or products being falsely advertised, displayed or described.

Employer's responsibilities

The employer's responsibility under the Act is to make sure that all staff are properly trained and understand the products they are using and the services they are giving.

Employee's responsibilities

Your responsibilities under the Act are to:

- describe treatments and products accurately: you need to know your product information well so that you can do this
- not make any false claims about a treatment or product.

Activity

Make a list of the different ways products could be priced incorrectly or advertised to give a misleading impression. Discuss with your colleagues.

Prices Act

The Prices Act requires the price of products or services to be displayed clearly. A treatment price list needs to be visible and product prices need to be clearly marked either on the item or on the shelf where they are displayed.

Activity

Discuss with your colleagues offers that you have been interested in only to discover hidden costs. How did it make you feel?

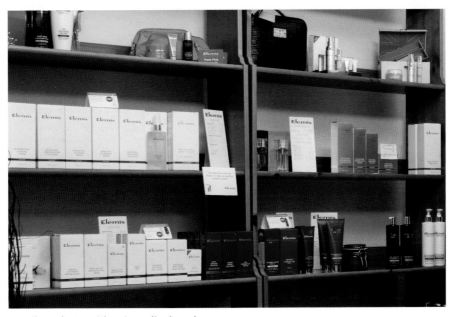

Retail products with prices displayed

Security in the salon

Stock displays

A salon stocks expensive items that are on display and can be tempting to thieves. Thieves will look out for opportunities (eg where stock is easily accessible and areas that are not always manned). Stock and product displays are usually found in the reception area, as this is where the till is located.

If possible, products and stock displays should be kept in locked cabinets so they aren't easily accessible. Any products on display should be dummy products (ie empty containers).

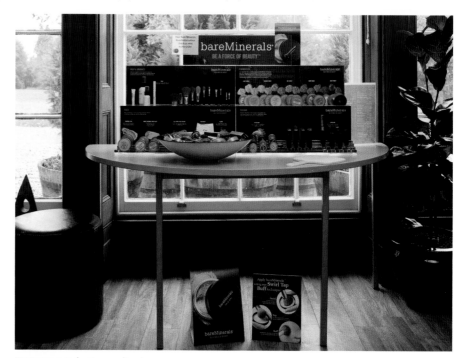

Dummy products on display

Personal and clients' belongings

Personal belongings may also provide an opportunity for a thief. The salon should provide lockers or safe storage areas for employees' belongings.

When seating clients in the treatment area, make sure their bags are stored away safely and that clients know where they are.

If a client removes their jewellery for a treatment, ask them to put it in their bag for safekeeping, so that you are not responsible for it. Your salon might have small plastic sealable bags that you can give clients so the item does not become lost or damaged in their bag.

When taking a client's coat to hang in a coat room, ask the client to remove all valuables and keep them in their bag.

Ask clients to put their valuables away in their bags to make sure that they are secure

Tills

If too much money is stored in the till, this could become a security risk. Make sure that the till is locked at all times and that the reception area is manned. Never leave large quantities of notes in the till; remove them regularly and put them in a safe place. When emptying the till, leave it open so that would-be thieves can see that it is empty.

Security in the salon

Follow the good practice security checklist:

- Never keep large sums of money in the till.
- Keep the till locked and the reception area manned.
- Keep tip boxes out of sight; store under the reception desk.
- When taking a client's coat, ask them if there is anything valuable in their pockets they wish to remove.
- Make sure a client keeps their personal belongings and clothing with them at all times, but make sure they are put away safely and securely when carrying out the treatment.
- Keep your personal belongings in your locker or a secure area.
- Don't leave any personal valuables in the salon overnight.
- Ensure windows and doors are locked when you leave the salon.
- Make sure product displays are dummies (ie use empty containers when displaying in accessible areas).
- If you notice anything suspicious, inform your supervisor or manager: do not ignore it.

Insurance

Within the beauty industry there are three types of **insurance** that an employer must have:

- public **liability** insurance
- employer's liability insurance
- product and professional treatment liability insurance.

Insurance provides protection both for the employer and the employee. It provides protection for the employer if a claim is made against them and they need to pay out compensation. It also provides protection for employees and visitors while they are on the premises.

INDUSTRY TIP

Make sure clients' bags are out of your way when you are working. Otherwise they could become a trip hazard.

INDUSTRY TIP

Don't bring expensive items to work with you.

INDUSTRY TIP

If you spot a thief, do not confront them yourself. Get help. Contact your manager and dial 999.

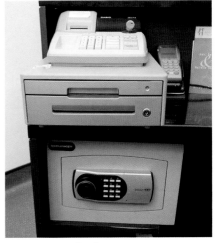

A salon till and safe

Insurance

Every year a business pays an amount (a premium) to an insurance company which will pay out compensation if a claim is made against the business.

Liability

Legal responsibility.

INDUSTRY TIP

Currently, the minimum cover available is £1 million, but the recommended amount to cover compensation costs is £2 million.

INDUSTRY TIP

Legally, businesses must be insured for at least £5 million. However, the industry standard is £10 million.

Public liability insurance

Public liability insurance is highly recommended when dealing with the public, especially in a salon environment. It covers claims made by members of the public or other businesses. For example, if a client injures themselves on the premises or is injured by a member of staff during a treatment, they can make a claim against the salon's public liability insurance.

Employer's liability insurance

By law, employers are responsible for the health and safety of their staff. Employer's liability insurance is a legal requirement for all businesses. It protects the employer against claims by employees for illnesses and injuries related to their work at the salon. It covers all members of staff who have a contract of employment, including apprentices.

Someone is considered to be an employee if:

- national insurance and income tax are deducted by the employer from the money they are paid
- the employer controls where and when they work
- the employer supplies work materials and equipment
- any profit made by the employee belongs to the employer
- they are treated the same way as other employees – for example, they do the same work under the same conditions as someone else.

If an existing employee suffers an injury or an illness associated with their work, such as an allergic reaction or a trip or fall, they might try to make a claim against the salon if they think the salon was responsible. The salon would be covered by its employer's liability insurance. If an employee has left the salon and becomes ill at a later date and believes their illness was caused by their work in the salon, they might also make a claim. Again, the salon would be covered by its employer's liability insurance.

Product and professional treatment liability insurance

Product and professional treatment liability insurance protects the employer and employee against claims from clients for injury or damage caused by treatments or products. It covers treatments and products that you provide to your clients. Even if you have carried out a treatment correctly, you may still be held responsible for damages and injuries that result from products you use. For example, if you do not carry out a skin test on a client prior to a self-tanning treatment and they then suffer an allergic reaction, you will be held responsible.

Activity

Look at the different treatments offered by your salon and identify any risks that need to be covered by insurance. For each of the risks explain why insurance is necessary. If you work in a salon that offers other services, such as hairdressing and nail services, include these areas too.

Activity

Research the different professional beauty therapy organisations that offer product and professional treatment liability insurance. Find out the cost of the insurance, the amount of cover and what treatments are covered.

Other relevant legislation

In this part of the chapter you will learn about the:

- Equality Act
- Employers' Liability (Compulsory Insurance) Act
- Copyright, Designs and Patent Act.

Equality Act

The Equality Act lays down laws to prevent discrimination against anyone on the grounds of:

- race or ethnic origin
- sexual orientation
- marriage or civil partnership status
- pregnancy
- religion
- beliefs
- age
- disability.

The Equality Act has replaced this older legislation:

- Sex Discrimination Act
- Race Relations Act
- Race Relations Act (Amendment) Regulations
- Equal Pay Act
- Disability Discrimination Act
- Employment Equality Regulations.

The Equality Act applies to both the employer and the employees within a business so it is important that everyone understands the effects of not adhering to it as they could be held liable. The Act includes protection against intimidation and bullying through **victimisation** and **harassment**.

HANDY HINT

Treat everyone as you would want to be treated – we all have the right to be treated fairly.

HANDY HINT

Look for the most recent amendment date (change) for the most up-to-date law if you need to check any legislation.

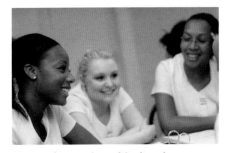

Beauty therapy is multicultural

Victimisation

When a person is treated less favourably than others.

Harassment

Persistent unwanted behaviour towards someone.

Employers' Liability (Compulsory Insurance) Act

If a business has employees it must have employers' liability insurance to comply with the Employers' Liability (Compulsory Insurance) Act. If an employee becomes injured or ill as a result of their work they have the right to claim compensation from their employer. Employers must have adequate insurance to cover any possible insurance claims. Most businesses would be unable to pay a claim outright so insurance is taken out to cover potential payments. The insurance must be with an **authorised** insurance provider. It might be part of a wider insurance package to meet the other liabilities, such as professional **indemnity** and public liability insurance.

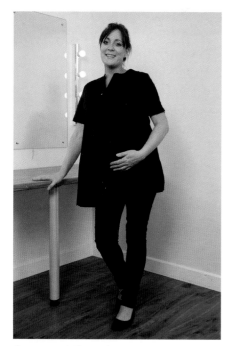

A pregnant therapist

Authorised

When a person or company has official power.

Indemnity

Insurance against damage or loss.

WHY DON'T YOU...
Find out more about the PRS or PPL licences by looking at its website.

HANDY HINT

Take a look at the UK government's licence finding website for licences required to play music.

PPL Licence

Photographic Performance Limited licence to play background music.

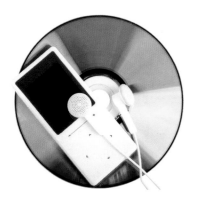

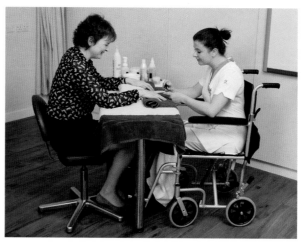

Disabled therapist at work

Copyright, Designs and Patent Act

Music being played in a salon can help to create the right atmosphere and ambience. Music can create an upbeat feel to a room or help listeners to feel calm and relaxed. In order to play music in the salon you need to hold a special licence to comply with the Copyright, Designs and Patent Act.

When we play music (even the radio in the staffroom) it becomes a public performance. Your employer must purchase a **PPL Licence** from the Performing Rights Society Ltd (PRS) in order to play music in the salon using a radio, TV, CD or MP3 player. The PRS works on behalf of artists, writers and publishers to collect and distribute a fee for a licence as royalties.

If you play recorded music or music videos in public, you will almost certainly be legally required to have a PPL licence.

Answers at the back of the book.

1 When should a risk assessment be carried out?

  a Every day

  b Annually

  c For each new client

  d Before using a new product or piece of equipment

2 What is the correct sequence for carrying out a risk assessment?

  a Decide who might be harmed, decide on precautions, identify hazards, implement, record findings, review assessment

  b Identify hazards, decide who might be harmed, decide on precautions, record findings, implement, review assessment

  c Identify hazards, record findings, decide on precautions, decide who might be harmed, implement, review assessment

  d Review assessment, identify hazards, record findings, decide who might be harmed, decide on precautions, implement

3 Which one of the following is not good security practice?

  a Keeping the till locked and the reception area manned

  b Keeping your personal belongings in your locker or a secure area

  c Ensuring that windows and doors are locked when you leave the salon

  d Leaving valuables in the salon overnight

4 Read the following two statements:

  Statement 1

  An obstruction to a fire exit is a hazard, but the risk of endangering someone's life is low.

  Statement 2

  Faulty electrical equipment poses a high risk to clients and staff.

  Which one of the following is correct for the above statements?

  a True True

  b True False

  c False True

  d False False

5 Read the following two statements:

  Statement 1

  A risk assessment identifies potential hazards and assesses the risks arising from these. Risks are categorised as high, medium or low.

  Statement 2

  A risk assessment is carried out to identify and minimise the impact of hazards.

  Which one of the following is correct for the above statements?

  a True True

  b True False

  c False True

  d False False

6 Which one of the following identifies the best course of action to take to lower the risk of contact dermatitis to staff?

  a Use aprons when in contact with chemicals

  b Take regular breaks when standing for long periods

  c Carry out a PAT test before microdermabrasion treatments

  d Use gloves when carrying out treatments

7 Read the following statements:

  1 Training needs for staff members

  2 An outline of staff responsibilities

  3 Pay scales for staff members

  4 Disciplinary proceedings for staff

  An action plan arising from a risk assessment in the salon may contain which two of these?

  a 1 and 2

  b 2 and 3

  c 3 and 4

  d 1 and 4

8 Which one of the following laws is concerned with the use of chemicals in the workplace?

a Management of Health and Safety at Work Regulations

b Workplace (Health, Safety and Welfare) Regulations

c Control of Substances Hazardous to Health Regulations

d Reporting of Injuries, Diseases and Dangerous Occurrences Regulations

9 Which one of the following is the legislation that requires a salon employer to carry out a risk assessment?

a Health and Safety (Information for Employees) Regulations

b Management of Health and Safety at Work Regulations

c Workplace (Health, Safety and Welfare) Regulations

d Health and Safety (First-Aid) Regulations

10 Poor posture can lead to which one of the following?

a Infections

b Infestations

c Contact dermatitis

d Musculoskeletal disorders

301
PROMOTE AND SELL PRODUCTS AND SERVICES TO CLIENTS

Promoting and selling products and services is an essential part of being a beauty/spa therapist. Selling is a way to increase business in the salon and an essential part of a service. Selling home-care products and additional services will help to enhance and maintain the effects of clients' treatments.

In this chapter, you will learn how to:

- understand the principles of promoting and selling products, services and treatments

- plan and create sales opportunities.

Why promoting and selling products and services is important to a business

Many people buy their beauty products from high street stores rather than buying them from a salon. This means that salons and spas lose valuable retail opportunities to recommend home-care products to the client and sell further treatments and products. A business is reliant on profit that is made through sales and services. If these are not promoted, the salon or spa loses the opportunity to **maximise** income. The therapist may also lose out if their wages include **commission** from product and service treatment sales.

Clients also miss out on an important part of their salon or spa experience. Information and advice on products and treatments could enhance the effects of the treatment and benefit their skin and well-being.

Maximise

Make large or use to its fullest.

Commission

An amount paid based on sales of products and treatments/services.

Successfully promote and sell products and services

Successfully selling requires good knowledge, understanding and commercial awareness of products and services. The **key skills** are:

- confidence in your ability and effective use of initiative and motivation
- professionalism in your appearance, behaviour, attitude in the workplace and in your client care
- effective communication skills and sales techniques that clients find acceptable and are well received
- problem solving when overcoming a client's **reluctance** to buy, and **adaptability** when successfully matching products/services to clients
- effective teamwork to share product/service knowledge and successful **ethical** sales techniques with colleagues
- the ability to manage stock and make the best of product displays and advertising material
- commercial awareness, which enables you to understand and create business for your benefit, the clients and your colleagues
- good literacy and numeracy to enable you to write clear client information and recommendations and to calculate service and products costs
- the ability to analyse and evaluate a sale to improve the business.

Key skills

Main job-related skills that employers look to find in an employee.

Reluctance

Unwillingness to do something.

Adaptability

The ability to adjust to different conditions.

Ethical

Describing right or professional conduct.

INDUSTRY TIP

A client's visit to a salon is a special experience for them. Clients need to trust and believe in the therapist's expertise and enjoy their time in the salon. It is therefore important to make sure that you look after your clients in the best possible way.

Promote and sell yourself in the future to new clients and employers

Similar techniques used in the promotion of products and services can also be used to promote and sell your skills to future clients and employers.

Many of the key skills, values and behaviours needed to promote yourself in a job application and interview are also the ones that are used to effectively sell products and services in the salon/spa and encourage new clients.

It is essential for you to be **work ready** in today's job arena, and to know how to make yourself employable and successful in your chosen career. This is called **employability**. It helps your colleagues and clients and, most importantly, benefits you when seeking future job roles.

Your professional standards should always be maintained when promoting and selling. They form the basics of the industry and are the foundation of what you need to know, do and understand, in order to sell and promote services and products competently and effectively.

Good practice in the workplace reflects standards. Standards are a level of quality and achievement which will be judged by your clients and colleagues alike. Your reputation as an excellent therapist is reflected in your standards. Good practice helps ensure a strong **client base** and sales performance as well as encouraging clients to return to the salon for further treatments and products.

Here are the key standards to ensure this happens:

- excellent standards of hygiene and safety
- strong knowledge of products and services
- excellent client care and the ability to form positive professional relationships with clients and colleagues
- attention to detail and time-keeping
- professional attitude, appearance and ethics
- listening well and communicating confidently
- strong work ethic and business skills.

Work ready

Having the necessary skills, knowledge and personal qualities to do a job.

Employability

Being capable of gaining and keeping a job or work.

Client base

Regular clients who purchase products and services and help keep your business up and running.

INDUSTRY TIP

Treat clients in the way that you would wish to be treated. View selling products and services as a great opportunity to educate your client and improve their well-being.

WHY DON'T YOU...

In groups, think about standards of client service and write down a list of poor client service skills that you have seen or experienced in daily life. Discuss with the group what made them poor and the effect they may have on a client's behaviour and loyalty to the salon in the future. Then discuss and list examples of good client service and their effects on a business.

Benefits to the salon of promoting services and products to the client

Promoting products and services helps to increase the salon's profit and turnover, giving the business money to buy new products and equipment. It:

- helps therapists reach their personal targets
- provides money for training and updating of staff skills
- encourages clients to try new products and services
- maintains the client's interest in the salon's service so they are more likely to return
- improves the professional image of the salon
- enhances the reputation of the salon, leading to new clients as a result of recommendations.

INDUSTRY TIP

Think of product and service promotion as part of your job and an opportunity to create business. The more your potential clients know about the products and services that you offer in the salon or spa, the more they are likely to try them and buy.

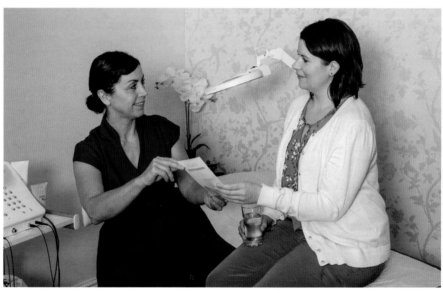

Promoting epilation services

Effective communication techniques for promoting and selling products and services

The way in which you communicate with clients will impact on your sales technique.

It is important to perform a consultation before a treatment but you can also do a consultation when a client shows interest in just purchasing products. A client consultation is essential to help the stylist or therapist identify:

- any concerns that the client has about their hair, skin or body
- products and services that will benefit the client at home

■ opportunities to **upsell** further treatments, rebook and **cross-promote** or **link-sell** other services.

A consultation form should always be used to record the information.

Verbal communication

When communicating with clients, it is important to speak clearly, use simple language and avoid the use of technical jargon so that the client understands what you are saying. Be professional and knowledgeable and use open and closed questions. A calm, unhurried manner is necessary when explaining products and services. Use a positive tone of voice and try to be keen, but not over-enthusiastic, about the products and services you are promoting. If the client is given clear and accurate advice it will allow them to decide whether or not they wish to try or purchase additional items or services.

Open and closed questioning techniques

Questioning techniques should include open and closed questions. Open questions should be used to get information from your client about their requirements. Closed questions have yes, no or one-word answers and should be used to confirm decisions.

Examples of open questions include:

■ What cleanser do you currently use?

■ Why did you book a body massage today?

■ What products do you use at home?

Non-verbal communication

Listening skills

Good listening skills are important to fully understand clients' answers to your questions. The clients' answers will contain valuable information that will allow you to select suitable home-care products or treatments for them.

Body language

Your body language should always be open, relaxed and professional.

Position yourself about a metre away from your client when talking to them. This is a comfortable distance for both of you..

Cross-promote/link-sell

Recommend another treatment or service from a different professional in your salon (eg if a client books a facial and you recommend an eyelash tint).

Upsell

Persuade a client to buy something additional or a treatment/service of a higher value (eg if a client books an eyebrow treatment and you recommend a facial).

VALUES & BEHAVIOURS

Communication is a key behaviour that applies to all beauty and spa treatments, not just to selling. Refer back to the communication section of the Values and behaviours chapter (pages 14–15) for more details on verbal and non-verbal communication.

INDUSTRY TIP

Ask the right questions to gain the information you need from the client. Try to use open questions beginning with what, why, when and how. The client will then give more information in their answers, which helps you to recommend products and treatments more accurately and more easily.

HANDY HINT

Your facial expressions, like your body language, give away a lot of information so remember to be welcoming with positive facial expressions. Maintaining eye contact shows that you are interested.

INDUSTRY TIP

Wearing a professional uniform presents a smart image and gives confidence to both you and the client, so look the part.

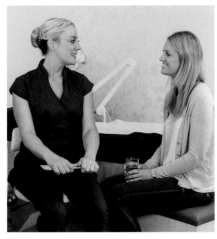

A therapist listening to her client and showing open body language

Personal appearance

A professional appearance sells! Before you can sell any products or treatments you need to be able to sell yourself. If you look clean and tidy and present yourself and your workplace in a professional way, it will give the client the confidence that you are professional and you know your trade

Product and service knowledge

To be able to promote products and treatments/services, you need to make sure you are familiar with what is available to clients in your salon. You therefore need to know:

- what treatments, services and products are available within your salon – if you are unsure, look at the salon's price list for treatments and products
- how much each product costs
- how much each treatment/service costs and how much a course of treatments costs
- the suitability of the treatment/service for the client
- what the treatment/service involves
- how long the treatment/service takes
- how long the product will last (ie its shelf life)
- how long a product will last with the correct usage (ie how long a product is likely to last the client if they use it correctly)
- what the features, benefits and results of the products/treatment are.

Keep up to date with industry trends

Be knowledgeable about your profession. It is essential to keep up to date with new trends within the industry and products that are new to the market.

- speak to account handlers (sales representatives) from product companies
- communicate with other therapists (eg social networking, online forums, industry and news websites)
- join an industry organisation so that you get newsletters
- visit salons and spas or look at their websites to see what they offer
- visit trade shows
- read trade magazines

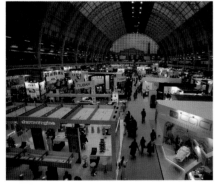

A beauty trade show

- collect price lists/treatment lists from salons
- do further training (eg workshops on new products and treatments).

By maintaining and updating your knowledge you are not only arming yourself with the information for selling but you are also engaging in continuing professional development (CPD). The beauty industry is fast-paced and ever-changing so it is vital to keep up to date with current trends and products. Keeping your knowledge up to date will mean that you can recommend and provide the best possible treatments and products to your clients and provide excellent home-care advice.

Knowledge of new products and treatments/services

You need to make sure you have a good knowledge of products and treatments/services to give clients confidence when you are selling. You will need to be able to answer the following questions about any new products and treatments/services you are offering or are planning to offer.

For each product:

- What does it do?
- What is its **unique selling point (USP)**?
- How much does it cost?
- What sizes are available? Are there both retail and professional sizes of the products?
- How exclusive is it? Will clients need to come to your salon to purchase it or is it available in high street stores?
- What **point of sale (POS) material** is available to help sell the product?

Unique selling point (USP)

The one thing that makes a product or treatment different from all others.

Point of sale (POS) material

Marketing and advertising materials that are provided to help you sell a product or service.

A manager carrying out product training with staff

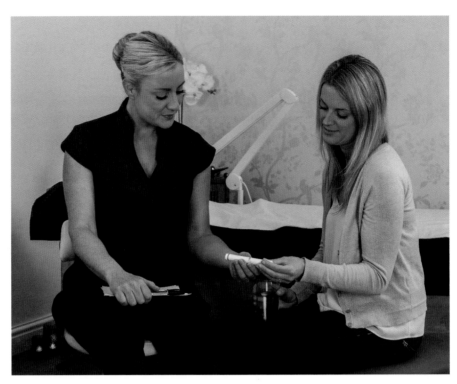

A therapist discussing a product with a client

Fad

A fashion or craze, usually short-lived.

Minors

Clients under 16, who must be accompanied by an adult when having a treatment.

Elderly

Clients who have reached their older years; some may be unable to make clear informed decisions about products and services.

Vulnerable adults

Clients who may have physical or mental disabilities that may prevent them from making clear informed decisions.

VALUES & BEHAVIOURS

Keep in mind the diversity of your clients when promoting products and services. Refer back to page 8 in the Values and behaviours chapter for a reminder.

Home-care products

Products recommended and sold to a client to help enhance or maintain the salon treatment/service they have received.

For each treatment/service:

■ Do clients really want the treatment/service? Is there a market for it?

■ Is this treatment/service just a **fad** or will it be around for a long time?

■ Is it appropriate to the client's needs? Make sure that you identify the client's needs appropriately. Consider the client's age and mental capacity (eg **minors**, the **elderly** and **vulnerable adults**). Consider their financial situation and their understanding of the service or product that you are promoting to them.

■ How often does the client need this treatment/service to achieve and maintain results?

■ Are you able to upsell other products/treatments/services to your client at the time of booking or get them to rebook for further treatments?

■ Can you cross-promote other treatments/services to your clients?

Consider any aftercare and maintenance required for the treatment/service:

■ What are the aftercare requirements for the treatment/service?

■ How expensive are the **home-care products** for maintaining the treatment/service?

■ Are there any before and after examples you can use to help sell the treatment/service or products?

For each piece of equipment:

- How expensive is it?
- What maintenance is needed?
- Are the **consumables**/items used with the equipment expensive?
- How many salons in your immediate area have this equipment?
- What are the trade reviews of the equipment like?

Consumables

Items that need to be used with the equipment (eg crystals for microdermabrasion and face pads for microcurrent treatment).

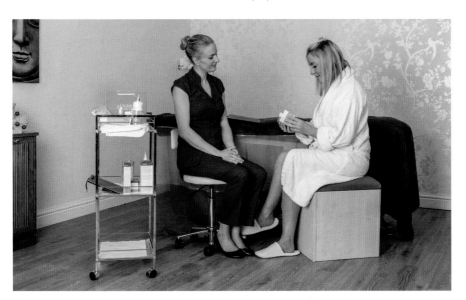

Advice and recommendations

Identify and plan selling opportunities

Throughout your working day, try to identify opportunities when you can naturally promote additional services or treatments or opportunities for upselling a treatment. For example:

- If a client is booked in for a massage, try to interest them in an extended treatment by explaining what it involves and the benefits. Some clients may not be aware that this service is available.
- If a client comments on a skin condition (eg dry skin), recommend a product or a treatment that will meet their needs.

Identify and interpret buying signals

If clients look at retail products or leaflets advertising products in the reception area while they were waiting, this could be a **buying signal**. It could provide you with an opportunity to discuss further suitable products. Other buying signals might include:

- a client enquiring about other treatments or products during a treatment

Buying signal

A visual or verbal indication from a client that they are interested in a treatment or product.

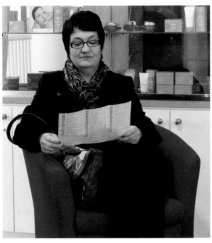

A client reading a treatment list is an opportunity for you to discuss any purchases they would like to make

■ a client focusing and enquiring about the price of a treatment or product.

■ a client holding their money/purse/wallet and discussing a price.

Use open questions to gain the client's interest. Consider whether they will benefit from purchasing products and services. Discuss their interests and/or concerns and then give them solutions by offering them suitable products or treatments.

If they show interest and confidence in purchasing the products, demonstrate the products and explain their benefits.

The diagram below shows the stages in identifying a buying signal and completing the sale.

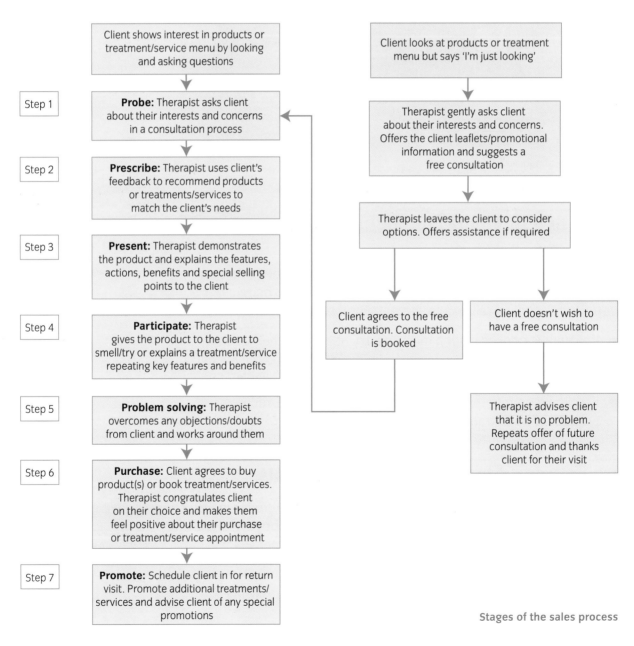

Stages of the sales process

THE CITY & GUILDS TEXTBOOK

Upsell

The key to upselling is to be knowledgeable, confident and assertive. However, remember that there is a difference between being assertive and being aggressive. Avoid using bullying tactics for the **hard sell**; it is intimidating and will lose the salon customers.

When clients visit the salon to buy retail products, try to find additional selling opportunities. For example, a client calls in to the salon to buy their usual cleanser. This provides you with an opportunity to offer them a consultation to see whether:

- the product was correct for their skin type
- they would benefit from additional products, such as a moisturiser
- their skin would benefit from a facial.

Hard sell

High pressure selling.

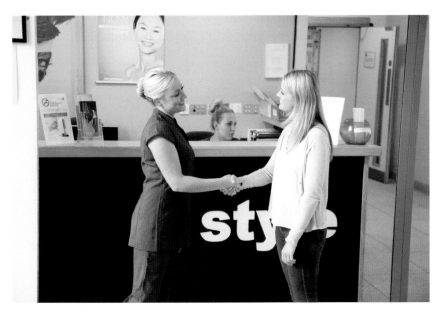

Sales opportunities begin the moment a client walks into the salon or reception area

HANDY HINT

Some clients will want to buy products because their friends use them, because celebrities endorse them or because they have used them for years. These products might not be the correct products for them.

INDUSTRY TIP

Don't be negative about products that a client might be using. It is unprofessional and the client may feel that you are challenging their opinions. Listen to the client and reinforce the benefits that your products would deliver.

Sales opportunities start from the moment a client walks into the salon. The receptionist can also try to upsell additional treatments/services. For example, if the client is booked in for a facial, the receptionist can ask if they would like to have an eyebrow shape as well.

Opportunities for upselling during a treatment

If the client is booked in for a treatment, explain the products you are using during the treatment and their benefits. This gives you an opportunity to show how they are being used. At the end of the treatment, after you have provided your recommendations, close the sale by asking them which size they would like to buy. If they are interested in booking another treatment/service, ask whether they would like a morning or afternoon appointment.

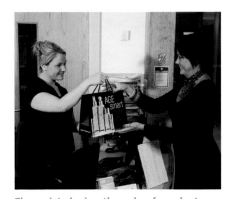

Therapist closing the sale of products with a client

Menu

List of treatments and prices available in a salon.

All companies use opportunities to upsell. Think about some of the places you visit. For example, in fast-food restaurants, they will always ask you if you want to 'go large' when ordering a meal or whether you 'want fries with that' if you order just a burger. They are identifying a sales opportunity and asking every customer. There is quite a high chance that customers will purchase extra items. It is not difficult to upsell just by asking a question. You are simply giving advice and information on the services and products that could match the clients' needs and interests.

Activity

Choose a beauty treatment (eg facial) from your college or local salon **menu** and write down the price. Select an extra treatment that you could upsell to a client (eg eyebrow shape) and a related product (eg moisturiser) and add these prices to the cost of the facial. Calculate the total cost of the three items and then the extra income generated by upselling the eyebrow treatment and the moisturiser.

Hard selling

We have all experienced hard selling. It makes us feel uncomfortable and puts us under pressure. Hard selling is when someone is pushy and does not consider the client's needs; they just want to make the sale or reach their target. We all hate having a wonderful treatment only to be pushed into buying a product before we leave. This is off-putting and might make the client reluctant to return. If the client says no or appears to be not interested, they may avoid eye contact, make excuses not to buy or look at several products without focus. You must accept this and not keep pushing them to buy something.

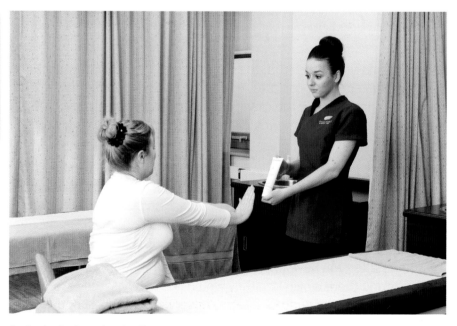

A client refusing a hard sell

Features, actions, benefits and special selling points (FABS)

When you have identified a sales opportunity, knowing the features, actions, benefits and special selling points (FABS) of a product or treatment will really help you to sell it. You will be able to inform the client about what the treatment or product is, and what it does.

Features

A feature is a description or characteristic of the product or treatment/service; for example, what ingredients a product contains or how much it costs.

Actions

This explains what can be achieved by the treatment/service or by using the product. It explains what the product or treatment/service does and how the client can use it.

Benefits

This explains the effects of the product or treatment/service, such as what it does for the client's skin. This is the most important information for a client and so the benefits need to be relevant to them.

Special selling points

This includes any special selling points to be aware of. Special selling points may be, for example, an ingredient found in a product (eg chamomile for soothing) or a particular benefit of a product (eg it smooths the appearance of fine lines).

Make sure you know the FABS of a product before you try to sell it to a client

The stages of the sales process

As well as knowing about the features, actions, benefits and special selling points (FABS) of products and treatments/services, you need to be familiar with the seven steps of the sales process (called the seven Ps of selling):

1 Probe

   To probe means to investigate. Probing is done by asking questions. Ask the client about:

   - previous treatments/services they have had
   - previous products they have used
   - the results these treatments/services and products have had.

   These questions should be used to begin the consultation looking at the client's home-care routine.

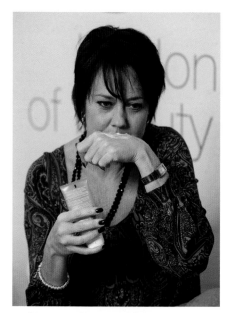

A client sampling a product

Unconscious

The part of your mind that you aren't aware of but that influences your feelings and actions.

Proactive

Anticipating and controlling a situation rather than reacting to it.

Reactive

Acting in response to a situation rather than expecting or predicting it.

Obstacle

Something that is in your way and is making it difficult to achieve something.

Pushy

Behaving in an unpleasant way to try to make someone do something.

2 Prescribe

Prescribing is using the information to make recommendations. By asking questions during a consultation process, the stylist or therapist is able to use the information to recommend suitable products, services and treatments.

3 Present

Demonstrating (ie presenting) the product to the client is important to allow the client to look at and try the product. For example, try the product out on the client's hands or explain in detail the treatment/service. Explain the features, actions, benefits and special selling points (FABS). Give them visual aids, such as promotional literature showing before and after pictures and explaining the results. Give the client clear explanations and think about drawing diagrams to help with your explanation. By educating the client about products and treatments they will understand the benefits more easily and will be more likely to follow your advice and buy.

4 Participate

If you are selling products, give the products to the client and allow them to use them and smell them. Let them participate in the process. Get the client to compare the results and repeat the features, actions, benefits and special selling points (FABS).

5 Problem solve

Be **proactive** rather than **reactive**. Try to think about any **obstacles** or objections to purchasing a product or additional treatment/service that a client might have and think of some possible answers to them that can be suggested in a professional way without appearing to be **pushy**. For example, if a client:

- cannot afford a product, advise them that it is available in a smaller size
- does not have enough cash with them, advise them of other payment methods that are accepted by the salon
- doesn't want to purchase right now, focus on rebooking them for a service or treatment and review the product recommendation at the next visit.

6 Purchase

If your client purchases a treatment/service or goods, reward them with a selection of product samples that will work well with their purchases. If they book a course of treatments, offer them a discount on home-care products. It is also good to congratulate them on their choices and make them feel positive about their purchases.

7 Promote

Make a record of the client's purchases and schedule them in for a return visit. If they have purchased products, this will give you an opportunity to review how the products are working. You can promote additional products and services at this stage and also advise the client of any special promotions within the salon.

INDUSTRY TIP

Always deliver excellent service to clients and congratulate them on their choice of products. Clients like reassurance from their therapist and to feel special.

Activity

Carry out a role-play to practise your knowledge of the features, actions, benefits and special selling points (FABS) of the range of products and treatments/services offered at your college or in your salon. Your friends and colleagues can be your 'clients'. Make notes and recommendations on a consultation form and use diagrams. Use the verbal and non-verbal communication techniques discussed earlier in the chapter to make sure you are asking your client relevant questions. Encourage them to give you clear answers. Recommend home-care products and further treatments from the range you have available at college or from products that you know. The more you practise, the more confident you will be!

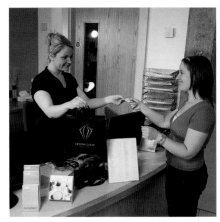

A client purchasing a product

Manage clients' expectations

It is important to manage the client's expectations of the treatment/ service or product during the probing stage/consultation stage. This can be done by explaining the results that the client is likely to see after two weeks or a month. Make sure that the client knows how to use the product and that they understand the instructions. Explain that they can only expect to see good results with regular use. Remember, you have to be realistic about the benefits and must not promise miracle results after a few days' use. If you do, the client is unlikely to see the results and they will lose faith in the product and you. In future, they may not take your advice or purchase from you. It is also important to manage your own sales performance, and together with your manager, be able to set realistic targets on what you are able to advise and achieve, with the knowledge and confidence that you have.

Legislation

When promoting and selling products and treatments/services, you must follow the relevant legislation:

- Data Protection Act
- Trade Descriptions Acts
- Sale and Supply of Goods Act
- Consumer Protection Act
- Prices Act.

For more on consumer protection legislation, see the section 'Laws relating to consumer protection' in the Health and safety legislation chapter.

The Prices Act – prices of products and services must be displayed clearly (eg a visible treatment price list or prices clearly marked on products or the shelf that they are displayed on).

The Consumer Protection Act protects customers against any products or treatments which may be dangerous or **defective**.

Evaluate the promotion of products and services

So far we have covered sales based around clients who are already attending the salon. However, you also need to know how to promote your salon so that you attract new clients and build a client base. A salon's business is based largely on **repeat custom**.

In this part of the chapter you will learn about:

- boosting sales through promotional events
- setting and agreeing sales targets
- reviewing and evaluating sales
- reviewing selling techniques and implementing improvements
- evaluating the effectiveness of advertising services and products to a target audience.

Boost sales through promotional events

The aim of product or treatment/service promotions is to boost sales of a particular product, treatment or service. Promotional events are also run to promote a new treatment, service or product and can also be used when opening a new business. Promotional events are often run at quieter times of the year to increase business. Promotional events can include:

- invitation-only evenings – customers are invited to the launch of a new product, treatment or service
- newspaper/magazine adverts or editorials on new products/ services launched in the salon
- posters, leaflets or flyers showing new products/services
- specific promotional evenings or discounted treatments/products aimed at specific customers, such as teenage clients, male clients or mature clients.

INDUSTRY TIP

The Consumer Protection Act covers misleading prices.

Defective

Faulty.

Activity

Write down and summarise in your own words two key points for each of the laws stated above. For each law, give an explanation of the consequences for the client if the salon/spa does not obey these laws.

Repeat custom

Customers who buy products and services again.

Other types of promotional activities include:

- offering in-store discounts when clients purchase a particular number of treatments, services or products in advance

- gift vouchers or discounts for clients who introduce friends and family

- offering free products or a **product trial** if clients purchase a less popular service or treatment

- newsletters (via email and text message or other social media such as Twitter or Facebook) to remind clients of special offers

- sending thank-you cards to repeat customers offering a discount

- customer loyalty schemes offering rewards such as a free treatment (eg have five treatments and receive a **complimentary** treatment).

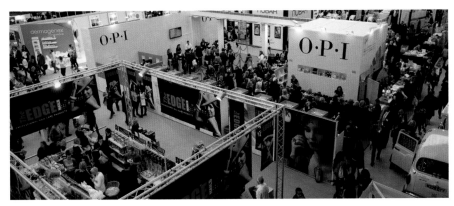
A promotional beauty event

Set and agree sales targets

Within a salon or spa environment, selling may make up part of your wage. This is called commission. **Productivity** and sales targets are often set by managers to encourage staff sales and for motivation. They also show the management and employees how much business is being created from product and treatment/service sales.

Targets should be agreed by staff to help develop their selling skills during the course of their career. They should be SMARTER:

- Specific – what exactly do you need to do/achieve?

- Measurable – how will you know you have achieved the target?

- Agreed – do both you and your manager agree on and understand what the target is that has been set?

- Realistic – are you realistically likely to be able to achieve the target and is it relevant to your role and ability?

- Time-bound – when do you need to achieve the target by?

- Evaluated – what is the date that has been set to evaluate progress so far?

- Reviewed – what is the date that has been set to review the outcomes?

INDUSTRY TIP

Make the free service/treatment one your client has not tried before as this may encourage them to try it again.

Product trial

Testing a product ahead of its release to give feedback on its results.

Complimentary

Free.

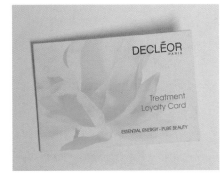

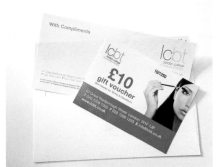

Loyalty cards and gift vouchers can be used by salons and spas

Productivity

A measure of how efficient a person or business is in producing goods/money.

Sales targets show who is selling well – healthy competition is important for both employees and management and should:

- motivate individual members of staff to do well by earning commission individually
- generate more profit for the business
- show what is selling well (ie which treatments, services and products are best sellers) and which products/treatments/services have done well as a result of a promotion (eg measuring the increase in the number of treatments/services and profit in response to an advert to promote treatments/services/products to teenage clients)
- indicate which products, treatments or services need promoting to ensure all stock and treatments are used effectively.

Review and evaluate sales

Different salons and spas have different methods for evaluating sales:

- Computer programs – some salons will have a computer program that will show each therapist's productivity and their sales achievements. Users have to log into the system so that it recognises them.
- Paper based-systems – other salons use a paper-based system where therapists write down everything that is sold.

Both of these systems will be reviewed by management to adjust targets if necessary, and to give out rewards for achievement.

Another way to review and evaluate sales is via client feedback and repeat business. You should also evaluate and analyse your sales performance.

Look at your strengths and weaknesses – which of them produce great sales and what part of your sales performance needs work (eg body language, communication, product knowledge)?

Are you aware if you are meeting your sales targets? Check with your line manager on how you are doing and what could be improved.

Review sales techniques and implement improvements

It is important for you to review your selling techniques on a regular basis with your manager to make sure that they are effective. Good sales techniques will increase the salon's/spa's business, increase your commission and result in satisfied clients. It is essential that the employer, manager or senior therapist create sales workshops either during or after work hours, to train staff in sales techniques, improve confidence and evaluate how they are progressing. These workshops often involve role-playing sales situations. The manager and employees

WHY DON'T YOU...
In groups within your class, set up a sales workshop. Role-play selling situations using the features, actions, benefits and special selling points (FABS) and seven steps to selling. Evaluate the group's performance. Ask colleagues to give feedback on your sales technique (ie what went well and what you need to change) and write down how you could improve this in the future.

visually and verbally demonstrate sales techniques on each other and act out different situations. The group completes an evaluation (written or verbal) of each other's techniques to help improve the team's sales techniques and performance.

There are three steps that lead to successful sales:

■ sell yourself – put yourself in your client's shoes and think like them

■ sell by asking not telling – asking questions helps you to find out what the client really wants

■ sell results – the client buys the benefits of the products or service, so tell them what it does and what results can be achieved.

Evaluate the effectiveness of advertising services and products for a target audience

It is important for a business to know how successful its advertising and promotions have been in attracting new business. A business needs to decide whether the promotion or advert has been effective so that it can decide whether to use that method of promotion again. The salon therefore needs to evaluate the promotion to see how much new business has been generated as a result of the promotion and whether it was effective. This can be done by:

■ client feedback – either verbally or by use of a form or questionnaire

■ reviewing and evaluating advertising and promotional material with colleagues to see what makes it effective and what type of clients were attracted (eg did it reach the right target audience – teenagers or mature males for example?).

The use of appropriate **verbiage** in posters, leaflets, videos, blogs and other social media is essential to reach the right target audience that your salon wants to attract. Verbiage should include:

■ nouns – name or identify something, eg 'facial treatment'

■ adjectives – describe nouns, eg 'fabulous facial treatment'

■ verbs – 'doing' words that describe an action, eg 'the therapist performs a fabulous facial treatment'

■ alliteration – repetition of the same letter at the beginning of words in a sentence, eg 'our fabulous facial treatment leaves you fresh and fragrant'; alliteration can be eye-catching in promotional material

■ simile – a figure of speech that compares two things, eg 'our fabulous one-hour facial leaves you feeling like a million dollars'.

This chapter has prepared you for the promotion and selling of products and services to clients. You should now be able to practise identifying retail opportunities within the workplace and evaluating your own methods of achieving sales and their success.

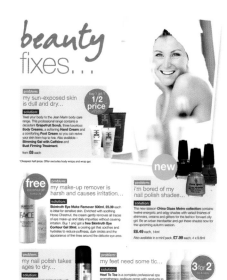

A promotional advert

Verbiage

Style of expressing something in words.

Activity

In pairs, select three beauty treatments and discuss and list examples of positive verbiage that could be used in promotional materials. Create your own advertisements for the treatments.

Answers at the back of the book.

1 Which one of the following Acts states that products must not be falsely described?

   a Supply of Goods and Services Act

   b Trades Description Act

   c Prices Act

   d Consumer Protection Act

2 Which one of the following Acts protects customers against products or treatments that may be dangerous or defective?

   a Supply of Goods and Services Act

   b Trades Description Act

   c Prices Act

   d Consumer Protection Act

3 How does promoting products and services benefit the salon?

   a Makes the staff feel good

   b Fills in time between treatment bookings

   c Increases the salon's profits

   d Keeps the salon owner happy

4 Which one of the following is a benefit of a treatment?

   a A description of the treatment

   b What equipment is used

   c What value it has to the client

   d The price

5 Hard selling will:

   a Make a client want to buy a product

   b Make a client feel uncomfortable and pressured

   c Help you reach your target

   d Make a client think you are knowledgeable

6 What is the term for the foundation skills that you need to know, do and understand for the beauty industry?

   a Sales skills

   b Hygiene and safety standards

   c Communications skills

   d Professional standards

7 Why is it important to evaluate promotions of products and services in the workplace?

   a To ensure that you don't repeat the same promotions twice

   b To see if you need to change the design and layout

   c To see how much new business was generated and whether it was effective

   d To decide if you and your colleagues liked it

8 What does the word verbiage mean?

   a Designing a poster or leaflet for a promotion

   b Promoting a product or service

   c Expressing something in words

   d A style of non-verbal body language

9 What does the word simile mean?

   a Another name for twins

   b A figure of speech that compares two things

   c A figure of speech that shows an action

   d Another name for the word similar

10 Which of these could be interpreted as a buying signal?

   a Client focusing on and enquiring about a treatment

   b Client avoiding eye contact and looking away

   c Client looking at several products without focus

   d Client holding their purse

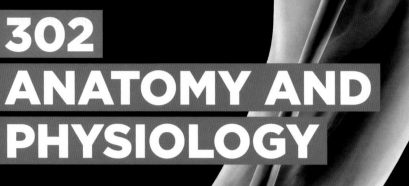

302 ANATOMY AND PHYSIOLOGY

Anatomy and physiology together are the study of the body – anatomy being the science of the structure of the body and physiology the science of the normal function of the body. It is important to have an understanding of anatomy and physiology so that you can understand what effects the treatments you are providing will have. It will also help you to become more knowledgeable about the treatments you carry out, making you a more effective therapist.

This chapter explores the anatomy and physiology that you are required to understand in order to be able to perform your treatments safely and effectively. In this chapter you will learn about:

- cells, tissues and organs
- skin, hair and nails
- the skeletal system
- the muscular system
- the cardiovascular system
- the lymphatic system
- the nervous system
- the respiratory system
- the digestive system
- the endocrine system
- the renal system
- the reproductive system.

At the end of each section, you will find a list of the common pathologies that are related to that system that you should be aware of. It is important that you know when a client should not be treated to avoid worsening a condition or because a condition is contagious.

Anatomical regions and related terms

Before you begin to learn about anatomy and physiology, there are some anatomical terms you need to know:

- anterior – front of the body
- posterior – back of the body
- lateral – away from the midline of the body
- medial – towards/closest to the midline of the body
- superior – above
- inferior – below
- proximal – close to the body
- distal – furthest from the body
- palmar – palm side of the hand
- plantar – sole of the foot
- frontal – forehead
- femoral – groin and inner thigh
- popliteal – behind the knee
- cubital – crease of the elbow
- thoracic – chest
- axillary – under the shoulder into the armpit
- brachial – arm
- cephalic – towards the head or pertaining to the head
- cervical – neck
- cranial – relating to the skull.

Cells, tissues and organs

Before looking at the different systems of the body, it is a good idea to understand about cells and tissues. Cells and tissues are the basic building blocks of each of the body's systems. Cells and tissues form organs which are the main **components** of the body's systems.

Components

Parts.

In this part of the chapter you will learn about:

- cell structure and cell division
- cell functions
- structure and types of tissues
- disorders related to the cells and tissues.

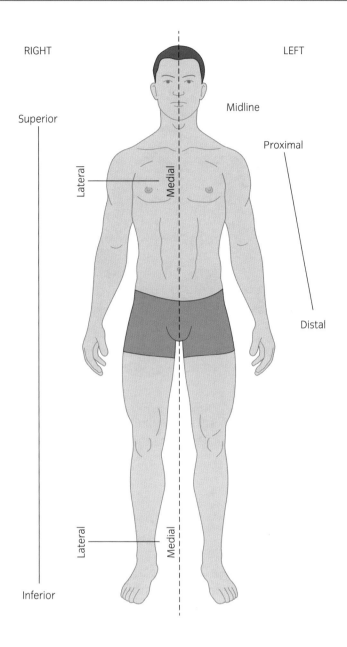

Cell structure

Cell membrane

This is a double-layer, semipermeable membrane that surrounds the cell, keeping its contents together and protecting it. It allows certain substances required by the cell (such as oxygen, nutrients, hormones and proteins) to enter the cell but keeps other substances out. Another important function of the cell membrane is to help maintain the shape of the cell.

Cytoplasm

Cytoplasm is a clear, gel-like fluid in which all the cell components, excluding the nucleus, exist. It is held in by the cell membrane.

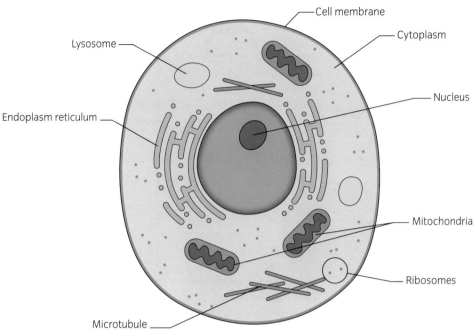

Lysosome

Cell membrane

Cytoplasm

Nucleus

Endoplasm reticulum

Mitochondria

Ribosomes

Microtubule

The structure of a cell

Intracellular fluid

The fluid between the cells is intracellular fluid and contains organelles. Organelles all have special functions that allow the cell to function properly.

Organelles

Nucleus

This is the largest organelle. It can be described as the control centre of the cell. It contains the body's genetic material. The nucleus of a cell consists of 46 **chromosomes** which are made up of **DNA** – deoxyribonucleic acid. The nucleus contains the nucleolus. The main function of the nucleolus is to **synthesise** ribosomes.

Mitochondria

These organelles have a sausage-shaped structure and are known as the powerhouse of the cells. They convert energy into forms that can be used by the cell for processes such as movement and cell division.

Ribosomes

Ribosomes are tiny organelles. They synthesise proteins and other materials that the cell needs.

Golgi apparatus

The Golgi apparatus is an organelle found in most cells. These are stacks of closely folded membranous sacs where molecules are sorted and packaged for transport to other components within the cell. The Golgi apparatus plays a role in the cell's storage of enzymes and the cell's metabolism.

Chromosomes

Thread-like strands of DNA.

DNA

Deoxyribonucleic acid – stores biological information (hereditary material).

Synthesise

Manufacture or create.

Endoplasmic reticulum

The endoplasmic reticulum is a series of canals in the cytoplasm. There are two types:

- smooth: synthesises **lipids** and is involved with detoxification
- rough: studded with ribosomes, and is the site of the synthesis of proteins including enzymes and hormones, which are exported out of the cell.

> **Lipids**
>
> A group of organic molecules that don't like water and prevent water entering the skin. They include fats, oils, waxes and fat-soluble vitamins.

Lysosomes

These are cellular organelles formed in the Golgi apparatus that act as the cell's digestive system. Lysosomes contain enzymes, which break down the fragments of organelles and other large molecules in the cell so that they can be recycled or removed as waste.

Cell division (reproduction of cells)

Cells are the building blocks of the human body. Cells are microscopic and have a slightly different structure and shape depending on their location and the function they have to perform in the body. Our body is always renewing cells to replace worn-out cells or cells that have done their job.

Cells are produced through cellular division, which is occurring constantly throughout our bodies. There are two types of cell division: mitosis and meiosis.

Meiosis

In meiosis reproductive cells called gametes are involved. In sexual reproduction these two gametes unite and combine their genetic material (chromosomes) during fertilisation.

Mitosis

During mitosis, a cell goes through a process of change before dividing and producing two exact replicas or daughters of the original cell. There are four stages to the process:

1 Prophase – the cell begins to double in size. The chromosomes replicate to form two identical copies of DNA. The chromosomes are now called chromatids and are connected by a spindle of fibres called a centromere. The nuclear membrane dissolves.

2 Metaphase – the centromere divides pulling the chromatids apart. These line up along the centre of the cell.

Interphase	46 chromosomes
Prophase	Chromosomes doubled to 92
Prometaphase	Nucleus dissolves and microtubules attach to centromeres
Metaphase	Chromosomes align at middle of cell
Anaphase	Separated chromosomes pulled apart
Telophase	Microtubules disappear, cell division begins
Cytokinesis	Two daughter cells form each with 46 chromosomes

Mitosis

3 Anaphase – the centromeres separate and one pair of chromatids (now 46 chromosomes again) move to opposite ends of the cell.

4 Telophase – a new membrane forms to surround each new set of chromosomes. The contents of the cytoplasm divide and two new daughter cells are produced.

Cell functions

Cells have many important functions including transportation of materials inside and outside the cell. Cells convert adenosine triphosphate (ATP) into heat or energy for mechanical and chemical activities when needed. Chemical reactions within the cell are responsible for the metabolic rate.

Cell transportation

The cell membrane has selective permeability, which means only certain specific molecules can enter and leave the cell. Transportation across the cell membrane can occur in different ways:

- Osmosis – the movement of water molecules from a weaker or more diluted solution through a semi-permeable membrane.

- Diffusion – diffusion is the movement of molecules in a solution from an area of high concentration to an area of low concentration.

- Facilitated diffusion – a special carrier protein attaches to a large molecule outside the cell membrane. The protein changes shape and is able to transport the substance inside the cell where it is deposited. When a cell is surrounded by a weaker solution, it will absorb water and swell. If the surrounding solution is stronger it can dehydrate and become distorted. It is vital that the fluid surrounding the cells remains in balance so that the cell structure is maintained.

- Active transport – the process by which dissolved molecules move across a cell membrane from a lower concentration outside the cell to a higher concentration inside the cell. As the particles are moving from a lower concentration to a higher concentration (ie against the concentration gradient), energy from the cell is used up.

Cell metabolism

Cell metabolism includes chemical reactions and processes, which are constantly taking place in every cell of the body. One example is the breakdown of chemical substances to provide energy to cells. When energy-providing molecules are broken down, adenosine triphosphate is formed and is used to provide energy or heat. The basal metabolic rate (BMR) is the rate of metabolism when at rest in a neutral environment, and when the body has not eaten for at least 12 hours.

Tissues

Cells are grouped together in specialised groups to become tissues. There are different types of tissues and each has a very specialised function. Tissues are **classified** by their shape, size and function. There are four main types of tissue in the body:

- epithelial tissue
- connective tissue
- muscle tissue
- nervous tissue.

Each of these four groups can be broken down into more specialised tissues.

Classified

Grouped or arranged by a particular category or type.

Epithelial tissue

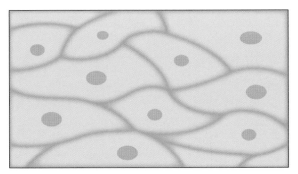

Epithelial tissue

This tissue covers the body (the skin) and lines the cavities, hollow organs, glands and tubes within the body. There are two types of **epithelial** tissue:

- simple
- stratified.

Epithelium (singular)/epithelia (plural)

Epithelium refers to a single layer of cells. Epithelia refers to two or more layers of cells.

Simple epithelial tissue

Simple epithelial tissue is made up of one layer of epithelial cells. There are three main types of simple epithelial tissue that are named according to their shape:

- Squamous or pavement epithelium has a flattened appearance and forms a paving-stone pattern. Squamous epithelium lines the heart and blood vessels.

- Cuboidal epithelium is made up of cube-shaped cells and is found in some glands. Cuboidal epithelium is involved in secretion, excretion and absorption.

- Columnar epithelium has a more rectangular appearance and lines many organs (eg the stomach).

Stratified epithelial tissue

Stratified (or compound) epithelium is made up of several layers of epithelial cells. There are four types of stratified epithelium:

- Stratified squamous epithelium has many layers of cells, which are mainly column shaped. As they grow towards the surface, they become flattened and are shed.

- **Keratinised** stratified epithelium is found in dry areas, such as the skin, hair and nails, and is designed to withstand wear and tear. The surface layer of keratinised stratified epithelium is made up of dead epithelial cells that produce a tough, protective, semi-waterproof layer protecting the living layers underneath.

- Non-keratinised stratified epithelium is found where surfaces need to be kept moist (eg the eyes and mouth).

- Transitional epithelium varies in appearance. It is similar to stratified squamous epithelium except the surface cells are not flattened. Transitional epithelium lines organs that need to be waterproof and those that need to expand (eg the bladder and the uterus).

Connective tissue

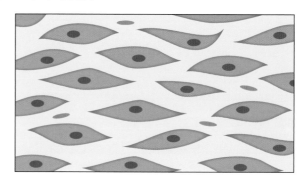

Connective tissue

Connective tissue is the most common tissue in the body. The function of connective tissue is to:

- protect
- transport
- insulate
- support.

The cells in connective tissue are more widely spaced than in epithelial tissue. In between the cells in connective tissue is a special substance called the **matrix**. This is a gel-like substance that contains fibres that provide support and protection. Types of connective tissue include the following:

- Lymphoid tissue – this tissue is found in the **lymphatic system**. It is an important part of the body's **immune system** and helps protect it from infection and foreign bodies. For more information on lymphoid tissue, please see page 209.

Keratinised

Describing cells that have become hard, flat and dead. This is caused by the production of a protein called keratin and the deterioration of the nucleus of the cell.

Matrix

The material (tissue) between cells in which more specialised structures are embedded.

Lymphatic system

Part of the circulatory and immune systems; consists of a network of lymphatic structures (including the tonsils, lymph nodes, etc) that carry lymph (a clear fluid) from the tissues back to the heart to recirculate.

Immune system

The system that protects the body against infection.

THE CITY & GUILDS TEXTBOOK

- Blood – for more information on blood, please see page 197.

- Bone – for more information on bone, please see pages 167-169.

- Fibrous tissue – fibrous connective tissue contains loosely packed **collagen** fibres in a thin matrix. **Fibroblasts**, which are the main active cells of connective tissue, are found within fibrous tissues. This tissue is found:

    - in ligaments

    - in the outer protective bone layer

    - around some organs for protection (eg the kidneys)

    - in muscle **fascia**, which extend to form the muscle tendon.

- Elastic tissue – elastic tissue is found where stretching of various organs occurs (eg in the walls of the arteries and the respiratory tract).

- Areolar tissue – areolar tissue is loose connective tissue. This tissue is semi-solid and contains fibroblasts, some fat cells, **mast cells** and **macrophages**, collagen and **elastin**. Areolar tissue provides elasticity and connects and supports other tissues.

- Adipose tissue – adipose tissue is a type of areolar tissue containing fat cells.

Collagen

A type of white protein that gives strength to tissues.

Fibroblast

A type of cell, found in connective tissue, that produces collagen.

Fascia

Thin sheets of connective tissue that wrap around muscles and organs. Its function is to connect tissues together and provide support.

Mast cell

A type of tissue cell of the immune system.

Macrophages

White blood cells within tissues; part of the immune system.

Elastin

Yellow protein fibres that are capable of considerable extension.

Muscle tissue

Muscle tissue has the unique ability to contract and relax producing movement. There are three types of muscle tissue:

- skeletal/voluntary/striated

- smooth, visceral or involuntary

- cardiac.

Further information on muscle tissue can be found in the section on the muscular system (see page 184).

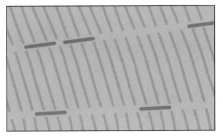

Muscle tissue

Organs

The organs of the human body (eg the heart) are groups of specialised tissues. Specific organs are grouped together to form the systems of the body. The organs of the body carry out many functions, such as transporting materials within the body, absorbing food into the blood, helping you move, protecting your body from infection and removing dead cells from your body.

Nervous tissue

We have two types of nervous tissue cell:

- neurones: a type of cell that carries information or signals to and from the brain and the rest of the body

- glial cells: supportive cells in the central nervous system.

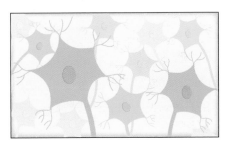

Nervous tissue

Further information on nervous tissue can be found in the section on the nervous system (see page 215).

Basement membrane

The basement membrane is a thin layer of connective tissues and forms a special type of extracellular matrix. It can surround tissues, form a sheet between epithelial cells or separate two sheet of cells. It underlies the epithelium of many organs and structures throughout the body. The basement membrane is the layer between the epidermis and dermis keeping the two layers tightly connected.

Tissue healing

The body is able to replace injured tissue with healthy and fibrous scar tissue. It can take several months for a damaged area to fully heal. It is worth remembering that while the body can heal, it will never be exactly the same as before the injury and often a visible scar is left as a reminder of the healing process.

Bleeding (hemostasis)

This is the first stage of healing and lasts a few hours. It is important to quickly stop and control bleeding. Platelets clump together to form a blood clot and chemical mediators are released. During this stage the blood flow must still continue to allow cells to carry out the healing process.

Inflammation phase

This is a coordinated response to cell and tissue injury, to heal and break down damaged or dead cells. Inflammation normally lasts up to four days. Common symptoms are pain, heat, redness, swelling and loss of function. Plasma and blood cells leak into the area to dilute harmful substances and support the cells. Chemical mediators infiltrate into the tissues to initiate a **vascular** phase (essential cells, antibodies, white blood cells, enzymes and nutrients move into the tissues) and a cellular response (cells deactivate and ingest bacteria).

Proliferation (healing) phase

Within two days, the **endothelial cells** near the edge of the dead tissue begin to **proliferate** into the area. Cells divide and seal the wound. A vascular network is formed to transport oxygen and nutrients while tissue healing is established. The next step is the removal of the damaged matrix. Approximately five days following injury, the wound, having been initially filled with a provisional matrix composed of fibrin, starts to change and fibroblasts synthesise new collagen, elastin and proteoglycan molecules. These cross-link the collagen of the matrix and produce granulation tissue. This has a distinctive grainy appearance. The tissue is further modified by

---

INDUSTRY TIP

Signs and symptoms of inflammation:
- swelling: oedema
- redness: erythema
- heat: increased temperature
- pain: pressure on the nerve ending due to increased fluid in the area.

Vascular

Relating to blood vessels.

Endothelial cells

Thin layer of cells that line the interior surface of blood vessels and lymphatic vessels.

Proliferate

Increase rapidly in number; multiply.

Inflammatory responses

Chemical mediators (some of these chemicals do more than one job)	Action
Prostaglandins, histamine, serotonin, bradykinin (chemical responders to inflammation)	Chemicals that cause **vasodilation**. Blood vessels dilate, and blood pressure falls.
Histamine, serotonin, bradykinin, leukotriene	Increase vascular permeability, making blood vessel leaky, so that plasma can enter the tissue and begin the healing phase. This movement causes swelling to occur in the area.
Leukotriene, which attracts polymorphonucleocytes	Increase movement of cells towards the injury.
Bradykinin, prostaglandins	Cause increased pressure on the tissues, leading to perception of discomfort or pain.
Cell mediators	**Action**
Thrombocytes (platelets)	Cells that cause blood to clot and are vascular mediators. Fibrinogen (a protein) is converted to **fibrin**, which forms an adhesive net between the thrombocytes that other cells stick together (clot).
Monocytes, lymphocytes, eosinophils, basophils, neutrophils (white blood cells)	These all fight infection and are vascular mediators. They have different functions and include macrophages, which are formed in response to an immune reaction. They are a type of phagocyte, which is a kind of cell that ingests **pathogens** and other cell debris (a process called phagocytosis). Neutrophils are the most common type of white blood cell, and are the first responders which both fight the infection and send out chemical messages to other white blood cells to help fight infection.
Fibroblasts (connective tissue cells)	When tissue is damaged, stimulated to start to reproduce.

Vasodilation

Relaxation of the muscles in the walls of the blood vessels, causing the blood vessels to dilate (get wider) and allow the blood to flow more freely.

Fibrin

Fibrous protein involved in blood clotting.

Pathogen

A collective term used to describe a type of microbe. It includes viruses, bacteria, fungi and parasites. A pathogen has the potential to cause harm.

fibroblasts. At first it is made up of **type III collagen**. This process takes about two to three weeks, during which time excess fluid is removed and the collagen matures. The new structure is at its weakest and vulnerable to bleeding at this point.

Collagen

Type III collagen: second most commonly found type of collagen and found in the skin and internal organs, muscles, with collagen type I. Composed of loose connective tissues, with reticular fibres, During wound healing there is higher proportion of type III collagen as it acts to bridge the wound to form a supporting framework.

Remodelling phase

This phase actually begins during proliferation and the two stages overlap. It can take between 21 weeks and two years, depending on the severity of the injury and age of the person, to fully remodel the tissues following injury. By week six the new circulation in the skin will match adjacent skin but sensitivity is reduced. By week 36, tissue function will be restored and be as close to normal as possible.

Collagen

Type I collagen: Most common type of collagen. Found in skin, tendons, ligaments and bones. Composed of loose, dense connective fibres. More type I found in injured skin. More resistant to tension than type III.

Fibroblasts continue to rebuild the extracellular matrix by providing a scaffolding-like framework. Epidermal skin cells in the top layer move down the sides of the wound to help fill the gap. Type III collagen is gradually replaced with **type I collagen**. The skin may continue to show a permanent reminder of an injury as scar tissue.

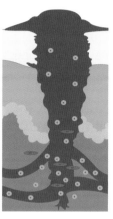

Damage to tissue, blood leaks out

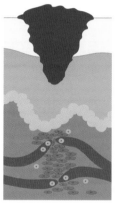

Scab formed on the skin

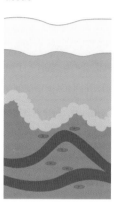

Skin healed with some surface change in skin tissue

Skin repair

HANDY HINT

Disease may also be called pathologies.

Disorders and diseases of the cells and tissues

Disorder	Description and cause	Contra-indications and general precautions	Advice for client
Cancer Normal cells / Cancer cells	A broad term covering over 200 different types of the disease. Each cancer has different symptoms depending on the organ or part of the body affected. Caused by uncontrolled abnormal cell growth. Metastasis is the migration of cancer cells from the primary site to another area of the body not directly in contact with the original site.	Many cancers will be contra-indications. If the client is having radiotherapy or chemotherapy that will restrict or prevent treatment. Chemotherapy reduces the efficiency of the immune system and make the client feel unwell. Radiotherapy causes tissue damage that you will not be able to see.	Seek medical advice prior to treatment.

Skin

The skin is the layer of tissue that covers the body and is the largest organ in the human body. The condition of the skin is subject to constant change and can therefore reflect the general health of an individual. The skin has two main layers, the epidermis and the dermis, and a third layer, the hypodermis, beneath.

In this part of the chapter you will learn about:

- the structure of the skin
- the functions of the skin
- the effects of ageing on the skin
- characteristics of the skin
- skin diseases and disorders related to the skin

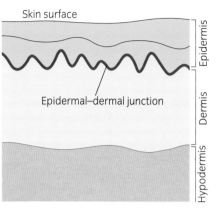

The three layers of the skin

Structure of the skin

The skin has three layers:

- the epidermis
- the dermis
- the hypodermis or subcutaneous layer.

The epidermis

The epidermis is made up of five layers.

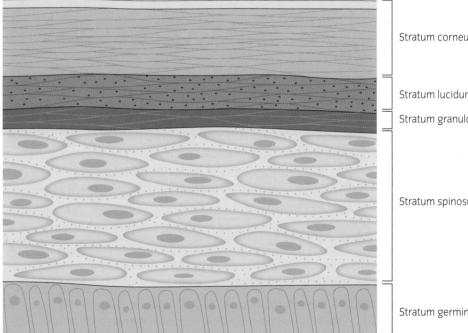

The five layers of the epidermis

Emulsion

A liquid evenly suspended in another so that neither can be distinguished.

Sebum

An oily secretion that lubricates the skin and hair.

Urea

The substance that urine mostly consists of.

Lactic acid

An acid produced in the muscle cells and red blood cells, a build-up of which can contribute to muscle soreness.

Amino acids

The building blocks of protein, found in your cells.

Pigment

Substance that adds colour.

Projections

Parts that stick out.

INDUSTRY TIP

There are two types of melanin:
- eumelanin: a brown or black pigment
- pheomelanin: a yellow or brown pigment.

Natural moisturising factor (NMF)

Water-soluble substances that absorb water from the air and combine it with their own water content to keep the stratum corneum hydrated.

Ceramides

Natural lipids (fats) that allow the skin to hold onto moisture keeping it hydrated.

Lubricant

A substance (such as oil) that reduces friction.

These layers are formed of sheets of cells that are held together by a special adhesive protein. There is still some ability for cellular movement between these tight junctions. Skin cells move upwards from the basal layer to the horny layer.

The average thickness of the epidermis is only about 0.12mm. It is thickest on the soles of the feet (1.5mm) and thinnest on the eyelids (0.5mm).

The surface of the epidermis is covered in complex substances, including:

- an acid mantle (or hydrolipidic layer) – a water-in-oil **emulsion** formed from a mixture of sweat and **sebum** making the skin's surface slightly acidic
- mineral and organic substances, including **urea**, **lactic acid** and **amino acids**.

Cells of the epidermis

There are different types of cells in the epidermis. Each has an important role to play:

- Keratinocytes – keratinocytes produce keratin. Keratin is an insoluble protein that makes the cell more resilient. The amount of keratin in a cell increases as the cell moves towards the skin's surface.
- Melanocytes – melanocytes are cells of connective tissue. They produce the **pigment** melanin, which gives colour to the skin and hair. The melanin forms in the melanocytes and is injected into the skin through finger-like **projections** (called dendrites).
- Langerhans cells – Langerhans cells are specialised white blood cells found circulating in the skin. They are a type of macrophage and alert the immune system to pathogens in the skin.
- Merkel cells – located in the basal layer, these are sensory receptor cells and are more abundant in areas where sensitive touch is required. Not all Merkel cells have contact with a nerve and may have other functions.

Stratum corneum (horny layer)

This is the outermost layer of the skin and its surface is in direct contact with the environment. The skin cells are hard and flat. The skin cells are also dead so they don't have a nucleus. They are very different from how they started out in the basal layer. One major function of the stratum corneum is to prevent dehydration of the skin. The **natural moisturising factor (NMF)** allows the stratum corneum to keep hydrated despite exposure to the environment. Lipids, which include **ceramides**, cholesterol and fatty acids (sebum), also help control water loss and prevent entry of water-soluble agents and harmful bacteria by providing a waterproof layer on the skin's surface. This surface **lubricant** also keeps the skin supple, preventing it from cracking and breaking, which would allow pathogens to enter into the skin and could cause the skin to become infected.

The thickness of the stratum corneum also varies with age. It gets thicker as we grow older. As it thickens, the signs of ageing can become more obvious.

Stratum lucidum (clear layer)

This layer is made up of flat transparent cells, hence the name clear layer. There is no melanin present in this layer. This layer controls the amount of water that can pass through the skin.

Stratum granulosum (granular layer)

As the cells lose their nuclei and begin to die, the cell functions begin to decrease dramatically. The cells take on a distinctive flattened shape and a **granular** appearance as a result of **keratinisation**. This is the start of the **keratinisation zone**. The keratin in this layer helps prevent water loss from the skin.

Stratum spinosum (prickle cell layer)

This layer includes the Langerhans cells (see page 128), which help support our immune system.

Keratin production begins in the stratum spinosum (prickly cell layer) and is injected into the living cells. The stratum spinosum is several layers deep. The cells have connection threads called fibrils which give the cells a prickly appearance.

Stratum germinativum (basal layer)

This is the deepest layer of the epidermis and forms a junction between the epidermis and the dermis. Skin cells are produced here by mitosis (see page 119) to produce new epithelial cells. The stratum germinativum also contains keratinocytes and melanocytes. The melanocytes help protect the skin against harmful UV rays. Eighty per cent of the moisture required for maintaining a healthy skin surface is found in this layer.

The dermis

The dermis is a layer of skin that is 3–5mm thick and lies beneath the epidermis. It is made up of tough extra-cellular tissue. The dermis has a high water content. It contains most of the living structures of the skin including blood vessels, sweat glands and sebaceous glands.

The main functions of the dermis are:

- to provide strength and flexibility
- to provide a system of capillaries to nourish the cells of the lower layers of the epidermis and to remove waste products
- to help control temperature and blood pressure.

INDUSTRY TIP

The NMF is water soluble and easily removed from the skin cells which is why repeated exposure to water makes the skin drier. It is therefore important to apply hand cream after washing your hands.

INDUSTRY TIP

If the dendrites that inject melanin into the skin become damaged, pigmentation is unevenly distributed causing a patchy skin tone.

Granular

Microscopic particles (grainy).

Keratinisation

The process by which living cells change into flat dead cells with no nucleus.

Keratinisation zone

The zone where cells begin to die and from where they are shed from the skin.

The dermis has two layers:

- the papillary layer
- the reticular layer.

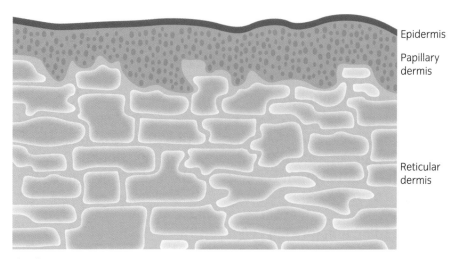

The dermis

The papillary layer

This papillary layer is made up of loose connective tissue. The surface of the papillary layer is covered with tiny, irregularly shaped projections called dermal papillae. These fit into the underside of the epidermis, forming a secure bond (eg like Velcro). They contain intricate networks of blood and lymphatic capillaries and nerve endings. These networks of capillaries nourish the lower layers of the epidermis and hair follicles, carry oxygen to the tissues and remove waste from the tissues. The papillary layer is rich with mast cells and macrophages (see pages 123 and 125).

The reticular layer

This is made up of thick tough fibrous connective tissue, which helps to support the dermis and hold the structures of the dermis in place. It is rich with fibroblasts, which form collagen and elastin. The reticular layer connects the dermis to the hypodermis/subcutaneous layer.

Cells of the dermis

The main cells of the dermis are fibroblasts, mast cells and phagocytic cells.

Fibroblasts (fibre cells)

Fibroblasts (fibre cells) play an important role in tissue repair following tissue damage. Fibroblasts produce two important proteins – collagen and elastin. Collagen provides strength and elasticity and elastin allows the skin to stretch. The production of collagen and elastin slows down as we age. This reduction, combined with damage caused by ultraviolet (UV) light, causes wrinkles and a loss of skin tone.

INDUSTRY TIP

If the skin is over-stretched, the elastic fibres break and stretch marks will appear. Elastin makes up 5% of the body's weight.

INDUSTRY TIP

Skin is looser around joints to allow movements without skin damage.

THE CITY & GUILDS TEXTBOOK

Mast cells

Mast cells release **histamine** in response to damage to local tissues caused by infections. Histamine causes the blood vessels to become dilated and allows fluid and cells of the immune system to leak out of the blood to the site of the infection to help in the healing process. White blood cells are also attracted to histamine, drawing them to the damaged tissue.

Phagocytes

Phagocytes are white blood cells that move through the skin's tissues destroying pathogens and other cell debris.

Structures of the dermis

Sensory nerve endings

The skin is packed with sensory nerve endings, which relay information about **tactile** sensation to the brain. Different nerve receptors respond to different sensations.

Nerve receptor	Sensation
Meissner's corpuscles	Tactile, light touch, vibrations
Ruffini corpuscles	Deep pressure, vibration and stretch
Pacinian corpuscles	Deep pressure and vibrations
Free nerve endings	Thermal, mechanical and **nociceptors**
Krause corpuscles	Thermoreceptors, sensations of cold

Histamine

A chemical that causes vasodilation.

INDUSTRY TIP

Hyaluronic acid is a naturally occurring substance in the skin that helps to keep the skin hydrated. It is also found as an ingredient in skincare products to help maintain hydration in the skin.

Tactile

Connected to the sense of touch.

INDUSTRY TIP

The most sensitive skin is on your lips.

Nociceptors

Free nerve endings are known as nociceptors. Nociception is the name given to something unpleasant or potential harm – it doesn't always mean that the sensation will be painful.

INDUSTRY TIP

Nociceptors respond to tissue damage and are responsible for the sensations that may be perceived as pain. Pain is a complex process whereby the brain reacts to tissue damage or injury. Pain is experienced when the brain perceives a sensation to be a sign of danger or a warning signal and this is why we experience pain differently and in unique ways.

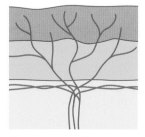

Free nerve endings

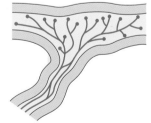

Ruffini corpuscle

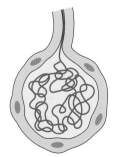

Krause corpuscle

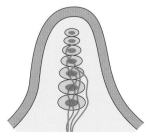

Meissner's corpuscle

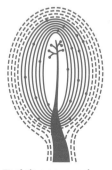

Pacinian corpuscle

Blood vessels

The dermis contains a rich, delicate network of blood vessels. The small blood vessels in the outer areas of the skin are known as the micro-circulation and are prone to vasodilation and **vasoconstriction**. Blood circulation brings oxygen and nutrients to the dermis (and epidermis) and removes waste products made during cellular activity.

Lymphatic vessels

A network of lymphatic capillaries nourish the cells in the dermis. These vessels allow lymphatic fluid to leave the network and move around the network of cells as tissue fluid. Tissue fluid moves back into the lymphatic vessels to take away waste from the extra-cellular tissues. (For more information on the lymphatic system see page 206.)

Sweat glands

The two main purposes of sweat glands are:

- to help control or maintain the body's temperature
- to help get rid of waste.

Sweat cools the body down by removing heat from the skin's surface. Sweat is excreted as a clear watery fluid. It removes waste substances (eg water, sodium and potassium chloride (salts), ammonia and urea) from the body.

There are two types of sweat glands:

- apocrine glands, found under the arms and around the groin
- eccrine glands, found all over the body.

Sebaceous glands

Sebaceous glands can be found all over the skin (but not on the palms of the hands or soles of the feet). Most sebaceous glands open into hair follicles where they secrete sebum but some open directly onto the skin. Sebaceous glands produce sebum (which is a lipid). Sebum is the skin's natural **emollient** and prevents the skin from drying out. It forms a barrier to keep moisture in. Sebum helps prevent the growth of bacteria as long as it does not become excessive. Excessive sebum will cause the skin to become oily and look shiny (particularly around the nose, chin and forehead). Very oily skin attracts surface debris, which may block the pores causing **comedones**, **papules** and **pustules**.

Arrector pili muscle

Arrector pili muscles are tiny muscle fibres that are attached to the hair follicle. When they contract they pull the hair up and away from the skin. These muscles cause goosebumps when we are cold or frightened. The raised hairs trap air next to the skin to keep it warm.

Vasoconstriction

Constriction (shrinking in size) of the muscles in the wall of the blood vessels, which restricts blood flow.

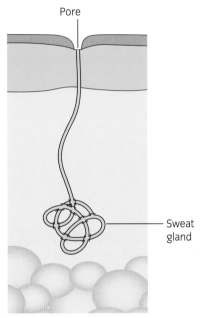

Cross-section of a sweat gland

Emollient

A substance that has a softening effect.

Comedone

Blackhead.

Papule

A small raised solid area of infected unbroken skin, which often develops into a pustule.

Pustule

A small amount of pus that is visible through a raised portion of the epidermis.

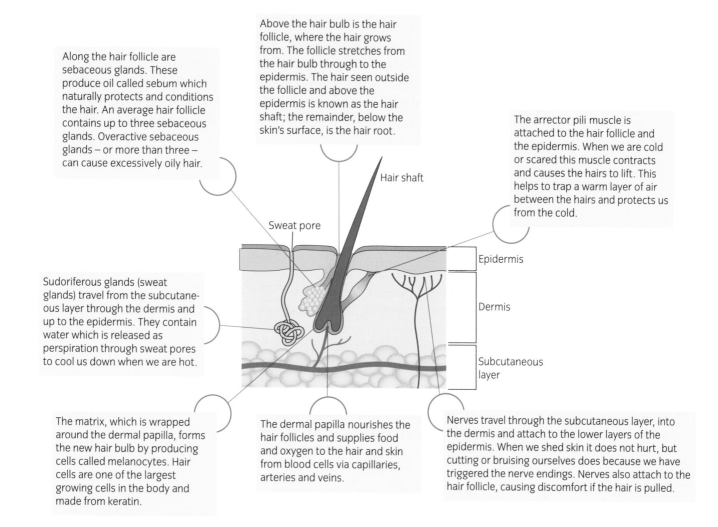

Above the hair bulb is the hair follicle, where the hair grows from. The follicle stretches from the hair bulb through to the epidermis. The hair seen outside the follicle and above the epidermis is known as the hair shaft; the remainder, below the skin's surface, is the hair root.

Along the hair follicle are sebaceous glands. These produce oil called sebum which naturally protects and conditions the hair. An average hair follicle contains up to three sebaceous glands. Overactive sebaceous glands – or more than three – can cause excessively oily hair.

The arrector pili muscle is attached to the hair follicle and the epidermis. When we are cold or scared this muscle contracts and causes the hairs to lift. This helps to trap a warm layer of air between the hairs and protects us from the cold.

Hair shaft

Sweat pore

Epidermis

Dermis

Subcutaneous layer

Sudoriferous glands (sweat glands) travel from the subcutaneous layer through the dermis and up to the epidermis. They contain water which is released as perspiration through sweat pores to cool us down when we are hot.

The matrix, which is wrapped around the dermal papilla, forms the new hair bulb by producing cells called melanocytes. Hair cells are one of the largest growing cells in the body and made from keratin.

The dermal papilla nourishes the hair follicles and supplies food and oxygen to the hair and skin from blood cells via capillaries, arteries and veins.

Nerves travel through the subcutaneous layer, into the dermis and attach to the lower layers of the epidermis. When we shed skin it does not hurt, but cutting or bruising ourselves does because we have triggered the nerve endings. Nerves also attach to the hair follicle, causing discomfort if the hair is pulled.

Hypodermis (subcutaneous layer)

The hypodermis forms a link between the structures below the skin and the dermis. It is made up of a layer of fat cells. It provides some cushioning from external pressure and some thermal **insulation**. It varies in thickness depending on the person's gender and the area of the body.

Insulation

Protection against heat loss.

Functions of the skin

The skin has seven functions:

■ sensation

■ temperature regulation

■ absorption

■ protection

■ excretion

■ secretion

■ production of vitamin D.

Sensation

The skin contains approximately five million tiny sensory cells. These sensory cells enable us to respond to sensations that are applied to the surface of the skin (eg touch, pressure and vibration). The cells respond to environmental changes and send information to the brain, where the sensation is perceived. Sensory nerve endings are located mainly in the dermis but some free nerves end in the epidermis.

Temperature regulation

The body needs to be maintained at a constant temperature of about 36.8°C to function correctly.

The skin responds to an increase in temperature by dilating the blood vessels in the dermis (vasodilation) to radiate heat away from the body where it is open to the elements. The skin begins to sweat. As the sweat **evaporates**, it takes the heat away from the skin's surface allowing the body to cool.

If the body gets too cold, the blood vessels constrict (vasoconstriction) to keep heat nearer to the **essential organs** of the body. Shivering makes the muscle contract. This muscle contraction produces energy to keep warm. Heat loss from the skin is affected by the environment and the amount and type of clothing worn.

Evaporate

To turn into vapour.

Essential organs

The organs that are essential to survival (the brain, heart, kidneys, liver, and lungs).

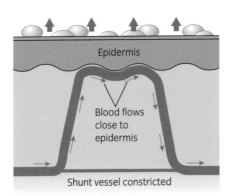
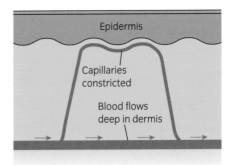

Temperature regulation: vasodilation (left) and vasoconstriction (right)

Absorption

The skin is not totally waterproof. It allows certain substances to be absorbed in a limited capacity. Some examples of substances that can be absorbed are nicotine, hormones and steroids.

Substances that can enter the skin are absorbed:

- between the cells of the epidermis
- through sweat glands
- through hair shafts.

Protection

The skin forms a water-resistant seal over the body. It is very hard-wearing and acts as a defence against chemicals, micro-organisms, dehydration and damage. Sebum, water and other substances are secreted onto the skin's surface to keep it waterproof, supple and flexible. The surface of skin is slightly acidic (**pH** 4.5–5.5), which prevents harmful bacteria growing. Melanin acts as a chemical filter absorbing and reflecting UV radiation.

The hypodermis (subcutaneous layer) cushions the underlying bones and organs to help prevent damage from external forces and pressure. The hypodermis and dermis together protect the body against temperature changes.

Excretion

Excretion is the process that our bodies use to get rid of waste or unwanted substances. The skin is a minor excretory organ. It excretes sweat, which contains water, sodium and potassium chlorides (salts), urea and uric acids and an aromatic substance which gives the body its personal odour. If we don't wash our skin or clothes regularly, bacteria break down our sweat causing unpleasant odours.

Secretion

Secretion is the process that our bodies use to release substances needed by the body. For example, sebum is secreted into the hair follicles and onto the skin. Sebum is an oily substance that keeps the hair and skin soft, supple and flexible. It can also give the skin and hair a shiny appearance.

Production of vitamin D

Vitamin D is produced in the skin as a response to exposure to ultraviolet B radiation (UVB). Cholecalciferol (a form of vitamin D) is produced when the sun penetrates the skin. Cholecalciferol is taken to the liver where it is made into calcidol and stored as vitamin D.

If you block UVB rays, you will prevent the production of vitamin D. Dark skin needs more exposure to UVB to produce the same amount of vitamin D than light skin because it contains more melanin, which restricts absorption of UVB rays.

pH

Potential of hydrogen – pH is a measure of the concentration of hydrogen ions in a substance. A low pH is acidic and a high pH is alkaline.

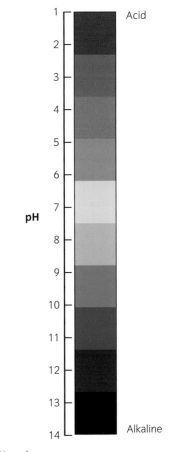

pH scale

HANDY HINT

Be careful to distinguish excretion and secretion. Excretion is getting rid of waste products. Secretion is the producion and release of substances our bodies need.

INDUSTRY TIP

The skin repairs and renews itself three times faster at night so it is important to get a good night's sleep. Specialised products to help repair the skin should be used at night.

INDUSTRY TIP

We all need to go outside into the sunlight for at least 20 minutes each day to make sure that we produce enough vitamin D. This does not mean sunbathing but general exposure.

The effects of ageing on the skin

Ageing is dependent on a variety of factors, which include internal and external influences. Some ethnic groups have a slower ageing process than others. The large amount of collagen in Afro-Caribbean skin prevents some of the effects of ageing. Caucasian (white) skin tends to be thinner and more prone to damage by the sun and the environment.

Age	Skin's appearance
Mid-twenties	The skin's **metabolism** begins to slow down.
	Skin renewal and repair to damaged cells are decreased.
	Each cell division passes on genetic information; however as we grow older, minute pieces of genetic information are lost. This means that the next generation of cells produced do not carry the same information as the previous generation of cells.
Mid-thirties	The skin's **contours** become less defined and the skin starts to sag.
	The structure of new collagen becomes more uneven.
	Elastin fibres show signs of cross-linking and hardening.
	The fat cells that plump out the skin begin to reduce, causing the skin to sag, thin and become crêpe-like.
	The skin retains less moisture, which means it begins to lose its plump appearance.
	The blood vessels of the dermis become more fragile and are more easily damaged.
	The production of sebum from the sebaceous glands declines, causing a reduction in the surface lipids and the skin becomes visibly drier.
Forties	Ageing becomes more obvious with lines deepening, particularly along the expression lines (ie lines caused by muscle movement).
Fifties	The skin is more wrinkled and a loss of elasticity is more noticeable, especially around the contours of the face.
	Older skins often have a more sallow or yellow tone caused by changes in the skin's brown pigment.
	Melanin is no longer distributed evenly throughout the skin. Instead, melanin becomes patchy leaving the skin with uneven pigmentation and **lentigines** (see page 140).

Metabolism

The chemical processes that occur within living organisms to maintain life.

Contours

Outline shape of the skin.

Lentigines

Small brown patches on the skin, typically as a result of ageing (plural: lentigines; singular lentigo).

Wrinkles

Whenever we smile, laugh or use our facial expressions, natural expression lines appear on our faces. Fine or deep lines are created as a result of muscular movement. Wrinkles are depressions in the skin's surface. Wrinkles occur as result of:

- a loss of skin thickness
- changes in the muscle density
- changes to the structure and position of elastin and collagen
- dehydration
- a decline in **hyaluronic acid**.

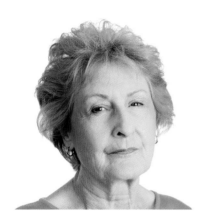 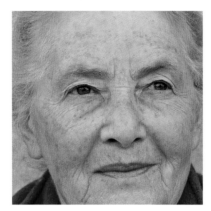

Skin appearance of women in their sixties and seventies

Hyaluronic acid

A key naturally occurring polysaccharide molecule found in the skin. It is a powerful humectant (moisturiser) and is responsible for the plumpness and suppleness of the skin.

INDUSTRY TIP

The hormone oestrogen has water-attracting properties and influences the amount of moisture held in the skin. Oestrogen levels drop following the menopause. This affects the skin's ability to hold moisture.

Characteristics of the skin

Skin tone

All skin has the same number of melanocytes but they have a slightly different structure and are more active in darker skins. Melanin, which gives skin its colour, is produced in a specialised area of the melanocytes called a melanosome. There is more melanin in the melanosomes in darker skin. The depth of colour depends on how the melanosomes are distributed in the epidermis. The melanocytes in darker skins have longer and thicker dendrites (see page 128) that distribute melanin differently. In Caucasian skin the melanosomes are smaller, rounder and surrounded by a membrane. The spaces between the cells give the skin a lighter appearance. There are three main skin tones:

- Afro-Caribbean skin
- Caucasian skin
- Asian skin.

The size and quantity of the sebaceous glands also vary between different skin tones. Afro-Caribbean skin has approximately 10% more sebaceous glands than Caucasian skin and they are larger.

Male skin

The male hormone **testosterone** stimulates fibroblasts to produce collagen at puberty, which means that male skin has a thicker dermis. On average, male skin has 32% more collagen than female skin. Men have higher levels of circulating **androgens**, making the skin secrete more sebum. This makes the skin more oily and the pores more obvious. The two combined give male skin a coarser texture.

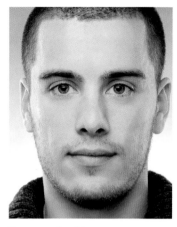
Young male skin appearance

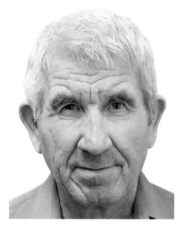
Older male skin appearance

Skin types

There are four main skin groups:

- balanced
- oily
- dry
- combination skin (a mixture of oily and dry).

Balanced skin

It is very unlikely that you will see a truly balanced skin in an adult. This skin is perfect. It is free from any blemishes or **imperfections**. It is neither dry nor oily as secretion levels are balanced. Pigmentation is even and there are no **abnormalities**. The skin is bright and appears healthy.

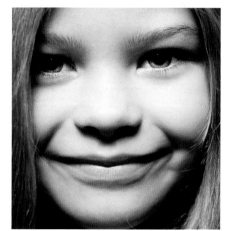
Balanced skin

Testosterone

Hormone produced in the male testicles (and to a lesser extent in female ovaries) that is responsible for male characteristics.

Androgens

Male sex hormones, including testosterone.

Activity

Create a table to show the differences between the different skin tones and types.

Give at least one example of how this may affect your treatments and recommendations.

Imperfections

Flaws in the skin (eg moles or skin tags).

Abnormalities

Things that are not normal.

Oily skin

Oily skin suffers from over-secretion of sebum. The skin appears shiny and sallow in appearance from the residue of surface oil. The skin cells do not exfoliate naturally as they stick to the oily surface. Very oily patches can give the skin a rough texture. Pores are relaxed and are more visible on the skin's surface due to over-active sebaceous glands. The skin can look like orange peel. There are usually comedones present and blocked pores. This skin can feel cool to the touch and have a tacky feel. The excess oil lowers the acidity levels of the skin making it easier for bacteria to multiply so it is prone to blemishes, papules and pustules. A skin with excessive oily secretions is called seborrhoeic.

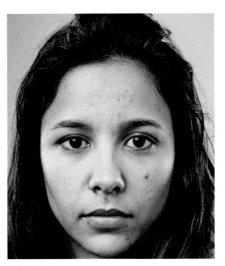

Oily skin

Dry skin

Dry skin lacks the natural lipids (including sebum), which are responsible for keeping the skin lubricated and hydrated. The surface cells appear more flaky and visible to the eye. The skin has a crêpe-like appearance. Dry skin will appear matte and feel warm to the touch. The lack of surface lubrication leaves the skin feeling tight. The skin is often more transparent and this means the circulation is more visible giving it a rosy appearance.

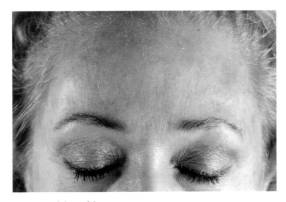

Dry sensitive skin

Combination skin

Typically combination skin type has an oily T-zone on the forehead, nose and chin where the sebaceous glands are more concentrated. The cheeks and neck are commonly dry. Around 75% of skin is combination skin.

Skin condition

The skin can also be described by its characteristics or condition, which might be:

- mature – showing signs of ageing
- dehydrated – lacking in moisture
- sensitive – reactive to touch or prone to allergic reactions.

Any skin type can have one of more of these characteristics/conditions.

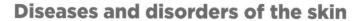

Diseases and disorders of the skin

It is important to be able to recognise common skin diseases and disorders to know whether or not treatments can be carried out (or modified).

Several common disorders can affect the pigmentation of the skin. Skin pigment can be lost, causing hypopigmentation, or increased, causing hyperpigmentation. In many cases the changes cannot be reversed. Avoiding sun exposure will help improve hyper-pigmentation. It takes a very long time for pigmentation to even out and, as most clients will not keep affected areas out of the sun completely, their skin won't have a chance to recover.

SPF

Sun protection factor. The number following it (eg 30), indicates the amount of protection a sunscreen will provide when the skin is exposed to UV light.

Disorder	Description and cause	Contra-indications and general precautions	Advice for client
Pigmented nevus or mole	A raised, pigmented skin growth. It is caused by a cluster of melanocytes cells between the epidermis and dermis or in the dermis. A mole can vary in size from a pinhead to several centimetres, and in colour from tan to bluish black. Some raised moles have hairs growing from them.	Contra-indication to microdermabrasion. Adapt treatment to avoid the area. Keep a note on the client's records and be aware of any sudden changes in colour or size or if the mole begins to weep or bleed. Avoid excessive stimulation over and around the mole.	Use sunblock over the mole for protection from UV.
Ephilides (freckles)	Clusters of melanin. These small areas of pigmentation become more prominent after exposure to UV.	Not a contra-indication.	Use sunblock or a high **SPF** sunscreen to minimise any further changes in pigmentation in the skin. Give advice on camouflage make-up if appropriate.
Lentigines (liver spots)	Also called age spots. Areas of darkened pigmentation about 1cm in size caused by an abnormality in the production of melanin. Skin is often slightly raised. Changes in the skin can be felt by touching the surface of the lentigines. Commonly found on the backs of the hands, face and upper chest of mature clients.	Not a contra-indication.	Use sunblock or a high SPF sunscreen to minimise further pigmentation changes. Give advice on camouflage make-up if appropriate. Recommend a course of microdermabrasion.

Disorder	Description and cause	Contra-indications and general precautions	Advice for client
Chloasma	A cluster of pigmentation in the skin. Commonly found on the upper cheeks, nose and forehead. Caused by hormonal stimulation (eg pregnancy, contraceptive pill). Sometimes disappears once hormones settle down but might be permanent. Skin can react to perfume and sunlight and cause hyperpigmentation.	Not a contra-indication.	Use sunblock or a high SPF sunscreen to minimise further pigmentation changes. Spray perfume onto clothing instead of directly on the skin. Give advice on camouflage make-up if appropriate.
Vitiligo	A lack of skin pigmentation where the melanocytes have been destroyed. White patches of skin can be seen. Thought to be an autoimmune disorder (where the body attacks its own tissues) or triggered by stress or severe sunburn. Hair growing in the area will also be white. The skin around the edge of the area may appear darker due to the contrast with the surrounding darker skin.	Be cautious. Some treatments may be contra-indicated depending on the severity of the **vitiligo**. However, most treatments would not be contra-indicated.	Use a total sunblock in the areas affected as there is no melanin to absorb UV radiation and the skin will burn easily. Give advice on camouflage with make-up if appropriate.
Albinism	The near total or total absence of melanin means there is little or no pigmentation. The hair and skin will be white; eye colour may vary but is often pale blue.	Contra-indication, depending on treatment. Tanning treatments would be unsuitable. The skin is often very sensitive.	Avoid unnecessary exposure to the sun and use sunblock or high SPF sunscreen.

There are a wide range of disorders and conditions that affect the skin's circulation. Some of these changes are permanent while others come and go. Some conditions are hereditary and are present at birth (**congenital**, eg birthmarks). Others develop over time and are the result of ageing.

Vitiligo

A long-term skin condition caused by a lack of a pigment in the skin called melanin.

Congenital

Present at birth, something you are born with.

Disorder	Description and cause	Contra-indications and general precautions	Advice for client
Telangiectasia (dilated capillaries)	Permanently dilated capillaries visible through the skin. Repeated changes in temperature both internal (eg hot flushes) and external (eg air conditioning, central heating and extremes of weather) all **aggravate** the condition. Also aggravated by lack of skin care, eating hot spicy food and alcohol.	Not a contra-indication but take care with some treatments (eg steaming and skin warming, exfoliation, vacuum suction treatments and microdermabrasion). Avoid extremes of temperature.	Can be treated and removed using advanced electrolysis techniques. Keep the skin protected with a good moisturiser. Give advice on camouflage make-up if appropriate.
Rosacea	A chronic skin disorder commonly affecting the nose, cheeks and centre of the forehead (butterfly pattern). Signs include redness, swelling and enlargement of the **superficial** blood capillaries, often giving a mottled appearance. The skin's surface becomes thickened and is superficially dry and flaky in texture. Pustules and papules might be present in more severe cases and are thought to be caused by an immune response. It may also affect the eyes. The cause is often hormonal (affecting women during the menopause). It can also be caused by intestinal disorders, on-going sinus infections, high blood pressure and certain medication. It can be hereditary. Microscopic mites called demodex folliculorum can also cause rosacea. These are commonly found on the skin and are generally harmless but in rosacea there may be an abnormal reaction to the mites causing the blood vessels to dilate. Alcohol and spicy food will aggravate the condition.	Not a contra-indication. Not contagious. Treatment will depend on how severe the condition is. Treat the skin with care and avoid extremes of temperature and **over-stimulation**.	Avoid stress, smoking, spicy foods and alcohol. Use a gentle anti-inflammatory skincare range, with a protective moisturiser and high SPF.\n\nGive advice on camouflage make-up and make-up colours (reds and blues) to avoid if appropriate.

Disorder	Description and cause	Contra-indications and general precautions	Advice for client
Vascular **naevi** (singular: naevus)	Caused by an abnormality of the capillary blood vessels. These cluster together to form a very red raised area of skin. There are different types and most are congenital.	Not a contra-indication. Care should be taken. Avoid excessive stimulation over and around the naevi.	Use sunblock over the area. Give advice on camouflage make-up if appropriate.
Allergies	When an allergic reaction occurs, the immune system produces antibodies in response to **allergens** that most people would not find harmful. Common allergic conditions include hay fever, allergic asthma, urticaria, dermatitis and eczema. **Anaphylactic shock** is a dangerous allergic reaction.	Contra-indication depending on the allergy. Include allergies on the client's record card so that allergens can be avoided. Carry out a patch test. You may have to call for medical assistance if the client has an **acute** allergic reaction (eg anaphylactic shock).	Check product labels and make sure you avoid ingredients that you know the client's skin is reactive to.
Urticaria (hives)	Also commonly known as nettle rash. An allergic reaction characterised by red blotchy skin, **wheals** and severe itching. The skin will feel very warm.	Contra-indication. If the client is already suffering with an allergic reaction, allow the body to heal before treating the client. Carry out a patch/ sensitivity test. If this happens as a contra-action to a product used during a treatment, remove all traces of the products being used from the skin and wash the area with lukewarm water. Do not continue with any further treatment.	Check product labels and make sure you avoid ingredients that you know your client's skin is reactive to. Avoid excessive heat if there is a history of urticaria.

Naevi

Lesions of the skin (eg birthmarks).

Allergen

A foreign substance that can trigger an allergic response in the body.

Anaphylactic shock

A rare but severe acute allergic reaction.

Disorder	Description and cause	Contra-indications and general precautions	Advice for client
Dermatitis	Symptoms include: ■ redness ■ scaling/flaking ■ blistering ■ weeping ■ cracking ■ swelling. Irritant contact dermatitis (ICD) occurs when there is contact with either a strong **irritant** or a weaker irritant over long periods of time. Irritants found in the salon include hand washes, essential oils, dust and wet work (ie constant washing of hands to maintain hygiene). Allergic contact dermatitis (ACD) occurs when someone develops an allergy to something that comes into contact with their skin. Any contact with the allergen will cause an allergic response. Allergens in the salon include glue adhesives, nail polish and skincare products.	This will depend on symptoms and level of severity.	When washing hands make sure they are dried well. Apply moisturiser regularly. Use specialised creams when recommended by a medical practitioner.
Eczema	Areas of extreme dryness on the skin. Wet eczema is when there are **vesicles** present. The irritated skin is itchy. Can be caused by an internal irritant (eg a food intolerance) or by contact with an external allergen (eg animal hair or a product). Eczema can be inherited and is often linked to asthma.	Only a contra-indication if severe and the skin is broken. Avoid direct contact with any area where the skin is broken. Only use gentle products with a natural base. Avoid any abrasive products and over-stimulation.	Seek medical advice as medication can help to relieve the symptoms.

Acute

Sudden and short term.

Wheal

A raised fluid-containing area of flesh-coloured or white skin surrounded by a red area. It can look like a cat scratch.

Irritant

A substance, product or chemical that causes inflammation of the skin.

Vesicle

A small, raised blister containing a pale serum.

Therapists will see lots of common skin disorders. It is important that you can recognise these to know whether they are contagious or not.

Treatments can then be avoided or modified.

Activity

Make a list of all the items/products in the salon that could potentially cause an allergic reaction.

Skin disorders involving the sebaceous glands

Some of the most common skin disorders and diseases that a therapist will come in contact with will be linked to the sebaceous glands. These glands are very active during times of hormonal change, particularly during puberty. These conditions are often easily irritated by the use of incorrect products and incorrect skin care. It is important to treat the skin gently and not remove all the natural oils that the skin needs for protection.

Disorder	Description and cause	Contra- indications and general precautions	Advice for client
Milia	Milia are small **cysts**. They appear as white pearly lumps of skin and might contain uric acid or sebum. Common around the eye area and on skin which is very dehydrated. Might be caused by inappropriate skincare products.	Not a contra-indication.	Check that the client's skincare products are appropriate for their skin type and that they are not dehydrating the skin. Skin must be kept moisturised to prevent dehydration. Avoid mineral-based products around the eye. Advise on facial treatments to stimulate and improve the skin's functions and to keep the skin soft. Milia can be removed using advanced electrolysis or a micro lance, which gently lifts the skin so the milia can be easily extracted.

Oxidation

Interaction between oxygen molecules and other substances.

Cyst

A small rounded swelling that might contain fluid, semi-solid or solid material. It extends both above and below the surface of the skin.

Disorder	Description and cause	Contra- indications and general precautions	Advice for client
Comedone (blackhead)	A grey spot caused by sebum blocking a hair follicle. The change in colour is caused by the **oxidation** of keratin in the sebum as it comes into contact with the air. Further change in colour is also caused by the attraction of surface pollution to the oil.	Not a contra-indication.	Recommend deep cleansing and exfoliating treatments and a suitable home skincare regime.
Sebaceous cyst (steatoma)	Caused by a plug of hardened sebum in the sebaceous gland blocking the follicle and causing it to expand. There are two types of sebaceous cyst: ■ epidermal cysts that can appear anywhere on the skin ■ pilar cysts which are commonly found on the scalp.	Not a contra-indication unless the cyst is very large or infected, then the area must be avoided.	Recommend that the client seeks medical advice if the cyst is causing irritation or if they are concerned.
Acne vulgaris	A bacterial infection of the sebaceous glands of the face, neck, chest, shoulders, back, thighs and bottom. It can affect one or more areas. Facial acne normally starts around the nose and spreads out over the face. Usually caused by a hormonal imbalance that can be aggravated by stress and poor diet. It might also be caused by exposure to certain chemicals and the use of certain drugs.	Contra-indication. Avoid contact with the infected areas to prevent further spread of infection on the client's skin. Only use very limited facial treatment to avoid aggravating the condition.	Seek medical attention early to avoid scarring and to treat any skin infection. Advise on make-up application and the use of matte make-up and oil-free products to protect the skin where appropriate.

Disorder	Description and cause	Contra- indications and general precautions	Advice for client
Seborrhoea	Excessively oily skin. The skin is very shiny and tacky with a sallow grey tone to the skin caused by the oily surface residue. Lots of comedones. Caused by a hormonal imbalance. Can develop into acne vulgaris.	Not a contra-indication. Do not over-stimulate the skin during treatment.	Recommend deep cleansing and exfoliating treatments and a suitable home skincare regime.
Bromidrosis	An unpleasant body odour. Caused by bacteria reacting with sweat.	Not a contra-indication. Might be unpleasant to work on a client who has body odour.	If appropriate, discuss personal hygiene. Recommend a daily shower and washing clothes regularly to remove bacteria.
Anhidrosis	Sweat glands stop working causing a lack of sweating. Caused by a number of factors – damaged nerves, genetic factors, skin damage and certain medication. Can become very serious if it affects large areas.	Contra-indication.	Seek medical advice.
Hyperhidrosis	Excessive perspiration at normal temperatures.	Not usually a contra-indication. Might be a problem with treatments requiring close contact with the skin.	Seek medical advice.
Miliaria rubra (prickly heat)	Red skin rash which is very itchy. Caused by excessive sweating as the body tries to cool down in hot conditions. Sweat gets blocked into the pores.	Contra-indication.	Keep the skin cool. Wear light, loose clothing made of natural fabrics (eg cotton).

Therapists commonly see abnormal skin growths (eg thickening of the skin on the soles of the feet to abnormal skin tags) that are a nuisance to the client. A therapist is unable to improve these disorders directly.

Disorder	Description and cause	Contra-indications and general precautions	Advice for client
Keloid scar	A noticeable thickened scar caused by excessive collagen production as the skin heals. The condition is more common in darker skins. Keloid scars differ from hypertrophic scars as they are firm, hard growths and larger than the original wound.	Contra-indication to any treatment that causes damage to the dermis, eg earpiercing and microdermabrasion. Avoid deep scar tissue for six months.	Check with a medical practitioner if concerned about the scar and check with the medical practitioner as to whether it might be possible to work over scar tissue.
Seborrhoeic keratosis (senile warts)	A brown thickening on the surface of the skin. Range in size from 3mm to 35mm. Exact cause of is unknown. Not caused by exposure to UV.	Not a contra-indication.	Can be removed by a medical practitioner.
Skin tags	Tiny skin extensions. Many have no known cause. Others might be caused by surface stimulation (eg along a neck line or under a bra strap). Made up of loose fibrous tissue.	Not a contra-indication. If there are clusters, avoid stimulation and exfoliation over the area.	If the client is concerned, refer them to an advanced electrolysis practitioner.
Psoriasis	Skin cells are produced very quickly and build up on the surface of the skin leaving scaly, itchy patches. The skin can crack and bleed. The exact cause is unknown. It is linked to stress and can be hereditary.	Not a contra-indication. Not contagious. Can be treated safely. Avoid any affected areas to prevent irritation.	Recommend relaxing treatments that will help to reduce stress. Suggest your client seeks specialist medical treatment from a medical practitioner. Specialist treatments include specialised UV treatment, coal tar treatments and cortisone-based medicines.

Disorder	Description and cause	Contra-indications and general precautions	Advice for client
Hyper-keratosis	A thickening of the skin caused by an excessive amount of keratin. This thickening is often produced to protect the underlying tissue from rubbing, pressure and irritation. Commonly affects the elbow, knees, soles and heels of the feet.	Not a contra-indication.	Exfoliation and a course of microdermabrasion will help improve the skin's texture.
Corns and calluses	An area of hard skin produced by the body to provide additional protection from friction (eg from poorly fitting shoes). Corns are smaller and can be found on the top of toes or between the toe joints. Some people have a corn on the middle finger from holding a pen (writer's lump). Calluses are larger and flatter and occur on the heels and palms.	Not a contra-indication.	Choose shoes carefully. Regular pedicures and manicures will help soften the skin. Use a pen with a soft cushion design. Refer to a podiatrist.
Malignant tumours	A tumour may be benign (non-cancerous) or malignant (cancerous). Caused by cells that have lost their normal features and reproduce in an abnormal way. A tumour might be in, or on, the body. It might be contained in an area or it might have spread into the surrounding tissues and organs. Malignant melanoma – develops in the pigment cells and is associated with excessive exposure to UV radiation. Basal cell carcinoma – develops in the epidermis. Squamous cell carcinoma (or prickle-cell cancer) – develops within keratinocytes in the epidermis. A thick scab develops over a small area of inflamed skin. As the cancer spreads it looks more like an ulcer and may bleed.	Contra-indication. The client should not be treated during cancer treatment. It is not contagious.	A client having cancer treatment should seek medical advice before any treatment takes place. Advise clients about excessive exposure to the sun and sun protection.

Viral infections of the skin

Viral infections are very contagious and you should not feel under pressure to treat anyone you feel is unwell or treat any areas that show signs of a viral infection.

Disorder	Description and cause	Contra-indications and general precautions	Advice for client
Herpes simplex (cold sores)	Caused by a **virus**. Starts with itching or irritation in the area where the cold sore is going to occur. It develops into a red patch followed by blisters. These become a moist crusty patch. Tend to develop when the sufferer is run down, under stress or after over-exposure to the sun and wind. The virus remains **dormant** in the skin after the infection has cleared up.	Contra-indication. Contagious. Can be caught by **direct** or **indirect contact**. Do not treat the area around a cold sore. It is infectious when the blisters are present. If a client is having a facial treatment, ask them to return once the cold sore has gone so they can fully enjoy their treatment.	There is no cure but over-the-counter treatments might help relieve the symptoms.
Human papilloma virus (HPV) Wart Verrucae	The virus enters into the skin through a small cut or scratch. It can lie dormant in the skin for many months. Keratin is produced too fast and causes a hard, raised cauliflower-like growth of skin. The tiny black dots are tiny blood capillaries which get caught as the wart grows. The common wart: about 70% of warts are common warts. Can occur singularly or in clusters. Verrucae (**plantar** warts): occur on the soles of the feet. The weight of the body makes them grow inwards. Particularly contagious in damp, warm conditions. Transmitted through direct and indirect contact.	Contra-indication. Treatment should be modified to avoid putting feet into water or direct contact with the treatment area. Damaged warts are contagious as the viral spores are exposed. Area should be avoided during massage. Precautions should be taken when using spa equipment (ie using equipment such as saunas or steam rooms where footwear might not be permitted or needed). If there are many warts/verrucae treatment is completely contra-indicated.	Most people will develop a wart at some time in their lives. Usually the body develops an **immunity** to the virus and the wart disappears within two years.

Disorder	Description and cause	Contra-indications and general precautions	Advice for client
Verrucae filiformis	Small thin tags of skin. Commonly found in clusters around the neckline and bra line.	Contra-indication as the condition can be easily spread on the client's skin. Avoid any treatment that might irritate the skin (eg body scrubs) and spread the condition further.	Client should seek medical advice before treatment takes place. Can be treated using advanced epilation and specialist medical skin treatments.
Herpes zoster (shingles)	Caused when the chickenpox virus is reactivated after lying dormant in the nervous system. Symptoms include tingling and extreme sensitivity along the nerve pathways followed by pain, itching and blisters. The client may generally feel run down. Pain along the affected nerve may last for many months. The physical symptoms disappear after a week.	Contra-indication. Although shingles is not contagious, you can catch chickenpox from someone who has active shingles if you have not had chickenpox before.	Seek medical advice.

Virus

A micro-organism that multiplies within a living organism.

Dormant

Not active.

Plantar

Sole of the foot.

Immunity

Protection from or resistance to infection.

Direct contact

A disease is transmitted by direct contact with a person who has the disease or infection (eg by touching).

Indirect contact

A disease is transmitted through another object used by a person with the disease or infection (eg towels, spa bath, etc).

Bacterial infections of the skin

Our body is covered with millions of tiny **bacteria** at any given moment. Bacteria can be good as well as bad but some bacterial infections are very contagious and can cause nasty infections. You should be able to recognise the following common bacterial infections and you should not feel under pressure to treat any area that is infected with a bacterial infection. If you catch something you will risk passing the disease on and it may also prevent you from working.

Bacteria

Tiny single-celled organisms. Some are harmful to us and others are important for our health.

Disorder	Description and cause	Contra-indications and general precaution	Advice for client
Furuncles (boils) and carbuncles	A deep bacterial infection of the hair follicle. Starts as an inflamed, tender area which develops into a large painful pustule. Caused by staphylococcus aureus bacteria and linked with poor hygiene and stress. A carbuncle is a collection of boils with several pustule-like heads. A scar is often left once the area has healed.	Contra-indication. Contagious. Avoid area to prevent cross-infection.	Leave the area alone. Seek medical advice if appropriate.
Impetigo	Caused by staphylococcus and streptococcus bacteria. Commonly found on the face around the nose and mouth but can occur anywhere on broken skin. Raised red areas of skin, which quickly form small blisters, followed by honey-coloured crusts.	Contra-indication. Contagious. Can be transmitted by direct and indirect contact.	Seek medical advice.
Conjunctivitis	Caused by staphylococcus bacteria or occasionally a virus. Inflammation of the mucous membrane lining and covering of the eye. Eyes look red, swollen and will feel itchy and gritty. There might be some sensitivity to light. The discharge might contain pus causing the eyelids to stick together in the mornings.	Contra-indication. Very contagious. Transmitted by direct contact (eg by sharing make-up brushes).	Seek medical advice.
Hordeolum (stye)	A staphylococcal bacterial infection of one or more follicles of the eyelashes. A small red area on the edge of the eyelid causes irritation. It becomes a small red lump, which might contain pus.	Contra-indication. Contagious. Do not treat the area to avoid cross-infection.	Seek medical advice.
Folliculitis	A common result of poor hygiene. Can occur following waxing and shaving. Inflammation of one or more hair follicles. Commonly found around the neck, bikini line, beard and armpits. The hair may grow inwards causing further inflammation and a condition called pseudo-folliculitis.	Contra-indication. There is a risk of cross-infection. Give very thorough advice and recommendation.	Seek medical advice. Follow very thorough advice and recommend-ation.

Fungal infections of the skin

You should be able to recognise tinea pedis (athlete's foot). It is one of the most common conditions that clients will present to you.

Fungus

A tiny plant micro-organism.

Disorder	Description and cause	Contra-indications and general precaution	Advice for client
Tinea corporis (ringworm of the body)	Initially appears as a pink circular patch, with a defined red outer ring. The skin heals from the centre as the infection spreads outwards.	Contra-indication. Contagious. Transmitted by direct or indirect contact.	Seek medical advice.
Tinea pedis (athlete's foot)	Symptoms include irritation and sometimes a distinctive odour. The **fungus** lives on keratin and likes a moist, warm environment. White spongy-looking skin might crack, split and peel. Commonly found between the toes but can also affect larger areas of the foot.	Contra-indication. Contagious. Transmitted by direct or indirect contact.	Seek medical advice. Wash and dry the feet well, particularly between the toes. Change socks at least once a day. Wear breathable fabrics that keep the feet dry.
Tinea capitis (ringworm of the scalp)	As for tinea corporis but the hair becomes brittle and breaks away leaving short brittle stubs. The scalp becomes patchy, with white or grey scales.	Contra-indication. Contagious. Transmitted by direct or indirect contact.	Seek medical advice.
Tinea barbae (ringworm of the beard)	Small pustules at the tip of the hair follicle from which broken hair protrudes.	Contra-indication. Contagious. Transmitted by direct or indirect contact (eg dirty towels or contaminated razors).	See medical advice.

Infestations

You are unlikely to come across many **infestations** in the salon but it is still important that you are familiar with them and are able to recognise them. There is always a possibility that you might be exposed to them.

Disorder	Description and cause	Contra-indications?	Advice for client
Pediculosis corporis (body lice)	Caused by a tiny blood-sucking insect. It lays its eggs on clothing and feeds on the skin. Symptoms include Intense itching at the site of infestation, usually in the skin's creases (eg the elbows).	Contra-indication. Contagious. Transmitted by direct or indirect contact.	Seek medical advice.
Scabies (sarcoptes scabiei)	Small **parasites** that burrow into the skin and lay eggs. Burrowing mites cause intense itching that is worse at night. They also cause inflammation and irritation of the infected area and a small grey swelling. Commonly found between the fingers and on the wrists but can also be found under the arm and around the groin.	Contra-indication. Highly contagious. Transmitted by direct or indirect contact.	Seek medical advice.
Pediculosis pubis (pubic lice)	These tiny insects look like crabs or scabs. The females lay eggs that hatch after eight days. Pubic lice can be found under the arms, in beards and in eyebrows. Symptoms include intense itching at the site of the infestation.	Contra-indication. Highly contagious. Transmitted by direct or indirect contact.	Seek medical advice.

INDUSTRY TIP

If you have a Wood's lamp for carrying out a skin analysis/inspection, it can be used to see whether ringworm is present. The fungus glows under the UV light of the Wood's lamp.

INDUSTRY TIP

Clients can often seek medical advice from a pharmacist for minor conditions.

Hair

Hair is 70–80% protein. The protein is in the form of dead keratinised cells that form a thread-like structure. The rest of the hair is made up of a combination of water, minerals, lipids and melanin (the pigment that gives the hairs its colour). Hair grows out from the hair follicle as new cells are produced.

The main function of the hair is protection. Hair covers the head to keep the head warm but also to protect the head from injury and from overexposure to the sun. Eyelashes and eyebrows (supercilia) shield the eyes. They prevent objects from entering the eyes and catch perspiration.

Hair also provides a larger surface area for sweat to evaporate from to cool the body. When we are cold, the arrector pili muscle, which is attached to the hair follicle, pulls the hair up to trap air next to the skin to keep it warm. Tiny hairs in the ears and nostrils, called cilia, catch and filter out dust particles to prevent them from entering the body.

In this part of the chapter you will learn about:

- the hair follicle
- the structure of the hair shaft
- hair texture
- the hair growth cycle
- hair types
- changes in hair growth
- diseases and disorders related to the hair.

The hair follicle

The hair follicle is a complex structure that produces hair. It extends deep into the dermis. The follicle has two layers:

- the inner root **sheath**
- the outer root sheath.

Sheath

A cover (here around the follicle root).

Inner root sheath

The inner root sheath has three layers:

- the cuticle, which holds the hair in place
- the Huxley layer
- the Henles layer.

Outer root sheath

The outer root sheath is a continuation of the stratum germinativum and surrounds the inner root sheath. This sheath remains static in the skin and does not grow with the hair.

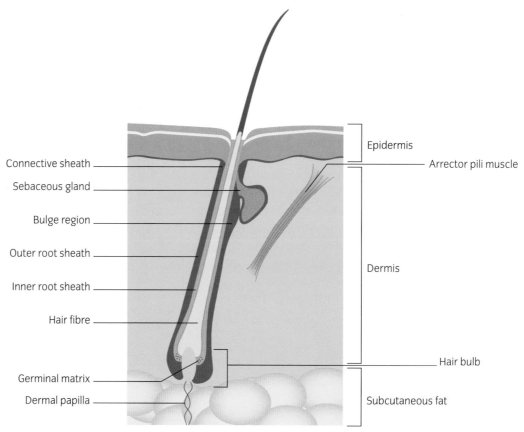

Connective sheath

Sebaceous gland

Bulge region

Outer root sheath

Inner root sheath

Hair fibre

Germinal matrix

Dermal papilla

Epidermis

Arrector pili muscle

Dermis

Hair bulb

Subcutaneous fat

Diagram of the hair

Connective sheath

This sheath surrounds the follicle and the sebaceous gland. It provides the hair with nerve endings and blood vessels.

Hair bulb

This is the enlarged part of the hair at the base of the hair root. It is surrounded by a mass of loose connective tissue called the dermal papilla.

Dermal papilla

At the base of the hair follicle is a mass of loose connective tissue that contains tiny capillaries to nourish all the cells of the follicle. Just above the papilla is a group of cells that produce the hair.

Germinal matrix

This is an area of cells around the dermal papilla where the cells divide by mitosis to produce new hair. It is also where melanin is transferred to the hair to give it pigmentation. This area is very active during the **anagen** stage of hair growth.

Anagen

The growing phase of a hair follicle.

Sebaceous gland

The sebaceous gland is usually located two-thirds of the way up the hair follicle. It produces sebum which is secreted into the follicle. In larger hair follicles there might be more than one sebaceous gland.

Arrector pili muscle

This is a small muscle that is attached to the hair shaft. It supports the hair follicle and, when we are cold, it pulls the hair upright so that the hair stands on end producing goosebumps.

Structure of the hair shaft

The hair shaft is the part of the hair that is visible above the skin. The part below the skin is called the root. The hair shaft is made up of three layers of keratinised cells:

- the medulla
- the cortex
- the cuticle.

Medulla

The medulla is the most central layer of the hair shaft. It is not always present in **vellus** hair (ie in fine body hair). It reflects the light, making hair look shiny.

Cortex

The cortex surrounds the medulla and creates the bulk of the hair. It contains melanin and gives the hair its colour. It is made up of elongated keratinised cells that are twisted together. These strands are able to stretch and flex and return back to their original shape.

Cuticle

The cuticle is the outermost layer of the hair shaft. It is made up of overlapping scales of keratinised cells which provide a protective coat. If you take a strand of hair and run your fingers towards the root you will feel these scales. The cuticle has no colour and is quite a thin layer.

Medulla

Cortex

Cuticle

Layers of the hair

Vellus

Short, fine, light-coloured hair that develops in childhood.

Hair texture

The texture or thickness of a hair depends on:

- the diameter and shape of the hair follicle
- the proportion of the cuticle around the hair.

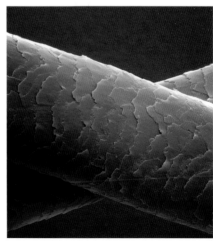

Smooth hair cuticles

In coarse hair, the cuticle makes up around 10% of the volume of the hair and the cortex around 90%. In fine hair the cuticle makes up around 40% of the hair and the cortex around 60%.

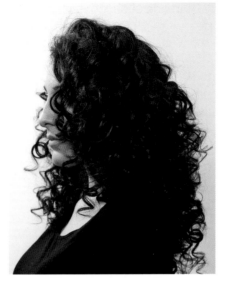

Curly hair

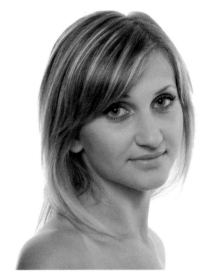

Straight hair

Hair growth cycle

The hair follicle has three stages of growth. These stages include periods of activity and rest and vary from person to person. The growth rate also varies in different parts of the body. The hair on the head has a growth cycle of between two to eight years while the growth cycle of the eyelashes is about four months. The three stages of the hair growth cycle are:

- anagen
- catagen
- telogen.

INDUSTRY TIP

The acronym ACT will help you to remember the hair growth cycle and its sequence.

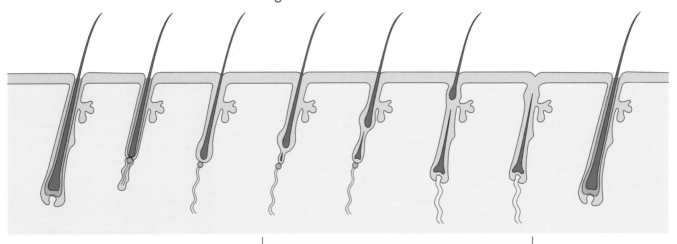

Anagen	**Catagen**	**Telogen**	**Early to mid-anagen**	**Anagen**
Growing phase	Transitional phase	Resting phase	Regrowing phase	Growing phase

The hair growth cycle

Anagen

During anagen the hair is in the active growth stage. The cells in the root sheath divide and grow down deeper into the dermis. At the same time cells grow up the follicle to form the inner root sheath and the hair itself. The hair becomes injected with keratin and becomes keratinised. As the hair matures the growth slows down. Around 80 to 90% of the hair on our head is in the anagen phase of growth at any one time.

Catagen

When the hair growth is complete, the hair goes through a state of change which lasts about two weeks. During this time the cell activity slows down until no new cells are produced. There is no melanin pigmentation so the hair produced in these final stages of growth has no colour. The hair bulb begins to wither and die and forms a club shape at its end. The follicle begins to shorten, shrink and becomes detached from the dermal papilla. A small cord forms between the dermal papilla and the club end of the hair. Around 1% of the hair on the scalp is in the catagen phase of growth.

Telogen

In this final stage, the hair is dead and is shed from the hair follicle. The follicle rests until it is stimulated to begin the cycle again. This stage lasts around three to four months. Sometimes a new hair begins to grow, pushing the old hair out of the skin straight away. Around 13% of hair on the head is resting in the telogen phase of growth.

WHY DON'T YOU...
Run your fingers through your hair and pull at the ends gently. Look at the hair that comes away. The telogen hair will have a distinctive white ball at the end and you will see the loss of hair colour towards the final hair growth. Compare this to a hair that has been removed from an eyebrow using tweezers.

Activity

Wax an underarm with hot wax. Turn the wax over and look at the hairs. Can you clearly see the different hair growth stages?

Activity

Discuss with your colleagues what impact waxing has on the hair growth cycle.

Hair types

There are three hair types:

- vellus
- terminal
- lanugo.

Vellus hair

This is the soft fine downy hair which is found all over the body with the exception of the soles of the feet and palms of the hands. It usually lacks any pigmentation. This hair has shallow roots.

Terminal hair

At birth, this type of hair is found on the scalp, eyelashes and eyebrows. During puberty it grows under the arms and in the groin areas. During male puberty it grows on the lower legs and chest and as facial hair. This type of hair has a well-developed root and bulb with a strong blood supply. The follicle extends deep into the dermis during anagen growth.

Lanugo hair

Lanugo hair is very soft fine hair that covers a baby in the womb and disappears a few months after birth.

> **WHY DON'T YOU...**
> Draw a table with two columns. Head one Vellus and the other Terminal. In the relevant column, write down the differences between vellus and terminal hair.

> **Activity**
>
> Ask some of your colleagues with different hair colours, degree of straightness or curl and thickness to brush their hair and collect any loose hairs. Compare the hairs. Discuss your findings.

Changes in hair growth

Hair growth and changes in hair growth can be caused by a number of different factors such as:

- hereditary/congenital factors (eg genetics will determine hair colour, type, amount and hair growth cycles)
- topical stimulation (eg from sunburn, waxing, scars)
- normal systemic changes (eg changes in hormones during puberty, pregnancy and menopause can cause excessive hair growth)
- abnormal systemic changes (eg diseases or disorders of the endocrine system)
- severe emotional trauma (eg stress can stimulate the adrenal glands which can cause the hair to become more coarse)

■ surgical changes and medication (eg some surgical procedures, such as removal of an ovary, and some medication, such as birth control pills or some steroids, can cause excessive hair growth).

Hirsutism and hypertrichosis

Hirsutism is excessive hair growth, usually in females. It is caused by an excess of the male sex hormone, androgen. The hair is usually dark and thick and grows on the face (upper lip and chin), chest, lower back and buttocks.

Hypertrichosis describes excessive abnormal hair growth on the body and affects both men and women. It can be hereditary or it can develop later in life.

Hair diseases and disorders

Parasitic infections of the scalp in hair growth

Parasitic infections of the scalp are very common. We tend to think of them affecting children but adults can get them just as easily.

Disorder	Description and cause	Contra-indications and general precautions	Advice for client
Pediculosis capitis (head lice)	Caused by a small wingless flat insect which feeds on blood. The eggs (nits) take 7–10 days to hatch. It takes 7–14 days for the lice to mature and mate. They survive for several weeks. Symptoms include intense itching at the site of infection. Nits look like grey-coloured beads attached to the hair shaft close to the scalp.	Contra-indication. Contagious. Direct contact is required for the lice to move from head to head.	Seek medical advice. Treatment must be ongoing for a minimum of 14 days. Use a special comb to loosen and remove nits and lice.

Scalp and hair conditions

While you do not generally deal with the head during treatments, it is useful to understand common conditions that affect the hair and scalp.

Disorder	Description and cause	Contra-indications and general precautions	Advice for client
Alopecia	Can be patches of hair loss (alopecia areata) or total hair loss (alopecia universalis). Can be caused by stress, shock, illness or medication (eg chemotherapy).	Not a contra-indication.	Stimulate the blood supply to the area to encourage healthy circulation. Recommend they see a **trichologist** for additional advice and treatment.
Fragilitas crinium	Very dry brittle hair causing the hair to split and break	Not a contra-indication.	Recommend conditioning hair treatments or masks, hot oil – leaving oil on the hair overnight. Indian head massage would be good with a suitable oil to nourish the hair and stimulate the scalp.

Trichologist

A person who specialises in hair and scalp problems.

INDUSTRY TIP

Androgenic alopecia is male pattern baldness in men and women. The hair growth begins to thin often starting at the crown and the hairline recedes. It can be hereditary or caused by hormonal changes. Androgens cause the hair growth to alter and the hair becomes shorter and finer until it stops growing, leaving the scalp hairless or with a fine covering of vellus hair.

Nails

A perfect healthy nail is smooth, unmarked and can be flexed without breaking or splitting. It is usually a delicate pink colour which shows that there is a healthy circulation to the nail bed. The nail is an extension of the stratum lucidum (clear layer). It is made up of dense keratinised cells, water, minerals (including calcium and zinc) and a small quantity of lipids.

In this part of the chapter you will learn about:

■ the functions of the nails

■ the structure of the nail

■ the growth cycle of the nail

■ diseases and disorders of the nail and their appearance and causes.

Functions of the nails

Nails have three functions:

- to protect the nail bed, and through the nail plate, to protect the soft sensitive fingers and toes
- to enhance the fingertips' sensitivity
- to assist the fingers when picking up objects or scratching.

Structure of the nail

The structure of the nail can be divided into three main sections:

- the matrix
- the nail plate
- the free edge.

There are several other important structures of the nail plate. Many form a tight seal around the nail plate to prevent entry of unwanted pathogens.

Matrix

The matrix is the living part of the nail structure and is an extension of the stratum germinativum. The matrix is sometimes referred to as the root of the nail and lies underneath the nail fold or mantle. It is nourished by an abundant supply of blood vessels. It is here that new cells divide by mitosis to produce the nail. Any injury to the area can cause damage to the nail's structure. The shape of the matrix determines the size and shape of the nail.

Nail plate

The nail plate is a modification of the normal epidermis. It is the visible part of the nail made up of compacted, translucent epithelial cells which have keratinised (80%). There are three distinct layers. The dorsal layer is the uppermost layer and is the hardest layer of the nail plate. The middle layer is called the intermediate layer. It is the thickest layer making up 70 to 75% of the nail plate. It is softer and more flexible than the dorsal layer. The ventral layer is the bottom layer; it is one to two cells thick and is composed of soft keratin.

Nails assist the fingers in picking up objects

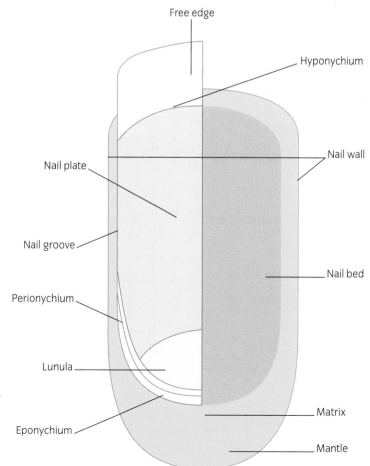

Free edge
Hyponychium
Nail wall
Nail plate
Nail bed
Nail groove
Perionychium
Lunula
Matrix
Eponychium
Mantle

Unlike the other two layers the ventral layer growth upwards and forwards from the nail bed and nail matrix. The ventral layer attaches the nail plate to the nail bed. These keratinised cells of the nail plate are bound together by sulphur bonds, moisture and fat. Unlike the skin, the nails cells cannot be easily exfoliated. The nail plate is dead and has no nerves or blood supply. The cells of the nail plate are able to absorb moisture but too much moisture can cause the nail to split or peel.

Free edge

This is the part of the nail plate that extends beyond the fingertip. It protects the hyponychium at the edge of the nail bed. This is the part of the nail that can be filed into shape.

Other structures of the nail plate

The hyponychium

The hyponychium is the part of the epidermis that is visible under the free edge of the nail. The hyponychium lies at the edge of the nail bed just beneath the free edge. It has a seal that protects it from infection.

The mantle or proximal nail fold

This is a fold of skin that protects the base of the nail and the matrix.

Nail bed

The nail bed lies under the nail plate. The nail plate is held in place by a series of ridges and grooves.

Nail grooves

These are tiny depressions at the side of the nail beneath the nail wall. They guide the nail as it grows up the nail bed.

Lateral nail fold or side wall

The skin along the sides of the nail folds back to form a protective wall and seal around the sides of the nail.

Lunula

This is the visible part of the matrix. It is the very pale pink area at the base of the nail plate. It is a different colour because the circulation is less efficient and also because the cells are not fully keratinised. Many people only have lunulae visible on their thumbs.

Cuticle

The cuticle is formed from thickened stratum corneum (the horny layer) and is constantly being shed. It is found at the base of the nail and grows up with the nail. The cuticle has two parts: the eponychium and the perionychium.

Activity

Look carefully under the free edge of one of your nails. Can you see the thickened area and some ripples in the skin's structure? This is the nail bed.

Lateral

On one side of the body or other.

Eponychium

The eponychium is the fold of skin that overlaps the lunula at the base of the nail plate. It forms a seal to prevent micro-organisms entering into the surrounding tissues. A healthy eponychium should be soft, supple and secure. This is the part of the nail that is freed from the nail plate during a manicure.

Perionychium

This covers the outer portion and sides of the nail.

Nail growth

The nail grows at a rate of about 3–5mm a month. It will take about three to five months to grow from the matrix to the free edge. Toenails grow at about half this speed. It will take about eight to nine months to grow a full new toenail.

> **HANDY HINT**
>
> Nail disorders are covered briefly as it is important to be aware of them. However, it is not necessary to cover them in depth, as you will not come across them in the chapters covered within this book.

Nail diseases and disorders

Disorder	Description and cause	Contra-indications and general precautions	Advice for client
Onychia	Bacterial infection of the nail fold causing the skin around the base of the nail to become red and inflamed. Pus might be visible.	Contra-indication. Contagious and can be cross-infected via poorly sterilised equipment.	Seek medical advice.
Paronychia	A bacterial infection of the cuticle. Symptoms include tenderness, redness and swelling in the infected area. A small pus-filled spot will appear if the condition is not treated.	Contra-indication. Avoid the skin around the infected toenail.	Consult a podiatrist who will remove the part of the nail with the disorder. If very infected, the client might need to seek medical advice.
Onychocryptosis (ingrown nail)	Symptoms include discomfort or pain around the side of the nail as well as redness and swelling. It is caused by poorly fitting shoes and incorrect nail care, in particular incorrect filing or cutting of the nail. It is often seen on the big toe.	Contra-indication.	Seek medical advice if infected or see a chiropodist for treatment.

Calcium

A mineral necessary for the healthy function of the heart, muscles and nerves and an essential part of the structure of bones and teeth.

Phosphate

A chemical compound containing phosphorous, a mineral that helps build bones and teeth.

Rigid

Unable to bend; not flexible.

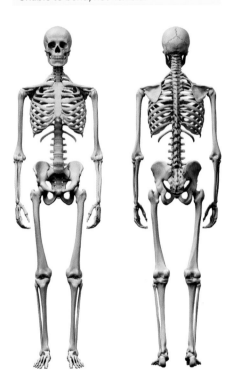

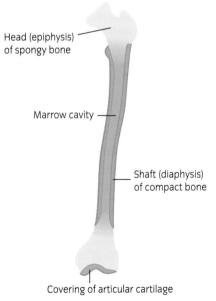

Head (epiphysis) of spongy bone

Marrow cavity

Shaft (diaphysis) of compact bone

Covering of articular cartilage

Long bone

Skeletal system

In this part of the chapter you will learn about:

- functions of the skeletal system
- classification and structure of the skeletal system
- location of bones of the skeleton
- types of joints and movement
- disorders of the skeletal system.

Bone is the hardest tissue in the human body. Bone is made from specialised cells called osteocytes which create a rigid non-elastic tissue. These cells are surrounded by a matrix of collagen fibres strengthened by **calcium** and **phosphate**. Bones have lots of hollow spaces within their structure which make them light and provide tiny spaces for blood vessels and nerves to supply the bone tissue.

Bone tissue is not completely **rigid**. If it is injured, it breaks down and rebuilds, renewing its shape and structure during growth and repair.

Functions of the skeletal system

There are five main functions of the skeleton:

- Protection – the skull protects the brain; the spine protects the spinal cord; the rib cage protects the heart and lungs.
- Support/shape – bones give support for the muscles of the body and give shape to the body contours and the characteristics of our face shape.
- Movement – bones have ridges where muscles attach to allow bones and joints to provide flexible movement.
- Formation of blood cells – all red blood cells and some of the white blood cells are made in specialised tissue called bone marrow.
- Storage and release of certain vitamins and minerals, including calcium and phosphorous.

Classification of the skeletal system

There are 206 bones in the human body and these are shaped according to the function they need to perform. There are five different shapes or types of bone:

- Long bones act as levers to raise and lower limbs. They have a shaft, made of compact bone with a central canal which contains bone marrow, and two ends, which have an outer covering of compact bone. Long bones contain bone marrow.

- Short bones often form bridges and are subject to pressure type forces (eg the wrist and ankle).

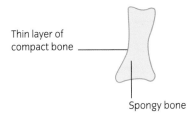

Thin layer of compact bone

Spongy bone

- Irregular bones often have complex shapes (eg the vertebrae).

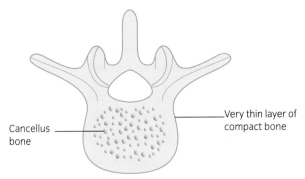

Cancellus bone

Very thin layer of compact bone

- Flat bones are good for creating protective shells (eg the bones of the cranium and sternum and scapula in the torso).

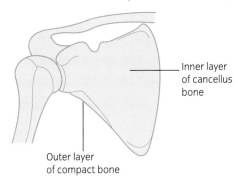

Inner layer of cancellus bone

Outer layer of compact bone

- Sesamoid bones are often rounded bones and sit inside tendons or synovial joints (eg the patella/knee cap).

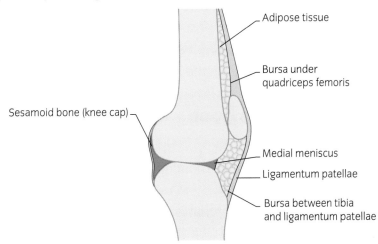

Adipose tissue

Bursa under quadriceps femoris

Sesamoid bone (knee cap)

Medial meniscus

Ligamentum patellae

Bursa between tibia and ligamentum patellae

Concentric

Circular shapes sharing the same centre.

Lamellae

Concentric layers of bone.

Haversian canal

The central passage of compact bone containing small blood vessels, lymph vessels and nerves.

Osteocytes

Individual bone cells.

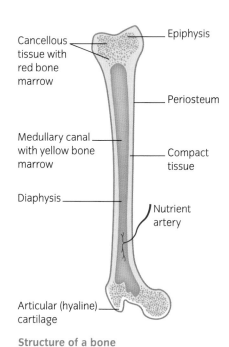

Cancellous tissue with red bone marrow

Epiphysis

Periosteum

Medullary canal with yellow bone marrow

Compact tissue

Diaphysis

Nutrient artery

Articular (hyaline) cartilage

Structure of a bone

Epiphysis

The rounded end of a long bone.

Diaphysis

The main shaft of a long bone.

Medullary canal

The central cavity containing fatty yellow bone marrow.

Structure of the skeletal system

There are two types of bone tissue:

- compact (hard) bone
- cancellous (spongy) bone.

Compact (hard) bone forms the surface layer of all bones and the tubular shafts inside long bones. It makes up around 80% of the bone in the body. Compact bone is made up of osteons. Osteons consist of **concentric** layers of bone called **lamellae** which surround a long hollow central passage (the **Haversian canal**). The central canal contains blood vessels, lymph vessels and nerves which supply the individual bone cells (**osteocytes**).

Cancellous (spongy) bone is sponge-like and is lighter than compact bone.

Bone marrow

Bone marrow is found inside long bones, flat bones and vertebra. Most of the cells in the blood are made in the bone marrow.

Erythrocytes

Erythrocytes are red blood cells. Red blood cells start as immature cells in the bone marrow. Once they have matured (after about seven days), they are released into the bloodstream. Red blood cells contain a special protein called haemoglobin. Haemoglobin is essential for transporting oxygen from the lungs around the body and for carrying carbon dioxide back to the lungs so that it can be exhaled.

Leukocytes

Leukocytes are white blood cells that help protect the body against diseases and fight infections. They include lymphocytes and granulocytes.

Thrombocytes

Also known as platelets, thrombocytes are tiny pieces of large bone marrow cells that are essential in the blood clotting process.

Structure of a long bone

A long bone has:

- two **epiphyses** that form the rounded ends of the bone. The inside is made up of compact bone
- a **diaphysis** – the main shaft that is made up from compact bone and forms the length of the bone structure
- a central space (cavity) called the **medullary canal** that contains special fatty yellow bone marrow

- a **periosteum** – a membrane that protects the bone; the periosteum contains **osteoblasts** and **osteoclasts** that are responsible for producing new bone and breaking down old bone respectively
- **hyaline cartilage** – a bluish-white type of cartilage found at the joints.

Bone formation

Ossification is the formation of bone by the activity of osteoblasts, **chondrocytes** and osteoclasts.

Chondrocytes can be found close to the end of the long bones. Chondrocytes multiply and become enlarged.

Osteoblasts can be found:

- in the periosteum
- in new bone
- at the ends of the diaphysis
- at the site of a bone fracture.

Osteoblasts begin laying down spongy bone. Calcium is deposited to form new, hardened bone cells. Once osteoblasts stop forming new bone they become osteocytes, which assist with blood flow through the bones.

Osteoclasts are cells that break down bone tissue and absorb it back into the body to maintain the skeleton. The maintenance of healthy bone is therefore a balance between osteoblast and osteoclast activity (ie osteoblasts create new bone and osteoclasts break down old bone tissue).

Effects of ageing on the skeletal system

As we age, our bones become more fragile. The calcium content of the bones decreases and as a result the bones become less **dense**, lighter and weaker. This means that bones break more easily. Any damage will take much longer to repair because bone growth and repair slow down with age.

Location of bones of the skeleton

The skeleton can be divided into two parts:

- the axial skeleton – there are 80 bones in the axial skeleton including the skull, the spine and the thorax
- the appendicular skeleton – contains 126 bones and includes the shoulder girdle, the arms and hands, the pelvic girdle and the legs and feet.

Osteoblasts
Cells responsible for bone formation.

Osteoclasts
Cells that break down bone.

Hyaline cartilage
A type of cartilage found at the joints.

Ossification
The process of bone formation.

Chondrocytes
Cartilage-forming cells.

Dense
Closely compacted.

Bones of the skull and face

The skull consists of:

- the cranium, which encloses and protects the brain
- the mandible – the jawbone.

The cranium consists of eight bones, which are fused together.

Bones of the cranium	Position
Frontal	Front of the cranium. Forms the forehead.
Occipital	At the back of the head. Forms the back of the skull.
Parietal	Two bones forming the sides and roof of the cranium.
Sphenoid	One bone forming the back of the eye sockets and the middle of the cranium.
Temporal	Two bones on either side of the cranium. They sit under the ears.
Ethmoid	One bone separating the nasal cavity and brain. Forms part of the eye socket.

HANDY HINT

The shape of the facial bones gives rise to our facial characteristics and individual features.

There are also 14 facial bones.

Facial bones	Position
Maxillae	Two bones forming the upper jaw.
Zygomatic arch	Two bones forming the cheekbones.
Nasal	Two small bones forming the bridge of the nose.
Mandible	Lower jawbone.
Palatine	Two bones forming the floor of the nose and the roof of the mouth.
Inferior conchae	Two bones forming the sides of the nasal cavity.
Vomer	One thin bone forming the nasal septum.
Lacrimal	Two small bones forming the middle wall of the eye sockets.

Sinus

A hollow cavity.

There are four air-filled spaces within the skull which form the facial **sinuses**. The sinuses:

- lighten the weight of the head
- protect the skull from impacts to the face
- give tone and quality to the sound of our voices
- secrete mucus to trap dust and germs that enter through the nose.

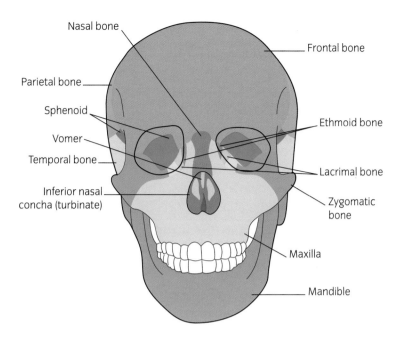

Front view of the skull

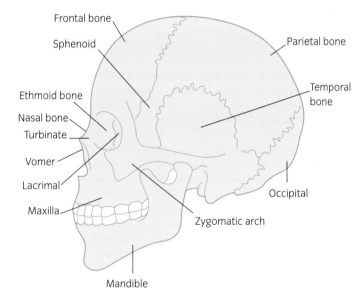

Profile view of the skull

The sinuses form one of the body's first lines of defence against infection.

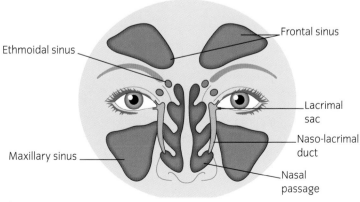

Sinuses

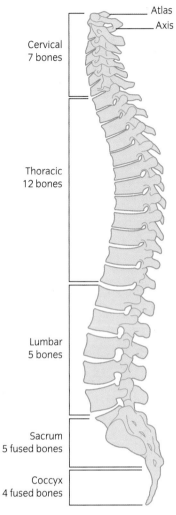

Atlas
Axis
Cervical
7 bones

Thoracic
12 bones

Lumbar
5 bones

Sacrum
5 fused bones

Coccyx
4 fused bones

Bones of the vertebral column

Vertebral column

The vertebral column is made up of 33 vertebrae bones. Of these, 24 bones are moveable.

Bones of the spine	Position
Cervical	Seven bones that form the neck. The first cervical bone is called the atlas. This sits on the second cervical vertebra known as the axis. The axis allows the head to rotate and the atlas supports the position of the skull.
Thoracic	Twelve bones. The ribs are attached to the thoracic vertebrae.
Lumbar	Five bones between the thoracic and sacral vertebra.
Sacral	Five fused bones at the bottom of the back located between the buttocks.
Coccyx	Four fused bones that form a small tail at the base of the spine.

Activity

Working with a partner, ask them if they would be willing to remove their top and lean forward so that their vertebrae stand out. Try to locate each of the different types of vertebra.

The functions of the vertebral column are to:

- protect the spinal cord
- provide a pathway for delicate spinal nerves to sit in while being protected
- allow flexion, extension and rotation
- support the skull
- absorb shock during movement to prevent tissue damage – there are soft intervertebral discs which sit in between the vertebrae to absorb shock during movement and prevent tissue damage
- provide attachment for other bones including the ribs, shoulder girdle, arms and pelvis
- provide attachment for muscles.

Bone structure of the torso

The thorax is the protective cavity for the chest and includes the ribs and sternum. The sternum runs down the centre of the chest and is commonly known as the breastbone. The ribs are long flat bones that run across the sides of the chest and there are 12 pairs in total. At the front of the body they are attached to the sternum and at the back of the body they are attached to the vertebrae.

The shoulder girdle includes:

■ two scapulae – the large bones at the top of the back that look like wings

■ two clavicles – the bones at the front that sit across the shoulders

■ the upper ends of the two humerus bones – the bones of the upper arm.

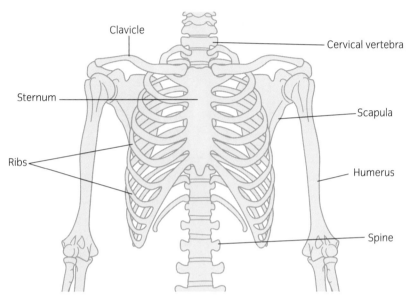

Front view of the chest, neck and shoulders

HANDY HINT

Be careful not to confuse the ilium (the largest bone in the pelvis) with the ileum (part of the small intestine).

The pelvic girdle is made up of:

■ the sacrum – the large, triangular bone at the base of the spine

■ the pelvis, which consists of two hip bones. Each hip bone is made up of three fused bones:

■ the ilium, the largest bone of the pelvis, which forms the synovial joint (sacroiliac joint) with the sacrum

■ the ischium, which takes the weight of the body when sitting down

■ the pubis – the pubic bones found between the legs.

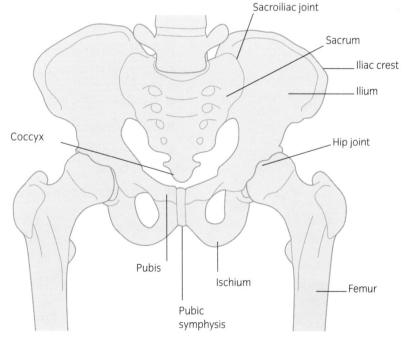

Pelvic girdle

The arms are made up of the:

- humerus (upper arm)
- ulna (forearm) – runs along the little finger side the forearm
- radius (forearm) – runs along the thumb side of the forearm.

The hands are made up of:

- eight carpals: triquetral, lunate, scaphoid, trapezium, trapezoid, pisiform, hamate and capitate (these form the wrist)
- five metacarpals (these form the palm of the hand)
- 14 phalanges (these form the fingers).

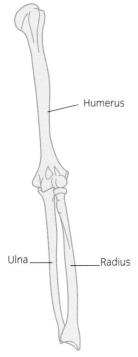

Bones of the arm

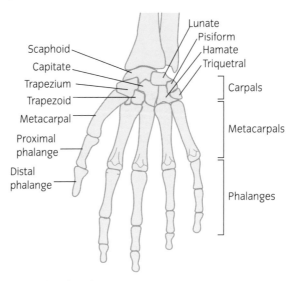

Bones of the hand

Bone structure of the lower limbs

The legs are made up of the:

- femur – forms the thigh and is the longest bone in the body
- patella – the knee cap
- tibia – on the big toe side of the lower leg and commonly called the shin bone
- fibula – on the little toe side of the lower leg.

The feet are made up of:

- seven tarsals: talus, calcaneus (or heel bone), cuboid, central cuneiform, medial cuneiform, lateral cuneiform, navicular (these form the ankles)
- five metatarsals (these form the main part of the foot)
- 14 phalanges (these form the toes).

WHY DON'T YOU...
Look at your bare foot. Can you make out any of the bones of the tarsals?

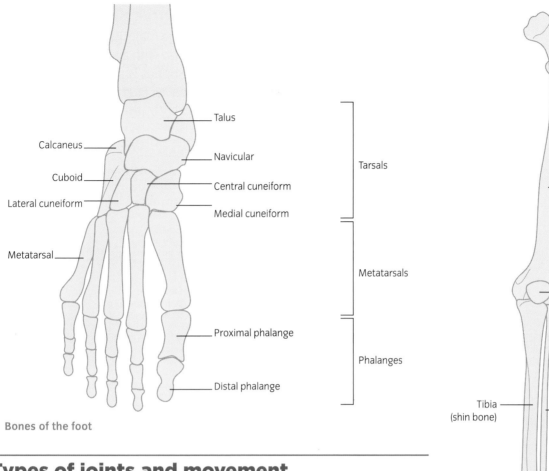

Calcaneus

Cuboid

Lateral cuneiform

Metatarsal

Talus

Navicular

Central cuneiform

Medial cuneiform

Tarsals

Metatarsals

Proximal phalange

Distal phalange

Phalanges

Bones of the foot

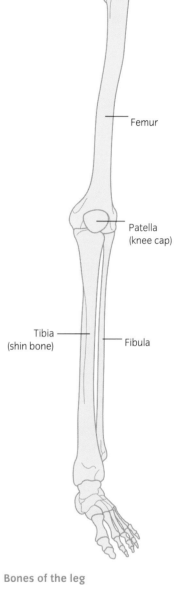

Femur

Patella
(knee cap)

Tibia
(shin bone)

Fibula

Bones of the leg

Types of joints and movement

A joint is where two bones meet. Muscles and tendons stretch across joints when they move. Joints are classified by their structure or by the way they move. There are three main types of joints:

- fibrous or fixed joints
- cartilaginous/slightly moveable joints
- synovial/freely moveable joints.

Fibrous/fixed joints

These joints are tightly linked with a tough fibrous material and have virtually no movement (eg the skull).

Cartilaginous/slightly moveable joints

These joints are formed by a pad of tough fibrous cartilage and have no movement or only a limited range of movement. The pad acts as a shock absorber (eg joints between the vertebrae).

Synovial joints/freely moveable joints

These joints have a range of movement. The majority of joints in the body are synovial. Each bone end is covered with a smooth coating of cartilage. In the small space between the bones is a liquid called synovial fluid, which is a lubricant. Around the synovial fluid is a capsule to hold the joint in place. Ligaments provide stability to the joint.

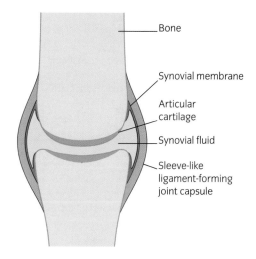

Bone

Synovial membrane

Articular cartilage

Synovial fluid

Sleeve-like ligament-forming joint capsule

Structure of a synovial joint

Convex

Rounded outward.

Concave

Rounded inward.

Type of synovial joint	Description	Movement range
Ball and socket	The rounded end of one bone fits into a neat cup-shaped cavity in another bone (eg the shoulder and hip).	Flexion, extension, adduction, abduction, rotation and circumduction. See page 178 for more details.
Hinge	The **convex** surface of the end of one bone fits into the **concave** surface of a second bone (or bones) (eg elbow and knee). (Think of the hinge of a door.)	Flexion and extension.

Type of synovial joint	Description	Movement range
Pivot	A pivot joint is where one joint rotates around another. The first two cervical vertebra (atlas and axis) pivot through a bony projection of the axis (C2), one vertebra with the ring shaped socket of another (C1). This joint allows the head to turn from side to side. Another example is the radioulnar joint at the elbow.	Rotation.
Gliding/plane	The surfaces of the bone are almost flat and glide over each other (eg tarsals and metatarsals).	Range is limited to a slight glide or small rotation.
Condyloid	This is a smooth rounded projection on a bone which sits into a cup-shaped depression on another bone (eg mandible and temporal bone, carpals and radius).	Flexion, extension, abduction, adduction and circumduction.
Saddle	The surfaces of the two bones that meet have both concave and convex surfaces. There is only one saddle joint in the body – at the base of the thumb.	Movement range is similar to condyloid.

Joint movement

Type of movement		Description
Abduction		A movement away from the body.
Adduction		A movement towards the body.
Flexion		A bending movement bringing two level joints together.
Extension		Straightening a joint (eg moving two levers away from each other).
Rotation		The movement of a bone in a circle around fixed points.
Lateral rotation		
Circumduction		The movement of a limb or finger with little movement where it is attached and greater movement at the end. For example, where the little finger is attached to the hand its movement is small but the fingertip can draw a large circle.

HANDY HINT

Dorsiflexion is flexion of the foot while plantar flexion is extension – think of planting the foot to the ground to help you remember.
Supination is turning the hand with the palm upwards; when standing the palm faces to the front. Pronation is turning the palm to face down.

Disorders of the skeletal system

Skeletal conditions can be easily overlooked as they are hidden away from view inside the body. It is important to remember that whether something is inside or not the body needs time to repair itself. Damage can be done if the body is not allowed time to heal properly. The conditions below will require you to **modify** your treatment. You should not work over the area directly around a sprain or broken bone.

Modify

Adapt or make changes to your treatment.

Displacement

Movement from its original position.

Compound break

An injury where there is a break in the skin around a broken bone.

Skeletal condition/disorder	Description and cause	Contra-indications and general precautions	Advice for client
Bunion	A **displacement** and inflammation of the big toe joint. Fluid collects around the joint. Caused by repeated pressure on the side of the first metatarsal, commonly from wearing tight, poorly fitting shoes.	Not a contra-indication. Take extra care as the joint might be very tender. Massage should be very gentle.	Seek advice from a medical practitioner or chiropodist if bunion is painful.
Broken and fractured bone	A fracture is a crack or break in the bone either across its width or diagonally across the bone shaft. A **compound break** or open fracture occurs when the bone breaks through the skin's surface. Closed fractures happen when the bone is still within the body. These can cause a lot of tissue damage in the area of the break. A greenstick fracture is where a long bone is fractured along the bone but not all the way through.	Contra-indication. Do not treat the area until fully healed to prevent further damage.	Rebook the treatment once area has healed.
Sprain	Occurs when a ligament is over-stretched or torn. A common area for sprains is around the ankle joint. A sprain can occur as the result of a fall when the full force of the body's weight is placed onto a joint.	Contra-indication. Do not treat until it is fully healed to prevent any further tissue damage or discomfort to the client.	Rebook the treatment once area has healed.

Skeletal condition/disorder	Description and cause	Contra-indications and general precautions	Advice for client
Rheumatoid arthritis	A **chronic**, **progressive** disorder of the immune system. The synovial joints and surrounding tissues become damaged and inflamed. Symptoms include inflammation of the synovial joints. The joints become deformed and painful and there is loss of movement.	Contra-indication. Avoid the affected area.	Seek medical advice.
Osteoarthritis	Causes restricted movement and pain in the affected joints. The **articular cartilage** thins and eventually the surfaces rub against each other. Symptoms include pain, swelling, stiffness and enlarged joints with some loss of joint movement.	Contra-indication. Treat joints gently and with extra care.	Seek medical advice.
Bursitis	Inflammation of the **bursa**. Usually the result of friction or slight injury to the membrane surrounding the joint.	Contra-indication. Avoid the affected area. Advise client to seek medical advice.	Seek medical advice and treatment.
Tendonitis	Inflammation of the tendon causing pain and possibly restricted movement.	Contra-indication. Avoid the affected area.	Seek specialist advice and treatment.

Skeletal condition/disorder	Description and cause	Contra-indications and general precautions	Advice for client
Osteoporosis 40 years 60 years 70 years Normal Reduced bone Osteoporosis	Bone **density** is reduced, making the bone weak and brittle. Bone is broken down at a greater rate than new bone is produced. The disease is associated with ageing, certain medication (eg steroids) and the menopause. There are no obvious symptoms.	Contra-indication to mechanical massage. Treat gently and lightly to avoid any damage.	Refer client to a medical practitioner. A bone scan will confirm diagnosis. Regular **weight-bearing exercise** will be beneficial as it helps to build and support the bones.
Rickets	Caused by a deficiency of calcium, phosphate and vitamin D in the diet. Causes a condition called **osteomalacia** in adults.	Treat with caution.	Seek specialist advice and treatment.
Hammer toes	A **deformity** of the tendons in the toe joints. Causes the toes to become bent.	Treat with caution.	Seek specialist advice and treatment.

Chronic

Long term.

Progressive

Increasing in severity.

Articular cartilage

Smooth white tissue that covers the ends of bones where they form joints.

Bursa

A fluid-filled sac between a bone and tendon that prevents friction.

Density

Compactness.

Weight-bearing exercise

Exercise that places weight on bones (eg walking).

Osteomalacia

A softening of the bones.

Deformity

Distortion or imperfection.

Disorders of the spine

Disorder	Description and cause	Contra-indications and general precautions	Advice for client
Scoliosis 	A **lateral** curvature of the spine in the thoracic region of the spine. May be caused by deformities of the bones and spine and poor posture. Signs of scoliosis include: ■ a difference in height between both ears and both shoulders. ■ twisted scapula and torso ■ curved spine ■ twisted pelvis with one leg shorter than the other.	Treat with caution. Might be visible when carrying out a full body consultation.	Seek professional advice from a medical practitioner or an alternative practitioner, such as an osteopath. Balancing and strengthening exercises and yoga and Pilates are beneficial.
Kyphosis 	Rounding of the shoulders and back in the thoracic region. The pectoral muscles become tight and the back muscles are over-stretched. Might cause back pain in the thoracic region. Causes include poor posture (eg as a result of leaning over a keyboard) and disease of the joints.	Not a contra-indication.	Seek professional advice from a medical practitioner or an alternative practitioner, such as an osteopath. Balancing and strengthening exercises and yoga and Pilates are beneficial.
Lordosis 	Curvature of the lumbar spine. Can be seen as a hollow in the lower back. The pelvis tilts forward and the **gluteal muscles** stick out.	Not a contra-indication.	Seek professional advice from a medical practitioner or an alternative practitioner, such as an osteopath. Balancing and strengthening exercises and yoga and Pilates are beneficial for correction of the pelvic tilt and to strengthen the abdominal, core and back muscles.

Disorder	Description and cause	Contra-indications and general precautions	Advice for client
Herniated or prolapsed disc 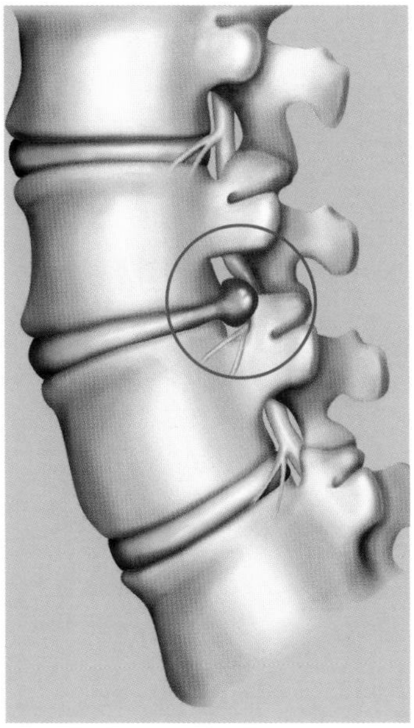	An intervertebral disc **protrudes**, placing pressure on the nerve. Often caused by strenuous activity. Can be part of the ageing process as the result of the wearing out of the discs.	Contra-indication. Avoid back area and mechanical G5 massage. Provide additional support for the client.	Seek medical advice.

Lateral

From side to side.

Gluteal muscles

Buttock muscles.

Protrudes

Sticks out.

Activity

Working with a partner, try to identify the curves of the spine. Make a note of whether the curve is natural, flattened or exaggerated.

Muscular system

Our muscular system includes all the muscle tissue in the body. Muscle tissue enables movement, maintains posture and is vital for the function of the organs of the body. All muscle tissue has four common properties. It can:

- respond to stimuli from the nervous system
- contract in response to a stimulus
- be stretched without damaging its structure
- return to its original shape after contraction (ie it is elastic).

In this part of the chapter you will learn about:

- the structure of the muscular system
- the functions of the muscular system
- locations and actions of the primary muscles
- disorders of the muscular system.

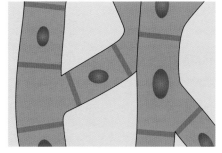

Cardiac muscle tissue

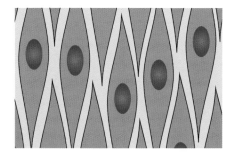

Involuntary muscle tissue

Conscious

When you are aware of what you are doing; deliberate.

Respiratory

Relating to the system for taking in oxygen and giving out carbon dioxide (ie breathing).

The structure of the muscular system

There are three types of muscle tissue:

- cardiac muscle
- smooth, involuntary muscle
- skeletal, striated or voluntary muscle.

Cardiac muscle

This is a specialised type of muscle tissue found only in the heart.

Smooth, involuntary muscle

This is not under **conscious** control and is found in the walls of hollow organs (ie blood and lymph vessels, the alimentary canal (digestive system), the **respiratory** tract, bladder, uterus and ducts of glands).

Skeletal, striated or voluntary muscle

These muscles are under conscious control. A tiny motor nerve carries messages from the central nervous system to the muscles to stimulate them into action. There are 650 named muscles in our body; 150 of these muscles are in the head and neck. Skeletal muscles make up about 40 to 50% of our body weight. Each muscle is made up of thousands of long narrow cells that look like fibres. These cells are surrounded by a tough sheath.

Muscles are covered in a layer called the **epimysium** or muscle fascia. The epimysium has a smooth surface that protects the muscle from friction against other muscles and bones and allows it to move easily against other structures.

Each muscle is made up of hundreds of small fibres called myofibrils. Myofibrils are made up of even smaller protein filaments called **actin** and **myosin**. Myosin forms thick filaments and actin forms thin filaments. It is bundles of the thick filaments and thin filaments that give muscle tissue its striped appearance. A sarcomere is the smallest unit of skeletal muscle that can contract. Myofibrils are made up of rows of sarcomeres.

Myofibrils are bundled together (in bundles of between 10 and 100 muscle fibres) to form a **fascicle**. Each individual muscle fibre within the fascicle is covered by a fibrous connective tissue called endomysium, which insulates the fibres and helps to keep the muscle in an organised structure.

The whole fascicle is also surrounded by a layer of protective tissue called the perimysium.

Nerves and blood vessels run along and through the layers of connective tissue to supply the muscle fibres. Each fibre is linked to the central nervous system by a tiny nerve.

Motor nerves carry messages from the central nervous system (brain or spinal cord) to the muscles to stimulate them to contract.

Epimysium

Sheath of tissue around muscle.

Actin

Thick muscle protein filament.

Myosin

Thin muscle protein filament.

Fascicle

A bundle of myofibrils.

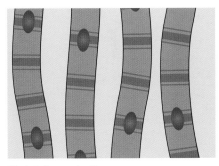

Skeletal muscle tissue

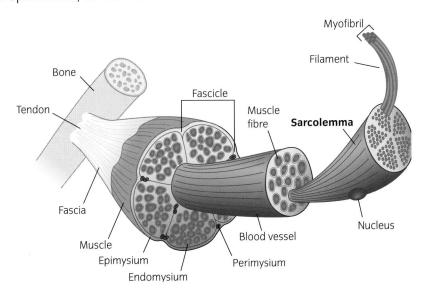

A cross-section of a skeletal muscle

Sarcolemma

Teh membrane surrounding myofiber.

The functions of the muscular system

The muscular system has several functions:

- Movement – movement happens as a result of the shortening (contracting) and the lengthening (relaxing) of muscle tissue.

■ Posture – some of the muscle's fibres are always contracted even when the muscle is at rest. Otherwise the body would not be able to function. This is essential for maintaining posture. This muscle tone is weakest when we are sleeping and in a relaxed state. Muscle tone makes sure enough blood supply reaches the muscles.

■ Creation of heat – muscular activity creates heat in the cellular tissues.

■ Assists with blood flow and lymphatic movement – muscular movement squeezes the blood and lymph vessels, which helps both blood flow and lymphatic movement.

■ Protection – some muscles also help to provide protection for some of the abdominal organs.

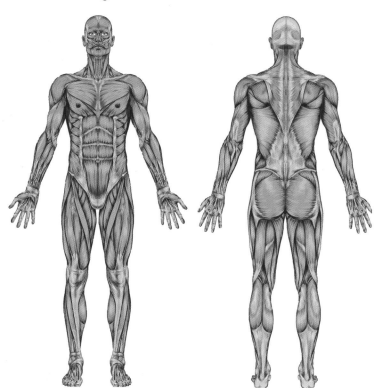

Anterior and posterior view of the muscular system

Muscle contraction

Muscle contractions occur every time we move. Muscles contract (shorten) when they are stimulated by a nerve. A stronger muscle contraction will take place when more muscle fibres are stimulated. Contraction needs energy in the form of adenosine triphosphate (ATP) which is made from glucose.

A muscle contracting and relaxing during exercise

Glucose from our food is taken to the muscles by the blood and stored as **glycogen** until it is needed. When muscles require energy, a metabolic process breaks down the glycogen to release energy. The glycogen is combined with oxygen from the blood and forms ATP to provide energy for the contraction. If there is not enough oxygen to keep this process going lactic acid is formed which causes tiredness (fatigue) in the muscles. Lactic acid can cause the muscles to ache and feel weak.

Glycogen

A polysaccharide (carbohydrate) stored in the liver and muscles. It is converted to glucose to provide skeletal muscles with energy.

Prime muscle mover

This is the main muscle that is producing a specific movement. The biceps brachii and triceps brachii of the upper arm are the prime movers (agonists) in flexion and extension of the elbow. Muscles usually work in pairs: the agonist muscle contracts to produce movement while the antagonist muscle relaxes to allow the movement to take place. In flexion of the elbow the biceps brachii is the prime mover while the triceps brachii is the antagonist. In extension these muscles would reverse their roles.

Synergistic muscles

Synergistic muscles work to stabilise a joint during movement and assist with movements. In flexion of the elbow the brachioradialis and brachialis assist the biceps. The origin of the agonist needs to be stable during movement and muscles called fixators achieve this. The example used here is the rotator cuff muscles at the shoulder.

Types of contraction

A muscle contraction occurs when tension is generated within muscle fibres.

There are two types of contraction: isotonic (concentric and eccentric) and isometric or static contraction:

- Isotonic muscle contractions – during isotonic muscle contraction there is equal tension which remains constant as a muscle shortens or lengthens.
  - Concentric muscle contraction (towards the middle) – this action makes the muscle shorter and moves the origin and insertion closer together.
  - Eccentric muscle contraction – the muscle does not actually lengthen but returns to its normal resting position. During eccentric movement of a muscle the muscle is often acting as a brake for resisting force to slow or control a movement.
- Isometric – here the prime mover and antagonist muscle remain under equal contraction. The muscles are held in either partial or maximal contraction against a force.

Muscle tone

Even at rest there is always a state of partial contraction in muscles fibres otherwise the body would not be able to keep upright when relaxed.

Poor muscle tone can be seen by under-developed muscles. These muscles tire easily when used and have a slow and/or weak contraction.

If a muscle has excessive tone it is over-developed and the muscle may shorten in length as a result. This may restrict the muscle's range of movement.

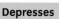

Locations and actions of the muscles of the body

Depresses

Pushes down into a lower position.

INDUSTRY TIP

If you confuse orbicularis oris and oculi, remember the i at the end of oculi for eye.

Muscles of the head and face

The muscles of our face define our features. They give us expression and show our age. You will find it particularly helpful to know the location and action of each muscle during massage treatments.

Facial muscle	Position	Action
Occipitalis	At the base of the skull at the back of the cranium at the base.	Moves the scalp.
Frontalis	Runs along the forehead.	Raises the eyebrows and helps you frown by wrinkling the forehead.
Temporalis	Side of the head stretching to the mandible (jaw).	Raises the mandible during chewing.
Orbicularis oculi	Surrounds the eye socket.	Closes the eyelids.
Corrugator	Between the eyebrows.	**Depresses** the forehead to frown.
Buccinator	At the sides of the cheek.	Squeezes the cheeks together during chewing.
Risorius	Found at the corners of the mouth.	Lifts the corner of the mouth into a smile.
Quadratus labii superioris	At the sides of the upper lip across the top of the maxilla and zygomatic bone.	Lifts the upper lip.
Depressor labii	Runs down the chin from the lower lip.	Pulls the lower lip down.
Procerus	Between the brows, extending down to the nasal bone.	Draws the eyebrows down in a frown and wrinkles nose.
Nasalis	Crosses of the bridge of the nose.	There are two parts to this muscle – one part dilates the nostrils and one part constricts the nostrils.
Triangularis	One each side of the chin.	Draws the sides of mouth down.
Orbicularis oris	Around the mouth.	Closes the mouth and pouts the lips.
Masseter	Sides of face in front of the ear.	Raises the lower jaw and helps us to chew food.
Zygomaticus major/ minor	Along the cheek.	Raises the corner of the mouth into a smile.
Mentalis	Over the chin.	Allows the lower lip to pout.
Sternocleidomastoid	Sides of neck.	When the muscles work singularly they help to rotate the head. Together they pull the head forward (chin down).
Platysma	From the chin down the front of neck.	Draws the corners of mouth down, lowers the mandible and maintains skin texture.

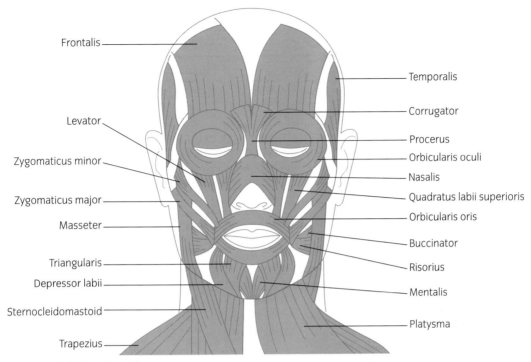

Frontalis

Temporalis

Corrugator

Levator

Procerus

Zygomaticus minor

Orbicularis oculi

Nasalis

Zygomaticus major

Quadratus labii superioris

Masseter

Orbicularis oris

Buccinator

Triangularis

Risorius

Depressor labii

Mentalis

Sternocleidomastoid

Platysma

Trapezius

Muscles of the head and face

Muscles of the shoulder, arm and hand

It is important to be aware of these muscles during body treatments that include the shoulders, arms and hands.

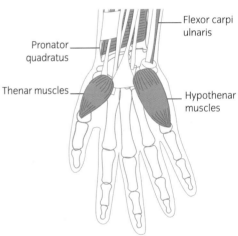

Pronator quadratus

Flexor carpi ulnaris

Thenar muscles

Hypothenar muscles

Muscles of the hand

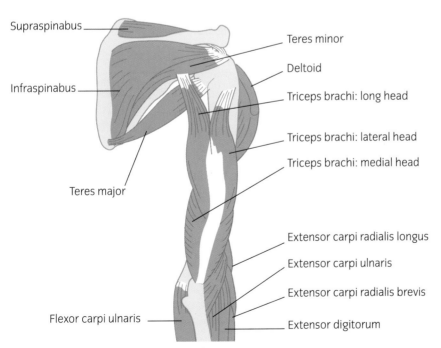

Supraspinabus

Teres minor

Deltoid

Triceps brachi: long head

Infraspinabus

Triceps brachi: lateral head

Triceps brachi: medial head

Teres major

Extensor carpi radialis longus

Extensor carpi ulnaris

Extensor carpi radialis brevis

Flexor carpi ulnaris

Extensor digitorum

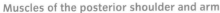
Muscles of the posterior shoulder and arm

Muscle of the upper arm	Position	Action
Coraco-brachialis	Front of chest to upper arm.	Adducts shoulder, flexes upper arm.
Brachialis	Upper arm.	Flexes elbow.
Biceps brachii	Front of the upper arm.	Turns and flexes the forearm, flexion of the elbow.
Triceps brachii	Back of the upper arm.	Extension of the arm at the elbow.

Muscles of the lower arm and hand	Position	Action
Pronator teres	Across inner elbow.	**Pronates** hand.
Brachioradialis	Crosses over elbow joint from upper arm to the wrist.	Flexes elbow, helps to pronate and **supinate** hand.
Extensor carpi radialis longus Extensor carpi radialis brevis	Back of forearm along the radius.	Extension and abduction of the wrist.
Extensor carpi ulnaris	Covering the back of the forearm.	Extends the wrist and adducts the hand.
Extensor digitorum	Back of the forearm.	Extends the fingers and extends the hand at the wrist.
Flexor carpi radialis	Front of the forearm.	Flexes and abducts the wrist.
Flexor carpi ulnaris	Front of the forearm.	Flexes and adducts the wrist.
Palmaris longus	**Medial** side of lower arm.	Flexes wrist.
Flexor digitorum superficialis Flexor digitorum profundus	Front and medial side of lower arm.	Flexes fingers.
Hypothenar eminence: Opponens digiti minimi Abductor digiti mini Flexor digiti minimi brevis	A group of small muscles located in the palm and around the little finger and medial side of the hand.	Controls movements of the little finger. Opposes the thumb – allows the little finger to touch the thumb. Abducts the little finger. Flexes the little finger.

Pronate

Turn face down.

Supinate

Turn face up.

Medial

Internal rotation to turn inwards.

Muscles of the thumb	Position	Action
Adductor pollicis	Palm of the hand.	Adducts the thumb.
Flexor pollicis brevis	Palm of the hand.	Flexes the thumb at the first joint.
Extensor pollicis brevis Extensor pollicis longus Abductor pollicis longus	Along ulna side of lower arm and hand.	Work together to flex, extend and rotate the thumb and help to abduct the wrist and flex the hand.
Flexor pollicis longus	Back of the lower arm and hand along radius.	Flexes thumb.
Thenar eminence: Opponens pollicis Abductor pollicis brevis Flexor pollicis brevis	A group of small muscles located in the thumb and lateral side of the palm of the hand.	Controls movements of the thumb. Opposes the thumb – brings it against the fingers. Abducts the thumb. Flexes the thumb.

Muscles of the thorax and abdomen

The muscles of the thorax and abdomen are involved in movement of the torso. It is important to be aware of these muscles during body treatments that include the back, chest and abdomen.

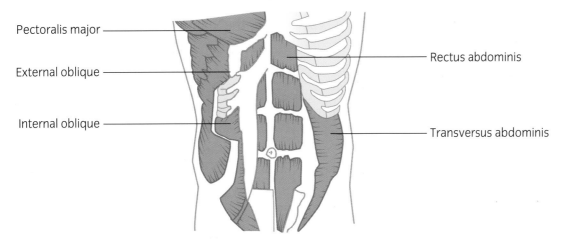

Pectoralis major

External oblique

Internal oblique

Rectus abdominis

Transversus abdominis

Muscles of the abdomen – front

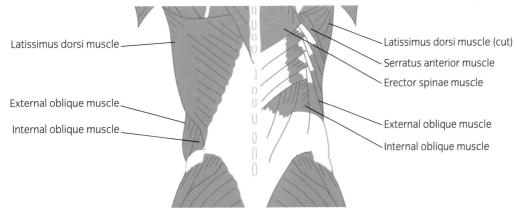

Latissimus dorsi muscle

External oblique muscle

Internal oblique muscle

Latissimus dorsi muscle (cut)

Serratus anterior muscle

Erector spinae muscle

External oblique muscle

Internal oblique muscle

Muscles of the abdomen – back

Muscles of the thorax and abdomen	Position	Action
Trapezius	A large diamond-shaped muscle that extends from the occipital bone to the vertebrae in the thoracic region.	Lifts and braces the shoulders and rotates the scapula.
Pectoralis major	Front of the chest.	Flexion, adduction and rotation of the upper arm. Draws the arm across the chest.
Sacrospinalis (erector spinae)	Group of muscles either side of the spinal column.	Rotates the body and extends the spine. Maintains posture of the trunk.
Serratus anterior	Starts on the upper ribs at the side of the chest along the side of the scapula.	Holds the scapula in position during movement. Pulls the shoulder forward. Rotates the shoulder.
Pectoralis minor	Front of chest.	Rotates and **protracts** scapula.
External intercostals	Between each rib in intercostal space.	Elevates rib so that forced respiration takes place.
Internal intercostals	Between each rib in intercostal space.	Depress rib and aids forced respiration.
Diaphragm	Dome-shaped muscle forming a partition between the thorax and abdomen.	Assists with inspiration by enlarging the thorax, drawing air into the lungs.
Rhomboid major and minor	Between scapula and thoracic vertebra.	Retracts and medially rotates scapula.
Serratus anterior	Upper part of trunk over the ribs.	Stabilises scapula during movement, pulls shoulder forward, rotates shoulder.
Quadratus lumborum	Forms part of the posterior wall of the abdomen.	Rotates arm, adducts trunk, extends the lower back.
External obliques	Either side of the rectus abdominis. Forms the sides of the abdomen.	Help maintain posture and **compresses** the abdomen. Allows rotation, flexion and sideways bending of the trunk.
Rectus abdominis	Forms the anterior wall of the abdomen. Runs from the pubis to the ribs.	Flexion of the spinal column and the trunk.
Internal obliques	A pair of muscles just below the external oblique muscles. Found at the sides of the abdomen.	Along with external obliques, help maintain posture and compress the abdomen. Allow rotation, flexion and sideways bending of the trunk.
Transversus abdominis	Wraps around the trunk from the front to the back. Extends from the ribs to the pubis.	Helps compress abdomen and internal organs. Stabilises the spine and helps with breathing.

Muscles of the shoulder	Position	Action
Levator scapula	Back of neck between the cervical vertebra and the scapula.	Lifts the shoulder and rotates the scapula.
Deltoid	Lies over the shoulder (like a shoulder pad).	Draws the arm backwards, forwards, rotates and abducts the arm.
Rotator cuff:	A group of muscles in the shoulder.	Rotates and stabilises the shoulder joint.
Teres minor	Over scapula.	Rotates shoulder outwards.
Supraspinatus	From top of arm over shoulder.	Abducts shoulder.
Infraspinatus	Over scapula.	Rotates shoulder outwards.
Subscapularis	Under scapula.	Rotates shoulder.
Teres major	Over scapula.	Adducts and rotates shoulder.

Muscles of the back	Position	Action
Sacrospinalis (erector spinae)	Group of muscles that lie either side of the spinal column.	Rotates the body, extends the spine. Maintains posture of the trunk.
Latissimus dorsi	Crossed back from lumbar region to the shoulder blade.	Draws arm backwards, adducts the upper arm. Rotates the upper arm.
Quadratus lumborum	Forms part of the posterior abdominal wall.	Helps extend and stabilise the lower back. Allows straightening of the spine (ie standing straight). Lateral flexion.

Protracts

Pull forward.

Compress

To squeeze or press.

INDUSTRY TIP

The rotator cuff contains four muscles (teres minor, supraspinatus, infraspinatus and subscapularis) that work together to stabilise the shoulder joint and the muscles involved in a frozen shoulder.

Muscles of the hip, leg and foot

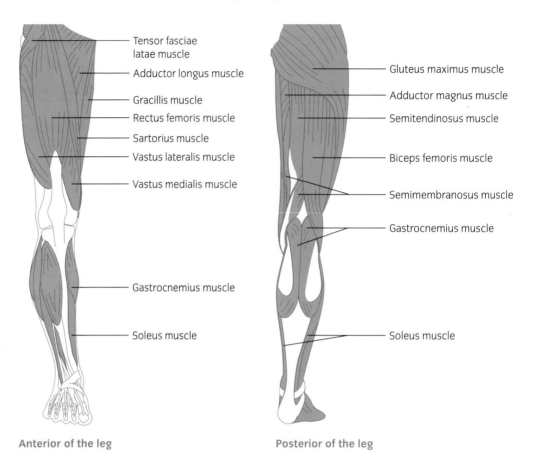

Anterior of the leg

Posterior of the leg

Anterior muscles of the leg and hip	Position	Action
Iliopsoas	Two muscles that cross from the lumbar and sacral vertebra to the femur.	Flex the hip and lumbar part of the spine, rotate the hip.
Piriformis	Across bottom under gluteals from sacrum to femur.	Rotates and abducts hip.
Tensor fasciae latae	Lateral side of the outer thigh. Runs from the ilium down into a tendon that attaches to the tibia.	Abducts the hip. Rotates the lower leg.
Sartorius	Runs diagonally across the front of the thigh from the hip to the inner knee.	Abducts thigh and hip, flexes hip and knee and external rotation of the thigh.
Hip adductors: Adductor longus Adductor brevis Adductor magnus Pectineus	Upper inner thigh.	Adducts hip and rotates thigh. Adductor magnus extends hip.

Anterior muscles of the leg and hip	Position	Action
Gracilis	Runs down the inner thigh from the pelvis to the top of the tibia.	Adducts leg and flexes knee joints.
Quadriceps: Vastus lateralis Vastus intermedius Vastus medialis Rectus femoris	Front of the thigh.	Extends the knee. Rectus femoris flexes the hip.

Posterior muscles of the leg and hip	Position	Action
Gluteals: maximus, medius	Form the buttocks.	Extend, rotate and adduct hip joints.
Hamstrings: Biceps femoris Semimembranosus Semitendinosus	Back of the thigh.	Extend thigh and hip and flex the knee.
Gastrocnemius	Forms the bulk of the calf at the back of the lower leg.	Plantar flexion of the ankle. Flexes the leg at the knee joint.
Soleus	Lies under the gastrocnemius.	Plantar flexion of the foot.

Muscles of the lower leg	Position	Action
Flexors of the toes: Flexor digitorium brevis Flexor digitorium longus Flexor hallucis brevis	The lower leg to the heel of the foot.	Flex the toes.
Extensors of the toes: Extensor digitorium brevis Extensor digitorum longus Entensor hallucis longus	The lower leg and the foot.	Extend the toes and plantar flexes the ankle.

Muscles of the lower leg	Position	Action
Tibialis anterior	Runs along the outside of the lower leg (tibia).	Inverts the foot, dorsi flexes the foot.
Tibialis posterior	Lateral side of the lower leg (tibia).	Plantar flexes the foot and lifts the medial side of the foot up (inversion).
Peroneus longus	One of three peroneal muscles in the lateral side of the lower leg.	Plantar flexes foot and lifts the lateral side of the foot.

Disorders of the muscular system

Disorder	Description and cause	Contra-indications and general precautions	Advice for client
Tendonitis	Pain and stiffness in the tendon of a muscle caused by inflammation as a result of injury.	Contra-indication. Avoid area in the early stages of healing.	Seek professional advice from a medical practitioner or an alternative practitioner, such as an osteopath.
Lower back pain	Pain in the lumbar region of the spine, usually due to the natural curve in the lower back, which takes a lot of muscle strain.	Treat with caution. Massage is often beneficial. Use extra cushions, bolsters to make sure client is comfortable.	Seek professional advice from a medical practitioner or an alternative practitioner, such as an osteopath, if the cause is unknown.
Repetitive strain injury (RSI)	Soft tissue injury (eg tennis/golfer's elbow, tendonitis, carpal tunnel syndrome) caused by over-use. Symptoms include pain, tenderness and weakness in the joint.	Not a contra-indication. Treat with caution. Massage is very beneficial.	Rest the affected area. Seek professional advice from a medical practitioner or an alternative practitioner, such as an osteopath.
Sprain	Over-stretching, twisting of a ligament during activity, falling awkwardly.	Avoid treatment while the area is inflamed or tender.	Avoid treatment to area. Seek medical advice if appropriate.
Cramp	Painful involuntary muscle contraction (spasm) commonly caused by muscle strain, fatigue. It is common during pregnancy and can also be linked with some medication for reducing cholesterol.	Not a contra-indication. Massage and stretch out the muscle with cramp.	It is not uncommon for the muscle to ache for some hours after the cramp has subsided. If cramp is a persistent problem, advise client to speak to GP.

Cardiovascular system

The cardiovascular system includes the heart, blood vessels and blood cells. The blood is the transport system of the body making sure that the body is provided with the essential **nutrients** it needs to function. The blood cells play a crucial role in fighting infection and providing immunity.

Nutrients

Substances that help us live and grow.

In this part of the chapter you will learn about:

- the structure and functions of the cardiovascular system, including:
  - blood vessels
  - heart structure and physiology
- the functions and composition of the blood
- the primary blood vessels of the body
- disorders of the cardiovascular system.

Blood vessels

The blood vessels are our transport system and are responsible for transporting blood around the body. They carry blood from the heart to the tissues and back to the heart again. There are three main types:

- arteries
- veins
- capillaries.

Arteries

Arteries are blood vessels that carry oxygenated blood away from the heart (with the exception of the pulmonary artery). The oxygen the blood is transporting is what gives it a bright red colour. Arteries are designed to withstand the high pressure exerted from the blood as it is pumped from the heart. Arteries vary in size but all have thick walls consisting of three layers of tissue. The middle layer is a thick layer of muscle. Arterioles are smaller blood vessels that branch out from an artery that lead to capillaries.

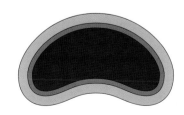

Artery

Veins

Veins are the blood vessels that transport blood to the heart and carry deoxygenated blood (with the exception of the pulmonary vein). The blood is a dark purplish red as it is no longer carrying oxygen. The walls of the veins are much thinner than those of arteries and they have less muscle and elastic tissue. Muscular movement and breathing help to

Vein

move blood along the veins in the body. The blood within the veins is not under pressure unlike the blood flow in the arteries. Most veins contain special valves which prevent blood from flowing back along the vein. The smallest veins are called venules.

Capillaries

Capillaries are the smallest blood vessels. They link the arteries (carrying blood away from the heart) back to the veins (to return blood back to the heart). Capillary walls are only a single cell layer thick, and are semi-permeable. Substances such as oxygen, vitamins, minerals, water and amino acids are able to move easily from the capillaries into the surrounding tissues to nourish and feed the cells. Substances such as carbon dioxide, cellular waste and water pass back into the capillaries to be removed. This simple process is known as capillary exchange. Due to their size, blood cells and large substances, such as plasma proteins, remain in the capillaries and cannot move out into the surrounding tissue unless the blood vessel is damaged.

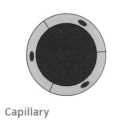

Capillary

Physiology of the heart

The heart is a powerful pear-shaped muscular organ that sits in the centre of the chest, tilted at its base slightly to the left side. It sits behind the sternum between the lungs. The heart wall is made up of three distinct layers of specialised tissue:

- The first layer is called the pericardium and is fibrous in structure.
- The second layer is a double layer (parietal and visceral pericardium) with special serous fluid between the layers to prevent any friction between the heart and the surrounding tissues.
- The lower layer is attached to the heart muscle.

The next layer is called the myocardium; this is the thickest layer and makes up the bulk of the heart walls. It is made up of specialised cardiac muscle. It has special conducting fibres embedded in the structure. These are responsible for keeping the heartbeat and contraction of the heart muscle regular. The final smooth layer is the endocardium and lines the chambers and valves of the heart. The four chambers of the heart vary in size according to the work being done. The atrium walls are very thin, as they only have to push blood into the ventricles. The ventricles are very thick as they have to push blood around the body.

> **HANDY HINT**
>
> When the left ventricle contracts, blood is pushed into the aorta. The pressure produced is known as the systolic blood pressure (systole = squeeze). This is around 120mmHg. When complete the heart rests; the pressure within the arteries is termed diastolic blood pressure (diastole = dilate). In an adult this is about 80mmHg.
>
> Blood pressure is written as systolic over diastolic, eg 120/80 (which is an example of a normal blood pressure).
>
> If the top reading goes above 140, it is classed as high blood pressure, and low blood pressure is if it goes below 90.

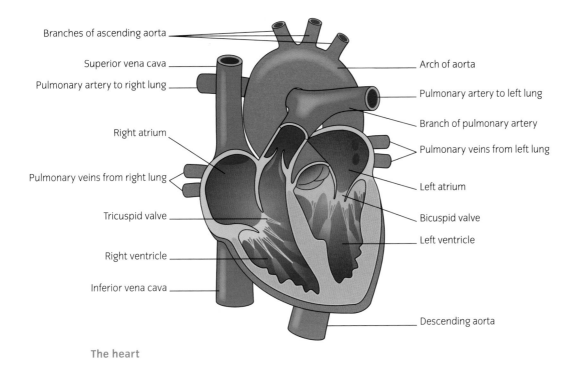

The heart

Blood vessels of the heart

The most important blood vessels in the **circulatory system** are:

- the vena cava, which carries blood from the body into the right atrium

- the pulmonary vein, which carries blood from the lungs into the left atrium

- the aorta, which carries blood from the left ventricle to the tissues on the left side of the body

- the pulmonary artery, which carries blood from the right ventricle to the lungs.

Circulatory system

The system that supplies blood to the heart muscles.

Functions of blood

Our blood can be described as our life force, making sure our cells have all the essential supplies they need and keeping **micro-organisms** at bay. The blood has several essential functions which are important for the body to survive. These functions can be divided into two main areas:

- transportation
- protection.

Micro-organism

A very small living thing that can only be seen through a microscope.

Transportation

Erythrocytes transport oxygen attached to **haemoglobin** from the lungs to the body's cells and return carbon dioxide from the cells to the lungs for **elimination**. Hormones and enzymes are transported from their cells of production to their target organs and tissues.

Haemoglobin

A protein that gives red blood cells their colour. Their main function is to transport oxygen from the lungs to the body's tissues.

Elimination

Getting rid of something.

Excretion

The process of getting rid of waste.

Invasion

Entering uninvited.

Phagocytic

Describing the process in which a **phagocyte** absorbs bacteria.

Phagocyte

A type of cell within the body capable of absorbing bacteria.

Antibody

Proteins produced in response to an antigen to neutralise it. (An antigen is a foreign body or toxin which stimulates an immune response in the body.)

Antitoxin

A protein produced in response to a toxin to neutralise it.

Conduction

The passing of heat or electricity from one object to another.

Convection

The movement of heat through a liquid or gas.

Superficial

On the surface; not deep penetrating.

Concentration

The amount of something within a liquid.

Homeostasis

The control of internal conditions. The body needs to maintain a constant state of internal balance. If one or more of the systems of the body gets out of balance, ill health and disease can occur.

The blood supplies nourishment to the cells. Nutrients are absorbed from the small intestine into the bloodstream and are transported to where they are needed.

The circulation removes waste products from the cells and surrounding tissues. These waste materials are transported to the liver to be prepared for removal and to the kidneys for **excretion**.

Protection

White blood cells defend the body against the **invasion** of micro-organisms and their toxins. They achieve this through:

- the **phagocytic** action of the white blood cells (called neutrophils and monocytes)
- the presence of **antibodies** and **antitoxins**.

Blood clotting prevents the loss of any body fluid and blood cells when the tissues are injured.

The blood helps to maintain the body's temperature. Chemical activity in the cells and tissues produces heat. This heat makes the blood warm as it circulates. If the body produces too much heat the blood vessels near the surface of the body dilate and heat is lost by radiation, **conduction**, **convection** and the evaporation of sweat. If the external temperature is cold, the **superficial** blood vessels constrict to prevent heat loss.

Composition and function of blood

Blood accounts for 7–9% of our total body weight and we have approximately 5.6 litres of this red viscous liquid flowing around our bodies. Around 55% of blood is plasma and the other 45% is made up from the different blood cells. The volume and **concentration** of our blood must be kept within narrow limits to maintain **homeostasis**.

Red blood cells (erythrocytes)

Red blood cells account for 45% of all the blood cells. They contain the molecule haemoglobin, which combines with oxygen to allow it to be transported around the body. Red blood cells are manufactured in the bone marrow of the short bones (ribs) and the ends of the long bones.

White blood cells (leukocytes)

White blood cells, also called leukocytes or white corpuscles, account for 1% of the blood. They vary in size, shape and function.

Granulocytes are the most numerous type of white blood cells. They are formed in the bone marrow. There are three different types of granulocyte. Each type has a specific function in response to injury and inflammation:

■ Eosinophils protect the body from foreign pathogens.

■ Basophils contain an **anticoagulant** (heparin) and histamine and are important in allergic reactions.

■ Neutrophils are attracted to the site being invaded by micro-organisms and ingest foreign particles and damaged tissue through the process of **phagocytosis**.

Agranulocytes account for 25–50% of all leukocytes. There are two types of agranulocytes:

■ Monocytes are formed in the red bone marrow. There are two different types of monocytes:

■ a phagocytic monocyte that engulfs and ingests pathogens and unwanted debris in the body (eg dead cells, dirt, germs)

■ a macrophage also ingests pathogens but also which has an important function in inflammation and immunity.

■ Lymphocytes circulate within the blood and are also found in lymphoid tissue. Unlike other blood cells they are also developed in the lymphoid tissue as well in the red bone marrow. Larger lymphocytes play an essential role in immunity and help the body to recover. Lymphocytes respond to specific antigens and produce antibodies. Antigens and antibodies work together. There are two different types of lymphocytes:

■ T-lymphocytes combat and destroy cells containing antigens

■ B-lymphocytes are involved in the production of the antibodies that neutralise antigens.

Plasma

Plasma is a transparent pale yellow fluid. If you remove all the blood cells from the blood, this is what is left. Plasma is made up of many important elements including:

■ water

■ blood proteins

■ salts and minerals (eg sodium chloride)

■ food substances (eg amino acids, glucose, fats)

■ waste (eg urea, uric acid)

■ gases (eg oxygen, carbon dioxide, nitrogen)

■ enzymes

■ antibodies

■ hormones

■ antitoxins.

Anticoagulant

A substance that prevents blood clotting.

Phagocytosis

Phagocytes absorb bacteria and digest them to help the body to dispose of unwanted matter such as dirt and dead body cells.

Activity

Discuss with your tutor or manager what effect you think poor circulation will have on a client and how this may be noticed during our treatment. Which treatments do you think will be beneficial and why?

Thrombocytes (platelets)

These are small fragments in the blood which play an essential role in blood clotting. When a blood vessel is damaged the blood vessels constrict and thrombocytes stick to the damaged wall. They form a thread-like mesh to prevent any further blood escaping.

HANDY HINT

If you feel the inside of your wrist and press gently with two fingers, you will feel the pulse of the radial artery.

Major blood vessels of the body

You need to be able to identify the location of the primary blood vessels as seen in the following illustration.

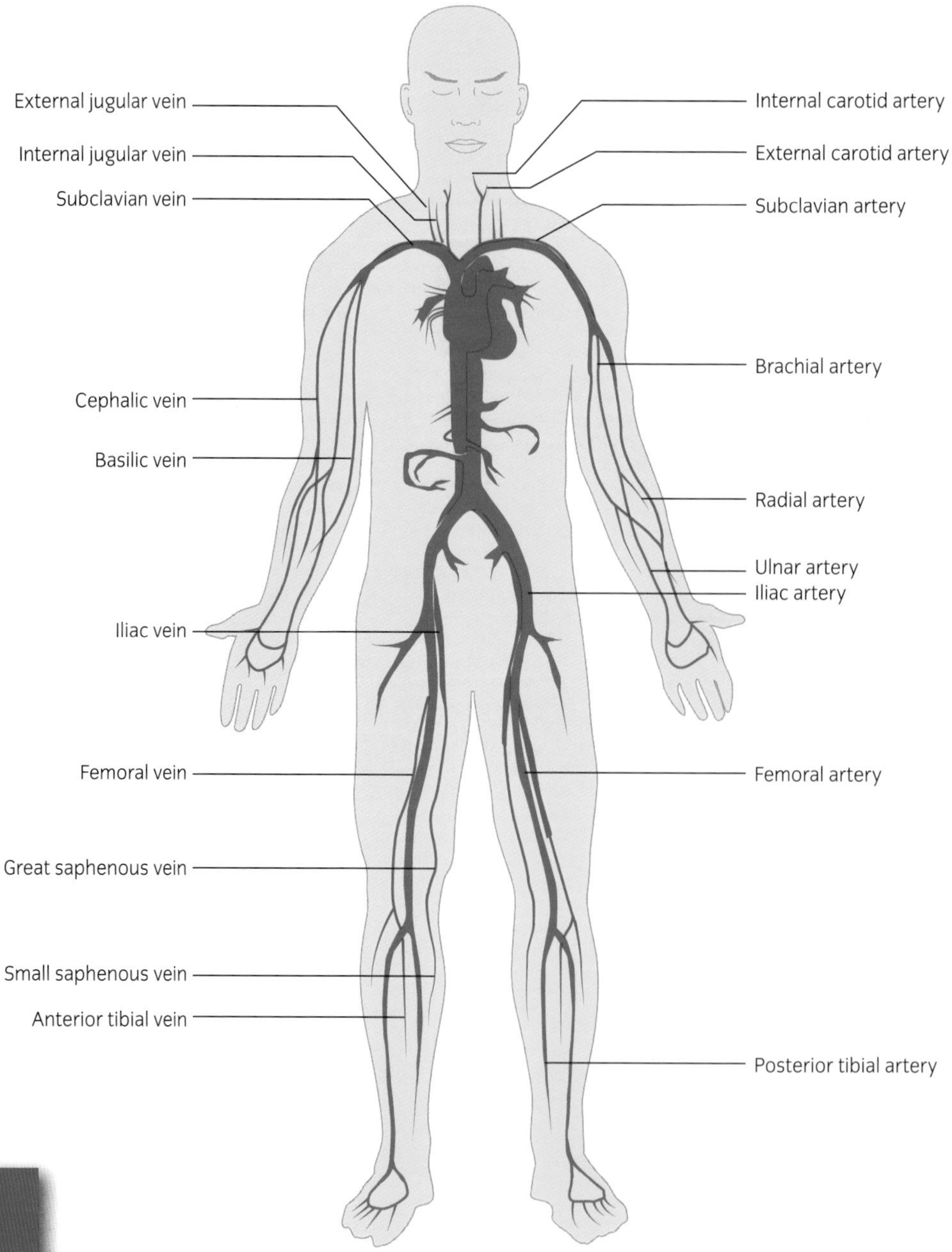

Activity

Using the diagram, make a list of the blood vessels that the blood would have to travel along from the heart and back for each of the following:

- the head
- the hand.

External jugular vein
Internal jugular vein
Subclavian vein
Cephalic vein
Basilic vein
Iliac vein
Femoral vein
Great saphenous vein
Small saphenous vein
Anterior tibial vein

Internal carotid artery
External carotid artery
Subclavian artery
Brachial artery
Radial artery
Ulnar artery
Iliac artery
Femoral artery
Posterior tibial artery

WHY DON'T YOU...
Find the pulse in your wrist or neck. Compare your pulse with those of other colleagues and discuss your findings.

Blood vessels of the head, face and neck

The following blood vessels supply and remove blood from the tissues in the head, face and neck.

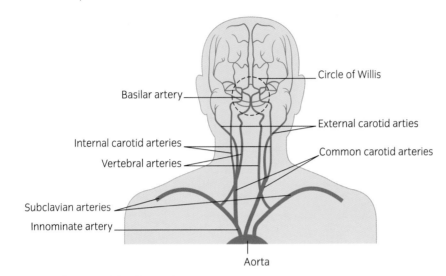

Position of primary blood vessels

HANDY HINT

If you feel the inside of your neck and press gently along the line of the sternocleidomastoid muscle with two fingers, you will feel the pulse of the carotid artery.

Blood pressure

Blood pressure is the force or pressure the blood exerts on the walls of the blood vessels in which it is contained. Normal blood pressure is dependent on several factors:

- the function of the heart
- the blood volume
- the elasticity of the artery walls
- the **venous return**.

Simple changes can make the blood pressure go up or down. Blood pressure will drop:

- if there is a loss in the volume of blood (eg from severe dehydration or blood loss)
- if you go into **shock**
- during deep relaxation.

It will increase:

- if there is fluid retention
- if there is excessive heat
- as a result of increased physical activity/exercise
- during vigorous massage.

Venous return

The blood flow back to the heart via the veins.

Shock

A condition that occurs when the body isn't getting enough blood flow.

Thrombosis

Clotting of the blood in the circulatory system.

Embolism

Blockage of an artery by a fragment of material travelling in the blood. This could be a thrombus (blood clot), air bubble or other fragment, such as bone.

Haemorrhage

An escape of blood from a ruptured blood vessel.

Arteriosclerosis

Thickening and hardening of the walls of the arteries in old age.

Disorders and diseases of the cardiovascular system

VALUES & BEHAVIOURS

If you suspect someone has had a stroke, think FAST:

- **F**ace – Is it dropped on one side? Can they smile or stick their tongue out straight?
- **A**rms – Can they raise their arms above their head?
- **S**peech – Can they speak clearly without slurring?
- **T**rouble – If they have trouble with any of these tasks, call 999.

INDUSTRY TIP

Erythema is increased circulation in the tiny capillaries near the skin's surface. It appears as a reddening of the skin. In combination with irritation and tingling, it can be a sign of an adverse reaction. If it appears before treatment, it might be sunburn. It can also be caused by massage or trauma following waxing or eyebrow shaping. If it is severe, it is a good idea to suggest the client rebooks the treatment for another time.

Disorder	Description and cause	Contra-indications and general precautions	Advice for client
Phlebitis	Inflammation of a vein. It can be seen as an area of inflamed, tender skin over a vein. Usually occurs in the lower legs. It can be caused by a blood clot (thrombophlebitis) or due to hormonal changes such as following pregnancy when the veins become more relaxed.	Contra-indication to treatment in the area.	Consult a medical practitioner. Rest the leg and keep it raised.
Low blood pressure (hypotension)	If blood pressure is too low, the vital organs will be unable to function properly. Can be caused by relaxation, heat, eating. Postural hypotension can be caused by getting up too quickly. There is a sudden drop in blood pressure as the body adjusts.	Not a contra-indication.	The client should take their time getting up or sitting up.

Disorder	Description and cause	Contra-indications and general precautions	Advice for client
High blood pressure (hypertension)	Blood is pushing against the walls of the arteries too strongly. There is an increased risk of damage to the blood vessels and a risk of internal bleeding. Often caused by a hardening of the artery walls due to ageing. Other causes include being overweight, a lack of exercise, eating too much salt and stress.	Contra-indication. There is a slightly higher risk of the client bruising more easily when they have high blood pressure. Make sure that their high blood pressure is being stabilised with medication before carrying out any treatments.	Seek medical advice if necessary.
Bruising	Damage to the blood vessels, allowing the blood to flow freely into the surrounding tissues. The skin tissue appears blue, black or yellow coloured. Caused by a sharp blow or by too much pressure being exerted on the body. Some medical conditions cause people to bruise more easily.	Contra-indication. Modify treatment. Avoid bruised area to allow the body to repair and to prevent any further blood vessel damage.	None.
Varicose veins	If one of the valves in the legs stops functioning properly, the blood will collect in the vein and become swollen. During muscle movement the blood seeps into the surrounding tissues.	Contra-indication. Avoid areas where there are visible varicose veins. Do not apply pressure to the area.	If client is concerned, seek medical advice before treatment. Raise the legs to help the blood flow return.

Disorder	Description and cause	Contra-indications and general precautions	Advice for client
Deep vein thrombosis	A blood clot that partially or fully blocks a blood vessel. Caused by changes in blood chemistry and long periods of inactivity.	Contra-indication. If the client is not on medication and the thrombosis occurred over a year ago, treatment may be given with caution.	Seek medical advice.
Stroke	Damage to the brain caused by the blood supply to the brain being disrupted by a **thrombosis**, **embolism** or **haemorrhage**. May cause some damage to certain body functions and weakness or paralysis on one side of the body depending on where the damage or reduced supply has occurred.	Contra-indication until medical advice has been given.	Seek medical advice before treatment.
Angina	Heaviness and pain in the chest. Caused by insufficient blood supply to the heart due to heart disease or **arteriosclerosis**.	Contra-indication until medical advice has been given.	Seek medical advice before treatment.

Lymphatic system

The lymphatic system is a network of lymphatic vessels and lymphatic organs that stretches throughout the entire body. It provides transportation of nutrients to the tissues and drains excess fluid from the spaces between cells. The lymphatic system is one-way; it returns fluid to the bloodstream but cannot collect lymph from the bloodstream.

In this section you will learn about:

- the functions and structure of the lymphatic system
- the structure and functions of the lymphatic organs
- the location of lymphatic nodes and ducts
- principles of immunity
- disorders related to the lymphatic system.

Functions of the lymphatic system

The main function of the lymph nodes is to filter lymph and prevent infection. The lymphatic system has a crucial role in immunity, producing T- and B-lymphocytes and antibodies in the lymph nodes.

The system also helps to remove fluids from tissue in the body and remove fat into the bloodstream. Special lymphatic capillaries, called lacteals, collect microscopic molecules of fat from the small intestine. The fat then travels through the lymphatic system and is slowly emptied into the bloodstream.

Structure of the lymphatic system

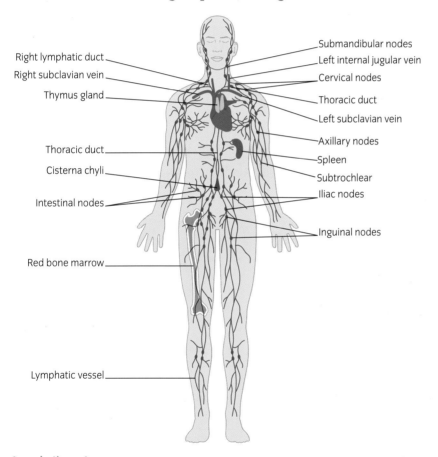

Right lymphatic duct
Right subclavian vein
Thymus gland

Thoracic duct
Cisterna chyli
Intestinal nodes

Red bone marrow

Lymphatic vessel

Submandibular nodes
Left internal jugular vein
Cervical nodes
Thoracic duct
Left subclavian vein
Axillary nodes
Spleen
Subtrochlear
Iliac nodes

Inguinal nodes

Lymphatic system

Lymph is a pale milky-coloured fluid that is made up of approximately 95% water and 5% lymphocyte cells. Lymph is also known as tissue fluid and it bathes the tissues of the body. It is formed from plasma seeping out of our blood capillaries. Lymph also contains additional substances that are too large to pass through blood capillary walls (eg debris from areas of infection and cells damaged by disease).

Lymph is a means of transferring nutrients such as food, oxygen and water and a means of collecting waste, such as urea and carbon

Activity

What signs are you likely to see if a client has a problem with their lymphatic system? Discuss your answer with your tutor or manager. What benefits will certain beauty treatments have for the lymphatic system?

dioxide. It creates the essential environment that cells need to survive. Most lymph returns to the bloodstream via the capillary walls, but the rest becomes lymph and enters the lymphatic system. Lymph moves very slowly as a result of contraction of the skeletal muscles and movement of the thorax during breathing.

Lymphatic capillaries

Lymphatic capillaries are located throughout the body. Each starts as a tube with a dead end **projecting** into the tissues. Their structure is similar to that of blood capillaries, in that they are composed of a single layer of cells. Their walls are more **permeable** and allow larger particles, such as cell debris and proteins, to be absorbed. They differ from blood capillaries in that a blood capillary has a venous end (an end connected to a vein) and an arterial end (an end connected to an artery), whereas a lymph capillary does not.

Lymphatic vessels

These vessels have thin collapsible walls and are similar to veins in structure. The lymphatic system, unlike the circulatory system, does not rely on the heart to pump the fluid along. Lymph is pushed towards the heart by the contraction of nearby muscles. Lymph vessels have many valves that prevent the backflow of lymph and make sure that the lymph moves in the right direction.

Lymphatic ducts

The lymphatic vessels gradually get larger and eventually form two large ducts called:

- the thoracic duct
- the right lymphatic duct.

The thoracic duct drains lymph from both legs, the pelvic and abdominal cavities, the left half of the head, the neck, the thorax and the left arm. The right lymphatic duct drains lymph from the right half of the head, the neck, the right arm and thorax.

Lymph is then returned to the bloodstream via the **subclavian veins**.

Lymph nodes

Lymph nodes are often referred to as lymph glands, even though strictly speaking glands usually secrete substances and lymph glands do not. Lymph nodes vary in size with some as small as a pinhead and larger nodes the size of an almond. These nodes are situated in specific locations throughout the body. Some are nearer to the surface and are called superficial; others are positioned deep in the tissues.

Projecting

Extending or reaching into.

Permeable

Porous, leaky.

Subclavian veins

A pair of veins, one on each side of the body, that return blood from the arms to the heart.

Lymph nodes are made up of reticular and lymphoid tissue that is enclosed inside a tough fibrous capsule. Each node contains a network of fibres and white blood cells called lymphocytes. Lymphocytes produce antibodies that destroy micro-organisms and fight infection. These cells work to filter and clean the lymph fluid before it is returned to the venous bloodstream.

INDUSTRY TIP

Efferent lymph vessels carry lymph *out of* the lymph nodes and afferent lymph vessels carry lymph *into* the lymph nodes.

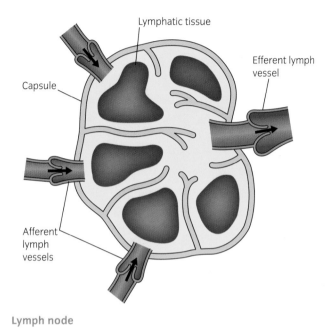

Lymph node

Lymphatic organs

Thymus

The thymus is a gland that is located beneath the upper part of the sternum close to the heart. It is very large in young children and keeps growing until puberty. The thymus gland produces T-cells which fight infection. By adulthood the thymus is much smaller. Its exact function in adulthood is not clear.

Spleen

This is the largest of the lymph organs. It can be found below the diaphragm between the stomach and the duodenum. It contains lymph nodes that produce lymphocytes and macrophages, which are phagocytic and fight infections. Blood passes through the spleen via a network of dilated blood vessels and is then taken to the liver.

The spleen's main functions are to:

■ break down and remove old red blood cells (erythrocytes) – the waste products, bilirubin and iron, are passed on to the liver

■ filter and remove white blood cells (lymphocytes), platelets and tissue debris

- store mature lymphocytes which are released when needed to fight infection

- store blood, which can be returned to the circulatory system at times of need.

Tonsils

The tonsils are masses of lymphoid tissue. There are two tonsils at the back of the roof of the mouth and a small pair of tonsils at the base of the tongue. They help to protect the throat and airways from infection. Together with the adenoids they produce antibodies against **ingested** or inhaled organisms attempting to enter the body through the nose or mouth.

Peyer's patches

These are patches of lymphoid tissue located in the small intestine. They react to pathogens which have been ingested.

Ingested

Taken into the digestive system through the nose or mouth.

The major lymph nodes of the body

There are many lymph nodes located throughout the body. The main lymph nodes are in the neck, armpit, breast, abdomen, groin, pelvis and behind the knee.

Major lymph nodes of the head, face and neck

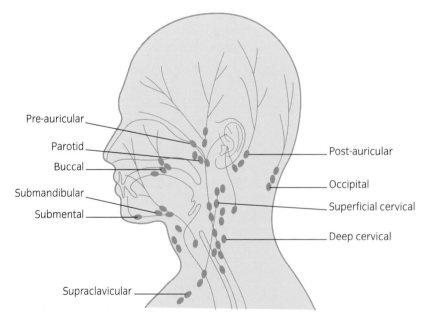

Pre-auricular

Parotid

Buccal

Submandibular

Submental

Post-auricular

Occipital

Superficial cervical

Deep cervical

Supraclavicular

Lymph nodes of the head, face and neck

Lymphatic node	Position	Function
Buccal nodes	In the cheek area next to the buccinators.	Drain the cheeks.
Mandibular and submandibular nodes	Underneath the mandible.	Drain inner eye, nose, cheek and upper lip.
Post-auricular nodes (mastoid)	Behind the ear.	Drain the scalp.
Occipital nodes	At the base of the skull.	Drain back of scalp and neck.
Anterior/auricular nodes (parotid)	In front of the ears above the jaw.	Drain scalp, upper face, eyelids, nose and cheeks.
Superficial cervical nodes	At the side of the neck.	Drain the scalp, occipital nodes and mastoid nodes.
Deep cervical nodes	Deep within the neck. Form a chain along the neck.	All lymph from the head passes directly or indirectly through these nodes. Drains the superficial nodes, tonsils and tongue.

Other major lymph nodes

Lymphatic node	Position	Function
Cervical nodes	Deep within the neck.	Drain the head, tongue and mouth.
Axillary nodes	Under the arms.	Drain the upper limbs and breasts.
Mesenteric nodes	In the walls of the intestines.	Drain the colon and upper part of the rectum.
Iliac nodes	In the lateral parts of the pelvis.	Drain the leg and buttocks.
Inguinal nodes	In the groin.	Drain the lymph from the limbs and abdominal walls.
Supratrochlear nodes	At the elbow joint.	Drain the lymph from the lower arm.
Popliteal nodes	Behind the knee.	Drain the lower limbs.

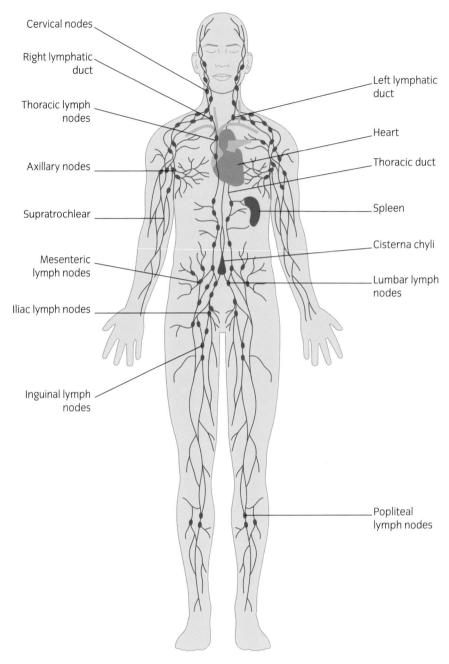

Cervical nodes

Right lymphatic duct

Thoracic lymph nodes

Axillary nodes

Supratrochlear

Mesenteric lymph nodes

Iliac lymph nodes

Inguinal lymph nodes

Left lymphatic duct

Heart

Thoracic duct

Spleen

Cisterna chyli

Lumbar lymph nodes

Popliteal lymph nodes

Major lymph nodes of the body

Immunity

One of the main functions of the lymphatic system is to create cells to help remove and destroy waste, toxins and debris. Immunity involves the interaction of antigens and antibodies.

Antigens

An antigen is a specialised protein that stimulates an immune response. Bacteria and viruses give off antigens which are recognised by the immune system as being harmful. The immune system then stimulates the production of antibodies.

Antibodies

Antibodies (immunoglobulins) are specialised **glycoproteins** that are secreted by white blood cells (lymphocytes) in the lymph nodes. They bind to receptors that protrude from the surface of the antigens and neutralise them.

Glycoprotein

Protein molecule that contains a carbohydrate.

Types of immunity

There are two types of immunity:

- Innate immunity – this type of immunity is present in humans at birth before they are exposed to pathogens or antigens.

- Adaptive immunity – this type of immunity develops when we have had contact with a pathogen. The body develops a defensive response and an army of immune cells attack the antigens given off by the pathogen. Our immune system remembers the pathogen for future responses.

Immunity to a specific pathogen can also be developed through immunisation. When we are immunised against a disease, the pathogen is deliberately introduced into the body. This causes an immune response in the body and antibodies are produced as a result of being immunised. For example, if you have the MMR immunisation, a very small amount of weakened versions of measles, mumps and rubella viruses are introduced into the body and the body fights the viruses. This should mean that you are protected against measles, mumps and rubella in the future.

INDUSTRY TIP

Remember the difference between the movement of blood (faster moving) and lymph (slower moving) as it might affect the technique you are using during your treatments. You might also be trying to target either the lymphatic system or the cardiovascular system during the treatment. You cannot make lymph flow faster but you can assist its flow.

Disorders and diseases of the lymphatic system

Autoimmune diseases

Antibodies are not always beneficial. The body can sometimes attack and destroy healthy body tissue by mistake. Rheumatoid arthritis is an example of an autoimmune disorder.

Lymphatic disorder	Description and cause	Contra-indications and general precautions	Advice for client
Swollen glands	Inflamed, tender lymph nodes are usually an indication that the body is fighting an infection. The nodes might swell even before the effects of the infection are felt (eg glands in the neck might become tender and sore even before a sore throat is experienced).	Contra-indication. The condition causing the swollen glands might be contagious. If the body is fighting an infection it should not be treated to allow the body to heal. Pressure over swollen nodes could affect the natural filtering of pathogens, forcing them through the nodes rather than being dealt with within the node itself by the lymphoid tissue.	Rest and recover.
HIV (human immunodeficiency virus)/AIDS (acquired immunodeficiency syndrome)	The HIV virus is a retrovirus that infects the T-lymphocytes. Causes defects in immunity. Symptoms might include unexplained weight loss, fever and swollen lymph glands.	Contra-indication to epilation and intimate waxing. As the treatments you are offering don't come into direct contact with blood (with the exception of epilation and intimate waxing), you should not be at any risk, unless you or the client has any open wounds.	Seek medical advice if needed.
Oedema	An abnormal accumulation of fluid in the body tissue. Associated with the lymphatic circulation but can also be due to problems with the blood circulation, heart or kidneys.	Contra-indication if you are unsure of the cause. Avoid treatment until you are sure of the cause.	Seek medical advice before treatment.
Fever (pyrexia)	Immune response to infection. A fever slows down the pathogen's ability to reproduce inside the body by raising the body's temperature. The symptoms of a fever of a high temperature (above 39°C) are a general feeling of being unwell, headache and shivering.	Contra-indication to avoid cross-infection or making a condition worse.	Refer client for medical advice if appropriate.

Allergies

Sometimes the immune system causes reactions that make the body very sensitive to a particular allergen that would not normally be dangerous (eg pollen). When this happens, we have an allergic reaction. Reactions can be so mild that they aren't noticeable or they can be life-threatening. An extremely severe allergic reaction is called anaphylactic shock. Anaphylactic shock can be caused by insect stings and nut allergies, for instance.

The lymphatic system's role in immunity and health means that any condition that a client has could have an impact on the lymph system and should be given time to recover.

There are many contra-indications that you will come across so it is important that you have a basic understanding of some of the common conditions. Insurance companies will expect you to carry out a full consultation before starting any treatment and the client should be referred to a medical practitioner before treatment if necessary. There are many conditions that can be treated with care and the treatment modified providing the client's medical practitioner has been consulted first. There are some conditions, however, that should not be treated.

Activity

Discuss with your manager or tutor what might happen if you were to treat a client with swollen glands or undiagnosed lumps.

Nervous system

The nervous system is responsible for receiving information from outside of the body and transmitting that information between different parts of the body. It is also responsible for transmitting information around the body. The nervous system works closely with the endocrine system to help maintain communication and homeostasis in the body.

In this part of the chapter you will learn about:

- the structure and functions of the nervous system
- disorders of the nervous system.

The structure of the nervous system

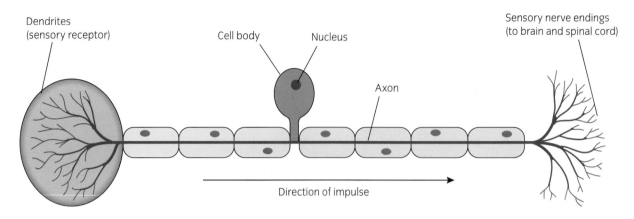

Dendrites (sensory receptor)

Cell body

Nucleus

Sensory nerve endings (to brain and spinal cord)

Axon

Direction of impulse

A nerve cell

Dendrite

Fine, branching extensions, which receive messages from other nerve cells.

Axon

A slender extension of the nerve cell which can be up to 100cm in length.

Nerve cell/neurone

A neurone is a specialised nerve cell designed to receive stimuli and transmit nerve impulses. Each neurone has a cell body, a central nucleus and special extensions called **dendrites** and **axons**.

The axon sends information one-way from the nerve cell to the axon terminal. The axon terminal is the point where the electrical charge being sent from a nerve cell is changed into a chemical signal.

Large axons are covered with a sheath of fatty material called myelin, giving them a white appearance. Myelin acts like an insulator and helps to speed up nerve impulses. There are breaks along the myelin sheath called nodes of Ranvier, and these help to transmit the nerve impulse. One type of nerve, C nerves, does not have myelin and transmits much slower impulses. Each nerve cell has only one axon, but the axon may have many branches.

There are three main types of neurones:

- Sensory or afferent neurones. These neurones are responsible for receiving stimuli from sensory organs and receptors. The impulse is then transmitted to the spinal cord and brain where the sensation is perceived. Sensations are transmitted by the different sensory neurones along different neural pathways and include heat, cold, pressure, touch, vibration, nociception, taste, smell, sight and hearing.

- Motor or efferent neurones carry impulses away from the brain and the spinal cord taking messages to muscles and glands.

- Association or connecting neurones connect sensory and motor neurones and are found in the brain and spinal cord.

HANDY HINT

Touch is transmitted along A-alpha (α) nerve fibres. The impulse travels faster than some unpleasant sensations from A-delta (δ) and C fibres, which is why rubbing something has a positive effect.

THE CITY & GUILDS TEXTBOOK

The transmission of nerve impulses

The function of a neurone is to transmit impulses. Neurones send messages throughout the body.

The nerve fibres of a neurone do not actually connect but have a junction called a synapse. Between each synapse is a minute gap called the synaptic cleft. Synapses cause nerve impulses to pass in one direction only. Nerve impulses are a change of electrical charge, which is carried down the axon fibre until it reaches the synapse. The electrical charge or action potential is generated by the rapid flow of sodium and potassium ions across the neurone cell membrane.

The impulse is relayed from one neurone to another by specialised chemicals called neurotransmitters. There are different neurotransmitters depending on the end effect. The effect can be **excitatory** or **inhibitory**. Neurotransmitters are stored in the postsynaptic membrane and are released when an **action potential** is successful in reaching the synaptic cleft. If the stimulus does not reach a certain threshold then the next nerve will not respond.

The motor point is a special kind of synapse. It occurs at the junction between a nerve and a muscle, where the nerve supply enters the muscle.

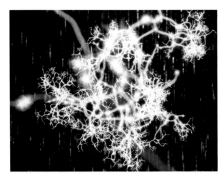

Transmission of nerve impulses

Excitatory neurone

Generates an action potential – simply, it opens the door to allow a nerve to send a positive charge.

Inhibitory neurone

Prevents an action potential – it closes the door and creates a negative charge response.

Action potential

A neurone's method of transporting electrical signals from one cell to the next.

The organisation of the nervous system

The nervous system can be divided into two parts:

■ the central nervous system (CNS)
■ the peripheral nervous system (PNS).

The central nervous system

The central nervous system, or CNS, consists of two parts:

■ the brain
■ the spinal cord.

The brain

Our brain is our consciousness and intellect. Our memories are stored here and it is the site of our ability to think, judge and reason. The human brain is a mass of complex nervous tissue lying within the protection of the skull. There are over 12 billion neurones and 50 billion supporting glial cells. The average brain weighs less than 1.4kg.

The brain is the central communication centre of the nervous system and its function is to receive all sensory information, process it, perceive and coordinate a response. This may be an instant action or a slow thought process.

The outer surface of the cerebral cortex (cerebrum) consists of grey matter and this contains the cell bodies of the nerves. Under this is the white matter of our brains containing myelin-covered axons.

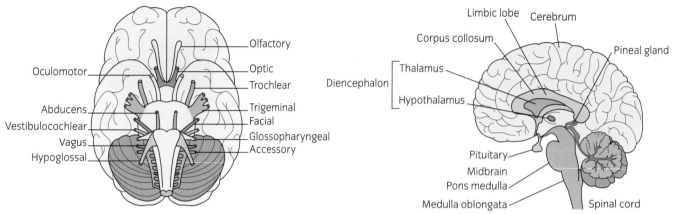

Structure of the brain

Structures in the brain

- Cerebrum – this is largest part of the brain and forms two distinct sections. The cerebrum is involved in mental activities such as those involving memory and is responsible for intelligence, sensory perception and voluntary movement.

- Cerebellum – this area of the brain is responsible for fine or precise movement, balance and posture.

- Hypothalamus – see page 237, on the endocrine system. This controls automatic body processes and is linked to the posterior lobe of the pituitary gland. It controls the hormones from both pituitary lobes to regulate the activity of other endocrine glands. The other functions of the hypothalamus include control of:
  - the autonomic nervous system
  - thirst and water balance
  - appetite and feeling of fullness
  - body temperature
  - emotions
  - biorhythms – sleeping and waking cycles.

- Thalamus – this acts like a relay station to sort, interpret and direct sensory information. It includes information about touch, pain and temperature and from the other senses.

- Brain stem – contains centres that regulate many basic survival functions (eg heartbeat, respiration, blood pressure, digestion and swallowing).

- Cerebrospinal fluid – a clear fluid which is produced and distributed all around the brain. It protects the brain from mechanical forces and infections.

- Meninges – these are a special tough membrane that cover and protect the brain and spinal cord.

INDUSTRY TIP

The blood supply to the brain is extremely important. The brain makes up only 2% of the body's weight but has 20% of the body's blood circulating through it.

The spinal cord

The spinal cord is an extension of the brain stem and extends from the base of the skull down to the lumbar vertebrae. The nerve cell bodies are grouped in the centre of the cord. Surrounding this are the axons running up and down the cord. Spinal nerves leave the cord to supply the body.

The spinal cord:

- relays impulses to and from the brain from both internal and external stimuli
- provides the communication link between the brain and the organs of the body
- is the centre for reflex actions.

Our reflex actions provide us with a very quick automatic response to external or internal stimuli, without involving the brain. They enable our body to respond extremely quickly without the need to think a process through, such as moving a hand away from a hot surface.

The peripheral nervous system

The peripheral nervous system is composed of the parts of the nervous system outside the brain and the spinal cord. It consists of:

- 31 pairs of spinal nerves
- 12 pairs of cranial nerves
- the autonomic nervous system.

The cranial nerves

There are 12 pairs of cranial nerves which connect directly to the brain and between them they provide a nerve supply to sensory organs, muscles and skin of the head and the neck.

The main facial nerves that you need to be aware of include the following:

- trigeminal nerves, which are the chief sensory nerves for the face and head and include the ophthalmic, maxillary and mandibular nerves
- facial nerves, which supply the facial muscles of expression
- olfactory nerves, which give us our sense of smell.

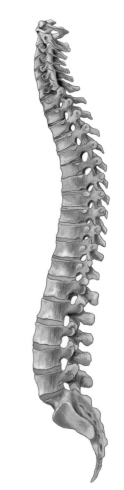

The spinal cord goes along the length of the spine

The spinal nerves

Spinal nerves receive sensory impulses from the body and transmit motor signals to specific regions of the body. Each spinal nerve passes out of the spinal cord to link with the autonomic nervous system. Each of the spinal nerves are numbered and named according to the level of the spinal column from which they pass out:

- 8 cervical
- 12 thoracic
- 5 lumbar
- 5 sacral
- 1 coccygeal.

Activity

Think of the last time you had a reflex action – write down what it was and how you responded.

Each spinal nerve divides into several branches to form a network of nerves, which serve different parts of the body.

The somatic nervous system

The somatic nervous system, or voluntary nervous system, is made up of nerve fibres that send information from the central nervous system to the muscles. It allows you to carry out voluntary actions (ie actions that you are aware of, such as picking up an object).

The autonomic nervous system

This is the part of your nervous system that makes sure that all your internal organs (including the cardiac muscle) and your glands function smoothly. This allows your body to carry out involuntary actions (eg your heart beating). The autonomic system is divided into two parts:

- the sympathetic nervous system
- the parasympathetic nervous system.

The sympathetic and parasympathetic nervous systems work together to regulate and balance the internal workings of the body but have opposite effects. For example, the sympathetic nervous system might increase your heart rate and breathing rate in a stressful situation whereas the parasympathetic nervous system will try to maintain your heart rate and breathing at a low level in a stressful situation.

Diseases and disorders of the nervous system

Disease	Description and cause	Contra-indications and general precautions	Advice for client
Epilepsy	Epilepsy can be described as uncontrolled electrical activity in the brain. This change can lead to a simple vacant expression with a lack of response or a grand mal seizure, which is when the individual becomes partially unconscious and suffers twitching and uncontrollable movements. Epilepsy often has no known cause but it can be triggered by a brain injury or a chemical imbalance. Some people with epilepsy have seizures that are caused by flashing lights, known as photosensitive epilepsy.	Not generally a contra-indication; however, it is a contra-indication to any electrical treatment. You might want to refer the client to a medical practitioner for advice. If the client's condition is controlled and they know what triggers their seizures, so that they can avoid the trigger, there is no reason why they shouldn't have safe treatments. As a therapist you need to decide whether you can cope with the possibility of an epileptic client having a seizure. This might be a frightening experience but if you are aware, prepared and take the right precautions you can treat these clients.	Suggest the client seeks medical advice before considering any treatment.
Bell's palsy	Facial paralysis caused by compression of the facial nerve. Symptoms include drooping of the facial contours and paralysis of the facial muscles on one side of the face.	Recovery usually takes a few months. Suggest the client seeks medical advice before any treatment is given. Avoid the use of electrical treatments in the area especially if the cause is unknown.	Suggest the client seeks medical advice before treatment.
Cerebral palsy	Cerebral palsy can affect body movement, balance and posture. It is caused by brain damage or abnormal brain development. The condition makes it difficult to control and coordinate muscles. The disease does not affect mental ability but can affect communication.	Contra-indication.	Suggest the client seeks medical advice before treatment.

Disease	Description and cause	Contra-indications and general precautions	Advice for client
Multiple sclerosis (MS)	A **neurological** condition that can affect memory and thinking. It can also have an impact on emotions. Symptoms include problems with vision, balance, muscle stiffness and spasms. The immune system attacks the substance that protects the nerve fibres. This damage causes scars or lesions on the nerve fibres.	Treatment might be possible in the early stages.	Suggest the client seeks medical advice before treatment.
Migraine	A migraine is a severe headache with other symptoms; these include feeling sick, vomiting and increased sensitivity particularly to sound and light. They are caused by changes to chemicals and circulation in the brain. Can be triggered by hormones, stress and food intolerances.	It is advisable not to treat a client while they are experiencing a migraine due to increased sensitivity.	Rebook for another time when they don't have a migraine so that they can get the maximum benefit/ enjoyment from their treatment.
Vertigo	Vertigo describes the sensation of the room moving or spinning around you. When it is severe a person will not be able to keep their balance and may be sick. It is usually a symptom of another condition such as an ear infection.	Avoid sudden movements with the client particularly involving the head.	Advise client to see GP for treatment to relieve symptoms. Rebook for another time when they don't have a vertigo so that they can get the maximum benefit/ enjoyment from their treatment.
Sciatica	Pain, numbness tingling, weakness along the path of the sciatic nerve. It can be localised to one side in the lower back or extend along the length of the nerve to the foot. It is caused by compression or irritation of the sciatic nerve.	Depends on severity of symptoms and cause. Sometimes massage can help to relieve muscular tension that is causing the sciatica.	Advise client to see GP for treatment to relieve symptoms. Suggest an alternative practitioner such as an osteopath or physiotherapist.

Neurological

Related to the nervous system.

Respiratory system

Everything we do is made possible by the air that we breathe. We need to breathe effectively to provide our body with sufficient oxygen to enable basic cellular activity. Oxygen is needed for the brain to function.

In this part of the chapter you will learn about:

- the structure and functions of the respiratory system
- disorders of the respiratory system.

HANDY HINT

During *inspiration* air is breathed *in*. During *expiration* air is breathed *out*.

INDUSTRY TIP

When you are carrying out treatments, make sure you breathe regularly and don't hold your breath. Often when we concentrate hard we hold our breath. You will suffer from fatigue if you don't breathe evenly.

The structure of the respiratory system

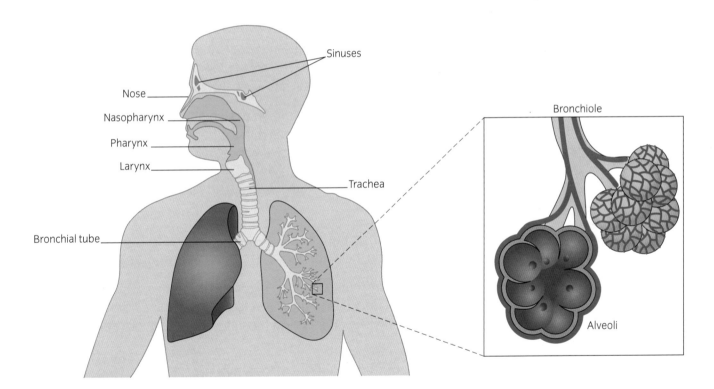

Upper respiratory system

Air is inhaled and exhaled through the nose and mouth. Tiny **cilia** line the nasal cavities and secrete mucus; this filters the air trapping dust and pathogens. As air is drawn in, it is warmed and moistened. When the demand for oxygen is high or if the nose is blocked, we breathe through our mouths.

From the nasal cavity the air is drawn into the nasopharynx, which contains the tonsils. The nasopharynx joins the oropharynx which receives air, food and liquid from the mouth and is part of the

Cilia

Microscopic, hair-like structures that move in a wave-like pattern to sweep away liquids and particles.

respiratory and digestive system. During swallowing the air is stopped. The oropharynx continues to the larynxopharynx where the larynx or vocal cords are situated. The larynxopharynx allows sound production and also moves upwards and forwards during swallowing, causing the epiglottis to block its opening.

Lower respiratory system

The trachea descends from the larynx making the connection to the lungs. The trachea is made up of dense connective tissue and smooth muscle, lined with epithelial cells that secrete mucus. They are also lined with epithelial cilia, which sweep particles upwards and away from the lungs.

The trachea divides at the carina into the left and right bronchi. The bronchi are composed of incomplete rings of cartilage and are also lined with mucous membrane. They divide progressively into smaller bronchi, which carry air from the trachea into the bronchioles.

The bronchioles filter particles and prevent them from entering into the delicate lung structures. The bronchioles carry air deep into the lungs, sub-dividing into small airs sac called alveoli.

Most of the lung tissues is made up of alveoli. These are delicate structures with walls a single cell thick. A dense capillary network surrounds each. Here gaseous exchange of oxygen and carbon dioxide occurs.

The lungs

There are two lungs: the left lung has two lobes, and the right has three. The lungs contain the alveoli and are the area where gases are exchanged.

The lungs are surrounded by the pleural membranes, which are made from elastic connective tissue. The pleural membranes protect the lungs, reducing friction between the lungs and the chest wall.

The following structures are needed to provide passageways for air to be transported to the lungs and then **exhaled**:

- nose
- nasopharynx
- pharynx
- larynx
- trachea
- bronchi.

Exhale

Breathe out.

Functions of the respiratory system

Gaseous exchange in the lungs

The main function of the respiratory system is the exchange of oxygen and carbon dioxide in the lungs. Oxygen, from the air that we breathe in, passes into the blood in the lungs. It is replaced by carbon dioxide, which has been released by the body as a waste product of cell metabolism. The carbon dioxide is then exhaled.

How respiration works

Air is breathed in through the nose and mouth and is transported into and out of the lungs by the combined action of the intercostal muscles and diaphragm.

Breathing is a passive process (ie we do it most of the time without even thinking about it). However, when we need more air our muscles can be stimulated to inhale or exhale more air. The rate at which we breathe is controlled by the respiratory centre in the brain and the levels of carbon dioxide circulating in the bloodstream.

Disorders of the respiratory system

Disorder	Description and cause	Contra-indications and general precautions	Advice for client
Influenza (flu)	Flu is caused by a virus which is spread in the air. It can be caught by direct or indirect contact with an infected client or a colleague. Symptoms include feeling very unwell, aching, headache and a high temperature. Other symptoms may include a runny or blocked nose, watery eyes, sneezing, **catarrh** and a sore throat. Symptoms can also include a stomach upset and gastric flu.	Contra-indication. Flu is a very contagious virus.	Advise client to go home and rest. Avoid contact to prevent further spread of the virus.
Sinusitis	Infection of the mucous membranes of the sinus cavities. Symptoms include headache, facial pain and congestion of the nose and sinuses.	Advise client to go home and recover.	Suggest client seeks medical advice.

Disorder	Description and cause	Contra-indications and general precautions	Advice for client
COPD (chronic obstructive pulmonary disease)	A group of diseases that all cause obstruction to the airways in the lungs. They are irreversible and cause progressive damage to the tissues in the lungs. They include **emphysema** and **chronic bronchitis**. Symptoms include coughing (with phlegm), shortness of breath and frequent chest infections	Not a contra-indication – consider how you position the client so that they are able to breathe easily, ie keep them slightly sat up. Avoid anything that may affect the breathing such as strong fragrances, sprays near the face (eg nail enamel fixers).	Advise client to see their GP if they are having problems with their symptoms.
Bronchitis	Inflammation of the bronchi. Caused by a viral or bacterial infection or can be caused by air pollution and smoking. It can also be present alongside other lung diseases. Symptoms include wheeziness, shortness of breath and a persistent, possibly painful, chesty cough.	Might be a contra-indication depending on the cause. Keep the client's head raised where possible to avoid irritation in the lungs.	Seek medical advice if symptoms are persistent.
Asthma	Attacks of breathlessness and wheeziness caused by inflammation of the bronchi. The inflammation causes the lining of the bronchi to swell which reduces the amount of air flow in and out of the lungs. Symptoms include breathlessness, wheeziness, a dry cough and a tight feeling in the chest.	Products with strong smells, dust, cold air and stress can all trigger an asthma attack. Make sure clients keep their inhalers close by.	Seek medical advice if the client has a severe attack.
Hay fever	Allergic reaction in response to hypersensitivity to pollen. Symptoms include sneezing, runny nose and itchy eyes.	Not a contra-indication but consider the treatment and severity of symptoms.	If the client's symptoms are severe, you may choose to advise the client to return when their symptoms have reduced so that they can enjoy their treatment.

Catarrh

Build-up of thick phlegm or mucus in the nose, sinuses, throat, ears or lungs.

Emphysema

A long-term, progressive disease of the lungs that causes shortness of breath.

Chronic bronchitis

An inflammation of the bronchial tubes that lasts longer than three months.

Digestive system

Most of the nutrients we eat are made up of complex substances that need to be broken down into smaller molecules that can be used more easily. The digestive system breaks down food using both physical and chemical processes. The body needs a constant supply of nutrients to continue to function, grow and repair and these are obtained from the food we eat.

In this part of the chapter you will learn about:

- the structure and functions of the digestive system
- the processes of digestion
- disorders of the digestive system

Basic dietary requirements

So that the body is provided with everything it needs to function and repair itself, we need to eat a balanced diet containing a variety of essential nutrients:

- water
- carbohydrates – including fibre (cellulose), sugar and starch
- proteins
- fats (or lipids)
- vitamins
- minerals.

Water

Water is an essential nutrient. Without it we would not survive more than a few days. Water is a major part of many foods and drinks. Water is essential in maintaining the body's fluid balance and for transporting fluids around the body.

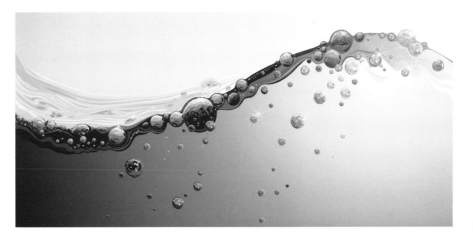

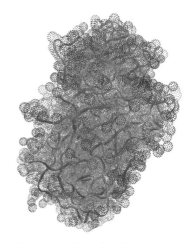

Pepsin – a protein molecule

Carbohydrates

Carbohydrates take the form of sugars and starches. These provide the body with its main source of energy. There are two types of carbohydrate:

- simple carbohydrates (or monosaccharides)
- complex carbohydrates (or polysaccharides).

Simple carbohydrates are simple sugars that are easily absorbed in the bloodstream.

Complex carbohydrates are more complex sugars (such as starch and cellulose (fibre)) that need to be broken down into simple sugars before they can be absorbed into the bloodstream. Cellulose and hemicelluloses form the main structure of plants' cell walls. Their fibrous structure gives plants their ridged form. These structures are so complex that our digestive systems cannot break them down. Fibre has the ability to absorb water as it passes through the digestive system. This increases bulk in faeces and encourages the large intestine to function more easily. A diet with good cellulose content is essential to prevent constipation and some digestive problems (eg irritable bowel).

> **HANDY HINT**
>
> Many cells, such as brain cells, need a constant supply of glucose to survive as glucose is used immediately. This is why our thinking skills and reactions become slower if we haven't eaten for a long time.

> **HANDY HINT**
>
> Unrefined foods such as wholemeal breads, cereals, grains, root vegetables and fruits can increase dietary fibre. Good sources are wholegrain flour, dried apricots and other dried fruit, peanuts, celery, peas (pulses), green beans, prunes, unrefined bran and potato skins.

> **INDUSTRY TIP**
>
> Most foods that are high in fibre are low in sugar and have little fat. Because fibre increases bulk it will reduce the space available and encourage a more satisfied feeling.

> **Activity**
>
> Eat a piece of wholegrain bread and chew until it is really liquid in your mouth. Can you now taste the sweetness of the sugars being broken down?

> **INDUSTRY TIP**
>
> A drop in sugar levels causing you to feel hungry, irritable and light-headed causes many food cravings. Sugary foods increase sugar levels rapidly but do not sustain them. Complex carbohydrates produce a slow release of sugars maintaining sugar levels, so it would be more beneficial to have a slice of wholegrain bread than a chocolate bar.

Protein

Proteins are necessary for the growth and repair of tissue. They are also used in the production of hormones and enzymes. Protein is found in fish, milk, meat and pulses.

During digestion proteins are broken down by the action of enzymes into amino acids. Protein is partly digested in the stomach. The enzyme pepsin breaks down large protein molecules into smaller ones. In the small intestine, other enzymes break the small proteins into amino acids. These are then absorbed into the bloodstream and transported to the tissues where they are rebuilt into other types of protein.

Fats (lipids)

Fats have a number of functions in our diet. They:

- transport and supply fat-soluble vitamins around the body
- improve the flavour of food
- provide energy and warmth.

There are two main types of fat:

- saturated fat (solid at room temperature – eg cheese and butter)
- unsaturated fat (liquid at room temperature – eg olive oil).

When fat is digested, it is made into an emulsion by the action of bile from the intestine. The enzyme lipase is released by the pancreas and digests the fat. The lipase breaks down the fat into **fatty acids** and glycerol, which are easily absorbed into the body.

Vitamins

Vitamins are organic substances that are needed in small amounts:

- for normal functioning of the body
- to help the body's resistance to disease.

Vitamins are divided into two types:

- Fat-soluble vitamins include vitamins A, D, E and K. These vitamins are carried in fats and are absorbed from the fat in the intestine and are stored in the liver or fatty tissue.
- Water-soluble vitamins include vitamins B and C. The body has a limited ability to store water-soluble vitamins and gets rid of any excess vitamins in the urine.

Minerals

Minerals have many functions and are vitally important in building bones and teeth. They also help to control the water balance within the cells and are also essential for the normal function of nerves and muscle tissue, hormone secretion and enzyme activity.

Fatty acids

Building blocks of fat for the body.

INDUSTRY TIP

Too much alcohol deprives the body of its vitamin reserves, including vitamins C and B, and causes dehydration.

INDUSTRY TIP

A deficiency in vitamin A can cause **hyperkeratinisation**.

A deficiency in vitamin B causes nerve damage.

A deficiency in vitamin B2 can cause cracks at the corner of the mouth.

A deficiency in vitamin C can cause premature ageing and can make wounds slow to heal. A severe deficiency in vitamin C can cause scurvy.

Hyperkeratinisation

The excessive production of keratin in the epidermis, causing an abnormal thickening of skin on the palms of the hands and soles of the feet.

The structure of the digestive system and the process of digestion

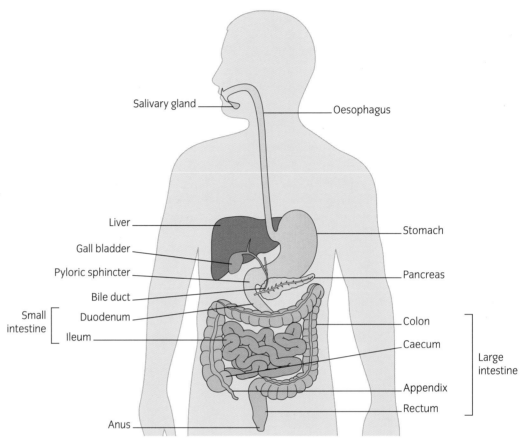

Salivary gland — Oesophagus

Liver — Stomach

Gall bladder

Pyloric sphincter — Pancreas

Bile duct

Small intestine — Duodenum — Colon

Ileum — Caecum

Large intestine

Appendix

Rectum

Anus —

The digestive system

Alimentary canal

Also known as the gastrointestinal tract.

The **alimentary canal** is a long tube which is about 9m in length. It starts at the mouth and ends at the anus. It includes:

- the mouth
- the pharynx and oesophagus
- the stomach
- the small intestine – the duodenum, jejunum and ileum
- the large intestine – the caecum, appendix, colon, rectum and anus.

The digestive system has organs that work alongside the alimentary canal and these are known as accessory organs. They include:

- the liver
- the gall bladder
- the pancreas.

The digestive process

Mouth

Digestion begins in the mouth, where food is broken into smaller pieces, chewed, and ground down by the teeth. This process involves several muscles, one of which is the tongue which moves the food around the mouth and mixes it with saliva to form a soft mass called a bolus.

The salivary glands

There are three pairs of glands that connect to the mouth and produce saliva. Saliva is a digestive fluid and is released in response to sensory nerves in the mouth and by the sight and smell of food. Saliva moistens food and makes it easier to swallow. It begins the digestive process helping to start to break down food. It also plays a key role in oral hygiene removing food particles and pathogens.

Pharynx

This is commonly known as the throat; it extends from behind the nose, mouth and larynx and is about 12–14cm long.

Oesophagus

This passes through the diaphragm down to the stomach. It is about 25cm long. Food is moved along by special intermittent muscular contraction called peristalsis.

Stomach

At the end of the oesophagus underneath the diaphragm sits the stomach. It is a J-shaped muscular bag that can extend and hold about 1.5 litres after a meal.

The main functions of the stomach are:

- to store food
- to begin protein digestion
- to control the entry of food into the duodenum. The stomach mixes food with gastric juices secreted by glands in the lining of the stomach to form chyme. It then churns this mixture of liquid and small particles.

Alcohol, water and glucose are absorbed into the blood directly from the stomach. After about four hours the partially digested food leaves the stomach and passes into the duodenum. Carbohydrates leave the stomach first, then proteins and finally fats.

Small intestine

This part of the digestive system includes:

- the duodenum
- the jejunum
- the ileum.

The small intestine extends to about 7m in length and is about 4cm in diameter. The main functions of the small intestine are to carry out digestion and absorption, absorbing some nutrients and water into the bloodstream. There are several digestive enzymes found in the small intestines and these include:

- bile
- pancreatic juice
- intestinal juice.

The inner wall of the small intestine is covered by millions of tiny projections called villi, which are essential for the absorption of fats and play a role within the lymphatic system.

Chyme (partially digested food) leaves the stomach and enters the duodenum. This is the first part of the small intestine and is a small C-shaped tube. Digestive fluids from the pancreas and bile from the gall bladder enter the duodenum. From the duodenum the digestive processes continue into the middle part of the small intestine called the jejunum. Enzymes produced here complete the process of digestion before finally moving food into the last part of the small intestine, called the ileum. The main function of the ileum is to absorb nutrients from the digested food.

Absorption of digested food

Absorption mainly takes place in the ileum. The inner surface area is greatly increased by villi. These contain a network of capillaries and lymph vessels called lacteals. The ileum's specialised structure helps to increase the surface through which nutrients from digested foods can be absorbed into blood and lymph.

The contents that are left move through into the large intestine for the final part of the digestive journey. The large intestine is wider than the small intestine. Within the large intestine are the:

- caecum
- appendix
- colon
- sigmoid colon
- rectum
- anal canal.

Gluten

The protein found in many grains including wheat, barley, rye.

The main function of the large intestines is to remove liquid from the contents to produce faeces. The caecum continues to become the ascending colon. At this point there is a junction called the ileocecal valve where the ileum feeds into the large intestine. At one end of the caecum is a fine tube that contains lymphoid tissue and is known as the appendix. Small amounts of digested food are still absorbed. The mucus produced in the large intestine helps to lubricate the movement of faeces. It also contains antibodies that help fight pathogens that may still be in the digested food. The colon also stores faeces until they are ready to be removed. Finally the faeces move into the last part of the large intestine – the rectum. This is a short space about 12.5cm long, which holds faeces. When the muscles contract, faeces are removed.

> **INDUSTRY TIP**
>
> Clients should be encouraged to drink liquids – water, fruit or herbal teas – following treatments to help aid the removal of waste from the body.

Accessory organs

The liver

The liver is the second largest organ and the largest internal gland in the body. It is located in the upper right-hand side of the abdomen sitting under the diaphragm. The liver has many essential functions within the body.

The functions of the liver are as follows:

- Regulation of carbohydrate metabolism – absorbs excess glucose and stores it as glycogen. Releases glucose if blood sugar levels falls.
- Regulation of fat metabolism – converts fats into a form that can be stored or broken down to release energy.
- Vitamin storage – several fat-soluble vitamins including A, D and B12.
- Mineral storage – iron and copper needed to make haemoglobin.
- Protein metabolism – amino acids are collected and used to make proteins. Surplus amino acids are broken down.
- Bile production – bile consists of water, mineral salts, mucus, bilirubin (a pigment which gives bile its yellow colour), bile salts and cholesterol. It is alkaline and breaks up (emulsifies) fat droplets.
- Detoxification of toxic substances – toxic substances are changed where possible into safer substances.
- Hormone breakdown – the liver removes hormones from the blood and breaks them down.
- Excretory function – breakdown of old red blood cells.
- Heat production – the activity of metabolism within the liver creates heat.
- Metabolises ethanol in alcohol.

Gall bladder

The gall bladder is a small pear-shaped muscular sac that is located underneath the liver. The gall bladder stores bile from the liver. When partly digested food enters the duodenum, the muscular sphincter at the opening of the bile duct relaxes and pumps bile into the duodenum. The functions of the gall bladder are to:

■ store bile

■ secrete mucus into the bile

■ release the stored bile through the pancreatic duct into the duodenum.

The pancreas

The pancreas is a pale grey-coloured gland, about 12–15cm long. It lies next to the duodenum and between the stomach, spleen and kidney. Its function is to produce pancreatic juices, which are rich in enzymes that break down carbohydrates, proteins and fats in the duodenum. These secretions together with those from the liver pass into the duodenum via the pancreatic duct. The pancreatic juices are alkaline and combined with those from the liver neutralise the acidic action of chyme.

The pancreas is also an endocrine gland and produces the hormones insulin and **glucagon**, which control the level of glucose in the blood.

Diseases and disorders of the digestive system

There are many common digestive problems. Most of them are not a cause for concern. However, there are a few that you will need to be aware of because in their more inflammatory stages they will cause discomfort and it would be best to avoid treatment during these times. Always ask the client how they feel and about their level of discomfort. Clients with contra-indications of the digestive system may prefer not to have the abdominal area massaged, for instance – although some light soothing effleurage might be beneficial.

Endocrine system

The endocrine system works alongside the nervous system to communicate, control and coordinate the body's activities. It produces hormones that control the body's metabolic processes.

Hormones are specialised chemical messengers that are stored and secreted by the endocrine glands. Hormones are transported to their target location via the bloodstream.

Glucagon

A hormone released by the pancreas when the level of glucose in the blood becomes low. It has the effect of converting gylcogen to glucose so that more glucose is released.

Acid reflux

A condition where stomach acid flows back up the oesophagus.

Jaundice

The yellowing of the skin and whites of the eyes due to build-up of bilirubin in the tissues of the body. Bilirubin is produced when the liver breaks down old red blood cells.

Disease	Description and cause	Contra-indications and general precautions	Advice for client
Crohn's disease	An inflammatory bowel disease. It affects the intestinal tract, causing inflammation and ulcers in the layers of the intestinal walls. It might also affect the lymph nodes in relevant areas. Symptoms include abdominal pain, tiredness, diarrhoea and weight loss.	Treat abdominal areas with care and avoid if painful.	Suggest client seeks medical advice.
Gallstones	Tiny stones of cholesterol that form in the gall bladder. There may not be any symptoms. When they do occur, they include abdominal discomfort, bloating and sickness.	Avoid treatment in the abdominal area if the client has gallstones.	Suggest client seeks medical advice.
Hiatus hernia	Caused when the stomach pushes through the diaphragm where the oesophagus passes through it. Can cause a lot of internal discomfort and **acid reflux**.	Caution. Avoid pressure over the upper abdominal area.	Suggest client seeks medical advice.
Irritable bowel syndrome (IBS)	Affects the large intestine or bowel. It causes an urgent need to open the bowels with loose faeces and/or constipation. Symptoms also include pain, bloating, discomfort and tiredness. It is commonly linked to stress and diet.	Avoid the abdominal area. If constipation is a symptom, massage can be quite beneficial.	Suggest client seeks medical advice if there are any sudden changes in the body's functions.
Gastroenteritis	Inflammation of the lining of the stomach and intestines causing vomiting and diarrhoea. Commonly caused by food poisoning or viruses such as norovirus.	Contra-indication	Client should consult GP.
Cirrhosis of the liver	Changes to the tissues of the liver due to long-term damage. Often associated with alcohol. The damage cannot be reversed and can be fatal if the liver stops working. In the early stages there are few symptoms, then there is a loss of appetite, nausea, skin irritation and **jaundice**.	Contra-indication	Client should consult GP for further advice before treatment.
Coeliac disease	An autoimmune disease caused by an adverse reaction to gluten. It damages the surface (villi) of the small bowel so that food is not properly absorbed. Symptoms include diarrhoea, bloating, abdominal pain, loss of weight, fatigue.	Check with client to see if their sensitivity also affects the skin. Caution with products that contain wheat or gluten.	No action required.

Hormones have an effect on or control the following bodily functions:

- emotions
- appetite
- sexual activity
- metabolism
- the sleep/wake cycle
- water (electrolyte) balance.

In this part of the chapter you will learn about:

- the structure, location and function of the endocrine glands.

The structure, location and function of the endocrine glands

HANDY HINT

The pituitary gland is often referred to as the master gland due to the effect it has on the other endocrine glands.

The endocrine system is made up of several ductless glands that release their hormones into the surrounding tissues. Most have a rich blood supply and lymphatic connection. Some glands form their own specific structure (eg pituitary gland) while others are contained within an organ as clusters of endocrine cells. The hormones released are chemicals which are capable of bringing about a change in another part of the body (target organ).

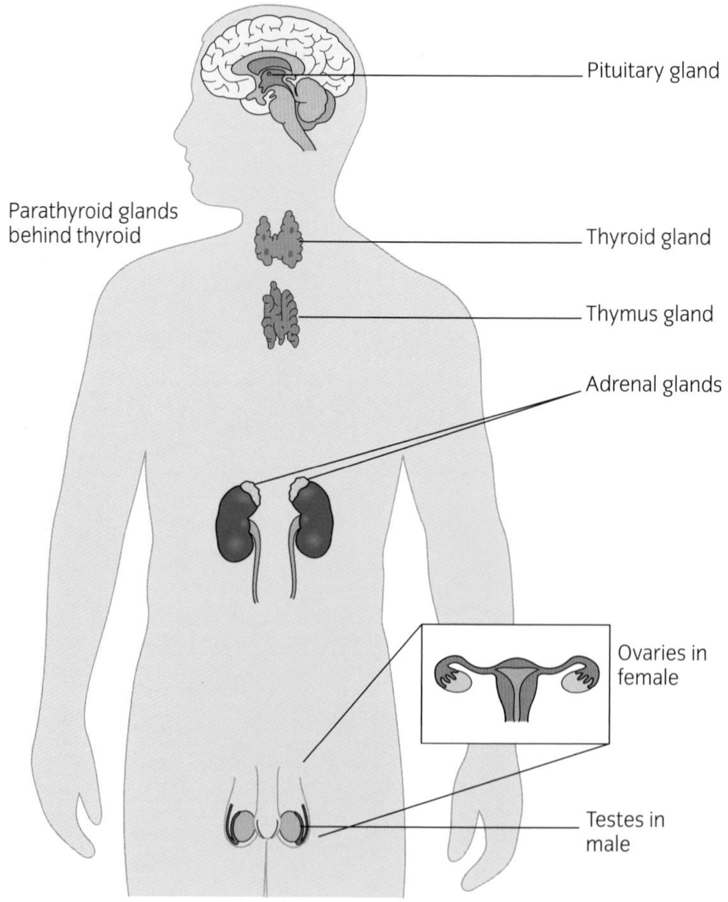

Location of endocrine glands

The hypothalamus and pituitary gland are located in the brain and work together regulating endocrine gland activity in the body. Stimulation of the pituitary gland is caused by releasing hormones produced by the hypothalamus. The pituitary gland lies below the hypothalamus and is attached to it by a stalk. The pituitary gland is found at the base of the skull and consists of two lobes:

- anterior
- posterior.

A network of nerve fibres is between the hypothalamus and anterior and posterior pituitary. The hypothalamus is the essential link between the nervous and endocrine systems.

INDUSTRY TIP

In some holistic therapies the pineal gland is also referred to as the third eye and is the place of the sixth chakra.

INDUSTRY TIP

Stimulation of the pituitary gland is caused by releasing hormones produced by the hypothalamus.

Endocrine gland	Releasing or inhibiting hormones secreted	Action	Target tissue/organ
Hypothalamus	Growth hormone releasing factor (GHRF)	Stimulates release of growth hormone from pituitary gland.	Pituitary gland – anterior
	Growth hormone release inhibiting factor (somatostatin) – (GHRIF)	Produced to reduce the release of growth hormone from the pituitary gland.	
	Thyroid releasing factor (TRF)	Stimulates release of thyroid stimulating hormone from pituitary gland.	
	Corticotrophin releasing factor (CRF)	Stimulates release of adrenocorticotrophic hormone from pituitary gland.	
	Prolactin inhibiting factor (PIF)	Produced to reduce the release of prolactin hormone from pituitary gland.	
	Luteinising hormone releasing factor (LHRF)	Stimulates release of follicle stimulating hormone from pituitary gland. Stimulates release of luteinising hormone from pituitary gland.	

Endocrine gland	Releasing or inhibiting hormones secreted	Action	Target tissue/organ
Pituitary gland (anterior)	Adrenocorticotrophic hormone (ACTH)	Adrenal cortex	Cortisol production.
	Growth hormone (GH)	All tissues	Controls growth of skeleton and muscles.
	Thyroid stimulating hormone (TSH)	Thyroid gland	Secretes thyroxine (T4) and triiodothyronine (T3) – regulates metabolism.
	Follicle stimulating hormone (FSH)	Ovarian follicles	Stimulates the development of the ovarian follicle. In males FSH stimulates the seminiferous tubules in testes to produce spermatozoa. Ovulation.
	Luteinising hormone (LH)	Formation of corpus luteum	Corpus luteum secretes progesterone. Progesterone levels rise, LH secretion is reduced. In males LH stimulates testes to secrete the hormone testosterone.
	Prolactin	Breasts	Stimulates milk secretion from the breasts following birth – lactation.
	Melanocyte stimulating hormone (MSH)	Skin	Skin pigmentation – regulates melanin production.
Pituitary gland (posterior)	Anti-diuretic hormone (ADH) or vasopressin	Kidneys	Regulates water re-absorption.
	Oxytocin hormone	Uterus	Stimulates contraction of the uterus – during and after childbirth.
		Breasts	Stimulates breast milk production for breastfeeding.

HANDY HINT

An example of a negative feedback mechanism is where FSH stimulates the development of an ovarian follicle; as it matures it secretes oestrogen. As a result, oestrogen levels rise and FSH secretion is inhibited.

HANDY HINT

The internal environment of the body is controlled and regulated partly by the autonomic nervous system and partly by hormones.

Endocrine gland	Hormone secreted	Target tissues/ organ	Action
Pineal The pineal gland is found near the centre of the brain, between the two hemispheres.	Melatonin	General body tissues	Regulates the natural biorhythms of the body.
Thyroid The thyroid gland is a butterfly-shaped gland positioned at the front of the neck. It is has two lobes. The lobes lie on either side of the larynx and on top of the trachea. There are four parathyroid glands that sit behind the thyroid gland.	Thyroxine (T4) Triiodothyronine (T3) Calcitonin	Cells and tissues within the body Kidneys, blood and bone tissue	Regulates metabolism – BMR. Regulates calcium levels in the blood.
Parathyroid (There are four parathyroid glands that sit behind the thyroid gland.)	Parathormone (PTH) or parathryn	Kidneys, blood and bone tissue	Controls the phosphorus and calcium levels.
Thymus The thymus gland lies in the upper part of the chest behind the sternum. It extends up towards the base of the neck.	Thymosin	Blood	Active during childhood and has an important role in developing a child's immune system. It produces T-lymphocytes.
Adrenal glands situated above the kidneys: Adrenal cortex	Glucocorticoids – cortisol, corticosterone	Liver, blood sugar	Regulates the metabolism of carbohydrates.
	Mineralocorticoids – aldosterone	Water content in tissues/renal tubules in kidneys	Maintain the balance of essential electrolytes, salts and water in the body by reabsorption of the kidney tubules.
	Sex hormones – androgens	Sex organs	Regulates the development and maintenance of the secondary sex characteristics.

Endocrine gland	Hormone secreted	Target tissues/ organ	Action
Adrenal medulla The adrenal medulla secretes adrenaline and noradrenaline. In times of stress these hormones work together.	Adrenaline	Bronchi, blood vessels, muscles, sweat glands	Prepares the body for fight or flight.
	Noradrenaline	Bronchi, blood vessels, intestine	
Pancreas – Islets of Langerhans are specialised cells. The pancreas has two functions: – to aid digestion by secreting pancreatic juice (an **exocrine** function) – secretion of insulin from the islets of Langerhans.	Insulin secreted by specialised beta cells in the pancreas	Bloodstream	Reduces the level of glucose in the blood.
	Glucagon secreted by specialised alpha cells in the pancreas	Bloodstream	Raises the level of glucose in the blood by converting stored glycogen back to glucose.
Ovaries The two ovaries are the female sex glands and are found beneath the kidneys. They produce ova and oestrogen and progesterone. They are controlled by follicle-stimulating hormone (FSH) and luteinising hormone (LH).	Oestrogen	Ovaries, uterus	Controls the development and function of the female reproductive system. Controls the development of secondary sex characteristics.
	Progesterone	Uterus	Prepares the uterus for pregnancy. Prepares the breasts for milk secretion.
Testes The testes are the male sex glands. They are located in the groin area and produce sperm and secrete testosterone.	Testosterone	Testes	Controls the development and function of the male sex organs. Produces male sexual characteristics.
	Androgens	Various body tissues, muscles, skin, etc.	Control the development of secondary sex characteristics.

Renal system

The **renal** system processes and gets rid of the body's normal metabolic waste. This waste includes excess water, urea, uric acid and mineral salts. The other main function of the renal system is to maintain homeostasis in the body by controlling blood pressure and volume. Water is introduced into the body through digestion but also through cellular activity. It is removed from the body through urine, **faeces**, sweat and our breath. Too much or too little fluid in the body can cause a variety of medical conditions. Approximately 80% of our blood is water and if this changes it can have an effect on the heart as it makes the heart work harder.

In this part of the chapter you will learn about:

- the structure and functions of the renal system
- disorders of the renal system.

Exocrine

The exocrine glalnds secrete products (eg sweat) through ducts. They are the opposite of endocrine glands which secrete products into the bloodstream.

Renal

Having to do with the kidneys.

Faeces

Waste that is removed via the digestive system through the bowel.

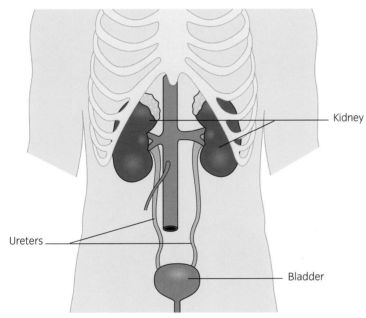

Structure of the urinary system

The structure and functions of the renal system

In this section you will learn about:

- the basic function of regulation of body fluids
- the general structure of the urinary system
- the functions of the urinary system.

The body will normally make changes to balance fluid levels such as making us pass urine to get rid of excess water or making us feel thirsty so that we replace the water we have lost. There is a complex interaction between both the nervous and endocrine systems to maintain these levels.

The renal system consists of the following:

- two kidneys, which secrete urine
- two ureters, which transport urine from the kidneys to the bladder
- the bladder, where urine collects and is temporarily stored
- the urethra, through which urine is removed from the bladder to the outside of the body.

The kidneys

The kidneys themselves are bean-shaped organs which lie on the posterior sides of the body near the abdominal wall and between the twelfth thoracic and third lumbar vertebrae. The kidneys are made up of fibrous outer capsules made up of connective tissue where fluid is filtered from blood. The kidneys have the following functions:

- to filtrate impurities and metabolic waste from blood
- to regulate water and the salts in the body, known as the **electrolyte** balance
- to maintain the balance of fluid in the circulatory system
- to produce urine.

Electrolyte

A chemical compound (eg of potassium, sodium) that ionises to produce an electrically conductive medium.

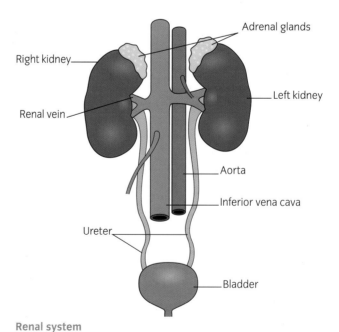

Renal system

The kidneys are responsible for regulating the amount of water and chemical compounds contained within the blood. If you have an excess of water in the blood, the blood concentration will be dilute, and the nerve receptors in the hypothalamus will trigger the pituitary gland to secrete the hormone ADH (anti-diuretic hormone) (see page 236). This carries a message to the kidneys to produce more diluted urine. If the blood becomes concentrated and we become dehydrated, the nerve receptors in the hypothalamus trigger the pituitary gland to send a message to the kidneys to produce more concentrated urine and reabsorb more water back into the body. The blood must also be kept at a constant pH of between 7.35 and 7.45: the kidneys help to maintain the chemicals in the circulation to keep blood pH within these narrow limits.

The kidney is composed of 1–2 million nephrons. Each nephron is an independent filtering and urine-processing unit. A nephron consists of:

- a renal corpuscle, which acts as a filter
- a renal tubule, which is a long tube that collects and processes the filtered fluid.

At the renal corpuscle a network of very tiny capillaries called the glomerulus makes contact with the closed end of the renal tubercle and acts as a sieve. The glomerulus is made up of a semi-permeable single layer of epithelial cells which allows selective molecules to move across from the blood supply by osmosis and filter into the kidney tubule to form urine.

Surrounding the glomerulus is the blind end of the tube, which forms a hollow cup-shaped structure called the glomerular capsule. There is a difference in pressure between the blood in the glomerulus and the filtrate now in the glomerular capsule and it is this difference in pressure which allows filtration under osmosis to take place. When blood pressure drops it affects this filtration process and the kidney function.

INDUSTRY TIP

The left kidney sits slightly higher than the right.

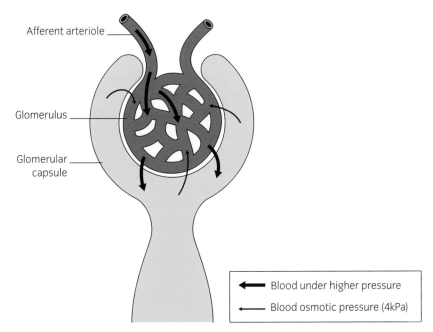

Filtration in the glomerulus

Urine is made of excess water, salt and protein waste. Urine has a pH of 4.5–7.8. Its colour varies according to its concentration and composition; the amber colour of urine is due to the presence of a pigment produced in bile by the liver. A healthy adult passes 1000–1500ml of urine per day.

As urine moves along the renal system is it further processed and selective substances (eg glucose, amino acids, mineral salts, vitamins and some water) that the body may need again are reabsorbed back into the bloodstream via the renal vein.

Urine is the waste product of filtration produced by the kidney. It collects in a funnel-shaped structure called the renal pelvis. Eventually the urine flows into a small tube called the ureter and into the bladder.

Activity

Discuss with your tutor how you think body treatments could affect urine output. In relation to the urinary system, what advice could you give your clients following body treatments and why would you give your clients this advice?

Activity

Next time you go to the loo, think about the colour of your urine. Does it indicate concentrated or weak urine? When do you think urine will be at its most concentrated?

Ureters

The ureters are tubes made of smooth muscle fibres that transport urine from the kidneys to the bladder. Muscles in the ureter walls tighten and relax and force urine downwards from the kidneys to the bladder.

Bladder

The bladder is a muscular balloon-shaped sac that is located in the pelvis. Its function is to store and remove urine through the urethra. In an adult, the bladder can hold up to 600ml of urine.

Urethra

This is a tube connected to the bladder through which urine is released from the body. The urethra is shorter in women than in men. In men it also has a reproductive function.

Autoimmune disease

A disease where the body's immune system attacks itself.

Oedema

Fluid retention in the tissues of the body.

Disorders of the urinary system

Disorder	Description and cause	Contra-indications and general precautions	Advice for client
Cystitis	An inflammation of the bladder. It can be caused by an infection or sensitivity to certain foods or chemicals. If it is not treated early enough it can travel up the ureter and infect the kidneys. Symptoms include a burning, stinging sensation or pain when passing urine and the urine may be dark and have a strong odour. There may also be discomfort in the lower back.	Contra-indication to body treatments. Caution is required. If the client is having a body treatment, suggest that they rebook once the condition has been treated. Any body treatment that makes the body work hard to eliminate waste will have an effect on the kidney and bladder and may further irritate the condition.	Suggest client seeks medical advice.
Nephritis	Inflammation of one or both of the kidneys. It can be caused by an infection or may be an **autoimmune disease**. Symptoms include reduced urine output, fluid retention, high blood pressure, tiredness and nausea.	Contra-indication. Any body treatment that makes the body work hard to eliminate waste will have an effect on the kidney and bladder and may further irritate the condition.	Suggest client seeks medical advice.
Renal failure	Chronic kidney disease (CKD) is a long-term kidney condition where the kidneys do not work properly. It will cause tiredness, shortness of breath, **oedema**.	Contra-indication.	Suggest client seeks medical advice.

Reproductive system

The reproductive system includes the internal and external organs that enable us to reproduce. There are very obvious different physical appearances between male and female organs. Adults produce specialised cells called gametes and in the male these are called spermatozoa and in the female ova. They contain the genetic materials which we call our genes or DNA and these enable us to pass on our characteristics to the next generation.

In this part of the chapter you will learn about:

- the structure and function of the reproductive system
- the key stages of the human reproductive cycle
- disorders of the reproductive system.

The structure and function of the male reproductive system

The scrotum

The scrotum is a sac made of fibrous and connective tissue along with muscle. There are two sections with one testis in each. The scrotum is suspended from the abdominal cavity and has a thin outer layer to keep the testes cool.

Testes

These are the reproductive glands in the male. They are suspended in the scrotum by the spermatic cords. Each testis contains special lobules within which are germinal epithelia cells called seminiferous tubules. Between the tubes are cells that secrete testosterone after puberty. Blood and lymph pass to the testis in the spermatic cord.

Sperm or spermatozoa are produced in the seminiferous tubules. Once these are mature they pass to the epididymis and are stored.

Urethra

The male urethra provides a pathway for both the flow of urine and semen.

The penis

The penis has two parts: the root and body. It contains erectile tissue and smooth muscle and is supported by a rich blood supply. At the tip of the body is an expanded structure called the glans penis. During ejaculation semen is propelled by powerful contraction of the muscles from the epididymis and through the deferent duct and along the urethra.

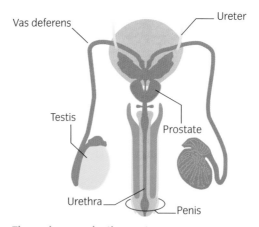

The male reproductive system

The structure and function of the female reproductive system

Female external genitalia

Female genitalia come in many shapes and forms, all of which are quite normal.

- Mons pubis or pubic mound – this is the padded area lying over the pubic bone where pubic hair grows.
- Vulva – this consists of the labia majora, labia minora, clitoris and vaginal orifice (opening).
  - Clitoris – erectile tissue located above the opening of the vagina containing sensory nerve endings.
  - Labia majora – two large folds encircling the vulva. The lateral sides are covered with pubic hair. They are composed of skin, fibrous tissue and fat and contain large numbers of sebaceous glands.
  - Labia minora – two smaller folds of skin between the labia majora.

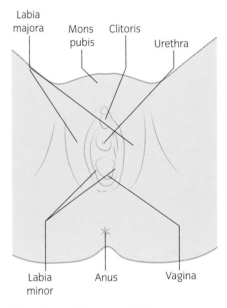

The external female genitalia

Female internal genitalia

Vagina

This is a muscular tube which extends from the external organs to the internal opening of the neck of uterus called the cervix.

The uterus

This is a hollow muscular organ which lies in the pelvic cavity. Its function is to nourish the ovum and the developing embryo and foetus during pregnancy. The uterus has a thick layer of muscle tissue, the inner layer of which is called the endometrium. This contains large numbers of mucus-secreting glands and a rich blood supply. The outer layer of the endometrium is shed during menstruation.

The uterine or Fallopian tubes

These extend from the uterus to the ovaries.

The ovaries

The ovaries are almond in shape and one lies on either side of the wall of the pelvis. Each ovary is attached to the uterus by the ovarian ligament and to the back by another ligament. The ovaries are composed of two parts: the medulla and the cortex. The cortex contains the ovarian follicles; each follicle contains an ovum or egg. Our ovaries contain thousands of immature ova (plural of ovum).

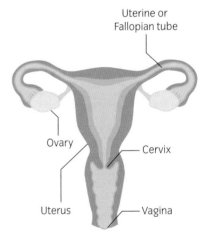

The female reproductive system

Puberty

Puberty typically begins between the ages of 12 and 14 at which time the reproductive organs begin to change and mature. Puberty is the start of the reproductive years.

- The breasts develop.
- Pubic and axillary hair begins to grow.
- The uterus, fallopian tubes and ovaries mature.
- The menstrual cycle begins to occur at regular intervals.
- Ovulation begins.
- The pelvis changes shape and there are increased deposits of fat around the buttocks and hips.

The menstrual cycle

During the menstrual cycle one ovum begins to mature and rise to the surface of the ovary. The ovum is contained in a follicle which eventually ruptures and releases the ovum into the Fallopian tube. The ovaries are stimulated by gonadotrophins from the anterior pituitary gland, FSH (follicle-stimulating hormone) and LH (luteinising hormone).

The menstrual cycle usually occurs regularly in females in 23–35-day cycles. It consists of three stages:

1 The first (follicular or proliferative) phase lasts approximately 10 days.
- The ovarian follicle is stimulated by FSH.
- Several follicles develop each with an egg; however, usually only one develops to maturity.
- The ovarian follicle produces oestrogen preparing the wall of the uterus.
- LH surges triggering ovulation.

2 The second (luteal or secretory) phase lasts approximately 14 days:
- Ovulation occurs and LH stimulates the egg to burst out of the follicle. The corpus luteum is what is left of the follicle once the egg is released.
- The corpus luteum secretes the hormone progesterone. Progesterone causes the uterus to become thick, vascular and ready for a fertilised egg to implant.
- Each egg is capable of being fertilised only for a very short time.

3 The third and final phase is the menstrual phase, lasting four days on average:
- High levels of progesterone in the blood prevent the activity of the pituitary gland and the production of LH is reduced.

■ The lack of LH causes the corpus luteum and progesterone to decrease.

■ The lining of the uterus begins to degenerate and the menstrual flow begins.

The anterior pituitary glands secrete FSH following menstruation causing the following:

■ New follicles develop in the ovary.

■ The ovary secretes oestrogen.

■ The walls of the uterus are repaired following menstruation.

■ Oestrogen begins to build up until it reaches a peak about two weeks following menstruation stimulating the anterior pituitary to produce LH.

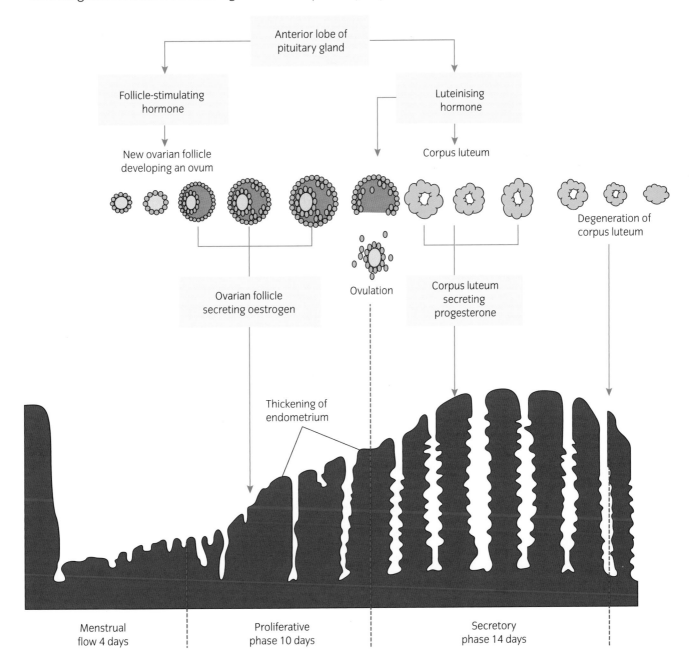

If the egg is fertilised, the corpus luteum starts to respond to the hormone hCG from the embryo. The corpus luteum continues as a result to produce progesterone. The corpus luteum disintegrates after about ten weeks. Progesterone continues to be produced during the pregnancy after this time but by the placenta.

Physical changes during the perimenopause and menopause

Perimenopausal is the name given to the changes that occur prior to the menopause. It is a natural progression and part of the ageing process. Symptoms start around the ages of 45–55 and may be experienced for several years. The menopause marks the end of the fertile reproductive years.

Hormone levels change and the ovaries become less responsive to FSH and LH. Eventually the ovaries become inactive and eventually the menstrual cycle ceases.

The physical changes of perimenopause include the following:

- There is a loss of subcutaneous fat.
- The ovaries reduce in size.
- The lining of the uterus becomes inactive.
- Axillary and pubic hair become sparse.
- The vagina narrows.
- Unwanted superfluous hair occurs.
- Susceptibility to osteoporosis.
- Skin becomes thin, dryer, scaly and inelastic.
- Breasts become flabby and lose fat content.

Some of or all of the following symptoms of the perimenopause may be experienced:

- headaches
- insomnia
- palpitations
- loss of bone mass (osteoporosis)
- menstruation changes – abnormal bleeding, irregular periods, periods stop
- fatigue
- numbness
- dizziness
- night sweats
- stress incontinence

- crawling/creeping sensation under the skin
- libido decreases, painful intercourse
- depression
- hot flushes.

Diseases and disorders of the reproductive system

Disease	Description	Contra-indications and general precautions	Advice to client
Endometriosis	A condition where the endometrial tissue grows outside of the uterus. This could be in the ovaries, Fallopian tubes and other pelvic organs. The endometrial tissue still behaves in the same way as the tissue that lines the uterus and responds to changing hormones at different times in the menstrual cycle (ie it grows during the menstrual cycle and bleeds). The endometrial tissue has no way of leaving the body which causes pain and swelling. Pain can be mild to severe. The condition can lead to infertility.	Carry out treatment with caution. A common condition and symptoms vary. Treatment over the abdomen should be avoided if there is discomfort.	Suggest client seeks medical advice before treatment if they are concerned.
STDs (sexually transmitted diseases)	There are several diseases that can be transmitted through sexual activity. These can be bacterial or viral. Examples include: HIV, chlamydia, genital herpes, syphilis, human papilloma virus. Each disease has different symptoms and they are the most common reasons for reproductive disorders.	Depends on the symptoms. It is more likely you will be unaware that someone has a STD.	Suggest client seeks medical advice before treatment if they are concerned.
Menstrual problems	These include: - painful periods (dysmenorrhea) - heavy periods - irregular periods - absence of periods (amenorrhea) - ovulation pain. There are many reasons for changes in hormonal cycles ranging from illness, disease, stress and the ageing process.	Not a contra-indication.	The client may need to avoid having treatments during their period if they have problematic symptoms.

Answers at the back of the book.

1 What is the name of the chemical released by the body that causes vasodilation?

a Histamine

b Erythrocyte

c Macrophage

d Pathogen

2 Which one of the following is not found in the acid mantle?

a Urea

b Water

c Sweat

d Sebum

3 Which one of the following is produced by fibroblasts?

a Histamine

b Collagen

c Pathogens

d Papillae

4 Meissner's corpuscles are nerve endings that are able to sense which one of the following?

a Pressure

b Pain

c Touch

d Temperature

5 The depth of skin colour is dependent on which of the following?

a How melanin is structured

b More active melanocytes

c The amount of melanin in the melanosomes

d How melanosomes are distributed

6 Which one of the following is a bacterial infection?

a Impetigo

b Shingles

c Milia

d Urticaria

7 What is psoriasis often caused by?

a Bacteria

b Virus

c Fungus

d Stress

8 What is the outer layer of the hair called?

a Medulla

b Shaft

c Cortex

d Cuticle

9 How many cervical bones are there?

a 4

b 5

c 7

d 12

10 Which one of the following is a characteristic of veins?

a They carry oxygenated blood

b Blood flow is under pressure

c The vessels have a thick layer of muscle

d The vessels have valves

11 Which one of the following is involved in the blood clotting process?

a Thrombocytes

b Leucocytes

c Erythrocytes

d Granulocytes

12 Which area does the thoracic duct not drain lymph from?

a Both legs

b Abdominal cavities

c Neck and left arm

d Right half of head and right arm

13 What is the name of the blood vessel that carries blood to the kidney?

a Renal artery

b Renal vein

c Aorta

d Vena cava

14 Filtration of blood in the glomerulus occurs by which of the following?

  a Active transport

  b Diffusion

  c Facilitated diffusion

  d Osmosis

15 Which of the following parts of the cell is commonly referred to as the powerhouse of the cell?

  a Mitochondria

  b Liposomes

  c Cytoplasm

  d Ribosome

16 Which one of the following occurs to skin cells during mitosis?

  a An exact replica of the original cell is produced

  b Two new but different cells are produced

  c Two new identical cells are produced

  d One new but different cell is produced

17 Which one of the following hormones regulates the metabolism?

  a Thyroid-stimulating hormone

  b Insulin

  c Glucagon

  d Adrenocorticotrophic hormone

18 Which one of the following hormones reduces the level of glucose and nutrients in the blood?

  a Insulin

  b Glucagon

  c Adrenaline

  d Thyroxine

19 Which one of the following hormones prepares the uterus for pregnancy?

  a Oxytocin

  b Progesterone

  c Oestrogen

  d Androgen

20 How many pairs of cranial nerves are there?

  a 8

  b 10

  c 12

  d 14

21 Which one of the following would happen in response to the parasympathetic nervous system?

  a Dilation of the bronchi

  b Decreased urine secretion

  c Increased cardiac output

  d Constriction of the blood vessels

22 What are fats made up of?

  a Monoglycerides

  b Diglycerides

  c Triglycerides

  d Polyglycerides

23 In which part of the digestive system are villi found?

  a Stomach

  b Large intestine

  c Small intestine

  d Colon

24 Which of the following occurs during inspiration?

  a Air is breathed out, diaphragm and intercostal muscles contract

  b Air is breathed out, diaphragm and intercostal muscles relax

  c Air is breathed in, diaphragm and intercostal muscles contract

  d Air is breathed in, diaphragm and intercostal muscles relax

25 Which one of the following is not caused by a viral infection?

  a Influenza

  b Sinusitis

  c Asthma

  d Bronchitis

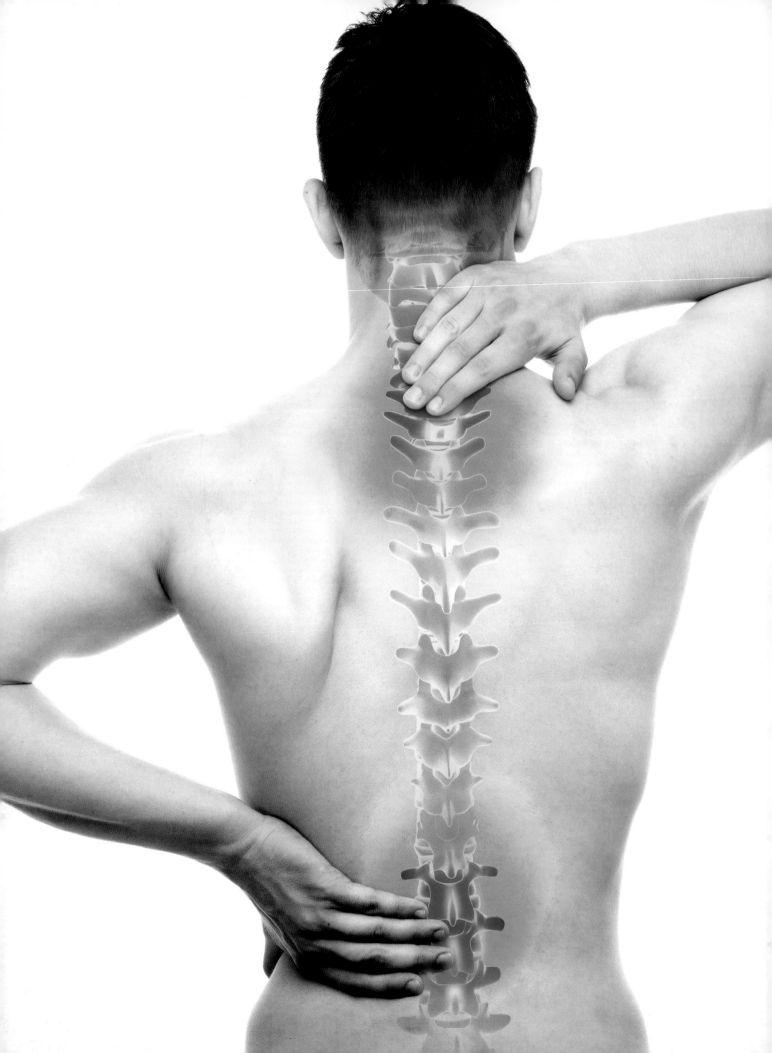

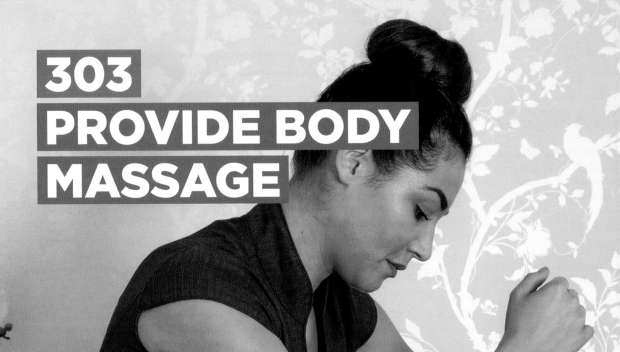

303 PROVIDE BODY MASSAGE

Massage is a wonderful, versatile treatment when applied professionally and appropriately according to the client's needs. It can be applied in various ways, using a range of techniques to achieve different effects. The origins of massage date back thousands of years and can be found within many longstanding traditions such as Chinese and Ayurvedic medicine. The power of touch cannot be underestimated and forms the basis of many healing systems.

This chapter also covers forearm massage techniques to minimise repetitive strain injuries and the use of pre-blended products as part of a massage treatment. The aroma and the effect of the essential oil blend as well as the different movements you use can add an extra dimension to the treatment and provide the therapist with an additional tool to customise the treatment to meet the individual client's needs.

In this chapter you will learn to:

- prepare for a body massage
- provide a body massage
- provide advice, recommendations, treatment and evaluation.

Philosophy of body massage

Massage is an art that is said to be as old as humanity itself. When we are hurt, our instinctive reaction is to rub an injured area or to apply pressure. Both help to provide comfort and relieve unpleasant sensations.

Ancient writings, some over 5000 years old, from China, Japan, India and Egypt illustrate different massage traditions. Priests or doctors originally practised massage in an almost ritual fashion. Many holy books describe massage and laying on of the hands to heal. Oils and herbs were used for bathing, healing and embalming. As the Roman Empire declined, massage began to be less associated with healing and more with the pursuit of pleasure. By the Middle Ages it had largely disappeared. In the early nineteenth century, Henrik Ling, a Swedish doctor, used his system of gymnastic movements to establish the benefits of exercises and keeping physically healthy.

Although we now associate the Swedish nationality with massage, massage as we know it today actually originated from the work of the Dutch practitioner Johann Georg Mezger in the nineteenth century. He was responsible for many of the techniques and the French terms we use today, such as effleurage and petrissage. Massage continued to develop and in 1899 Sir William Bennet opened a massage department at St George's Hospital in London. From here massage began to separate into different fields of expertise – physiotherapy along one route and some other prominent alternative therapies along others. Now we see many variations of touch or massage therapies and the techniques and tools used to support them including stones, crystals, wood, shells, bamboo and other massage tools.

Prepare for body massage

Preparation of the therapist

Proximity

Nearness.

As a therapist you will be working in close **proximity** to the client throughout this treatment. It is very important that you are dressed and presented in a professional manner. See the Values and behaviours chapter for more information.

Before you start any treatment you should make sure you are physically prepared and mentally focused. The client is paying for your time and attention and you should avoid any distractions.

Hand exercises

It is important that your hands are warm before you start the massage. This will help to prevent any injury or muscle strain. You can warm your hands up by placing them in warm water for a few minutes. It is also a good idea to exercise your hands regularly to increase their flexibility when you first start massaging. You can also use simple exercise to help prepare, warm up and loosen the joints before massage.

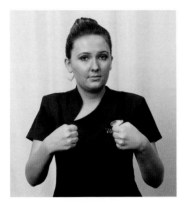

EXERCISE 1 Make a fist, clenching and then stretching out the fingers.

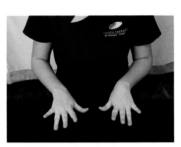

EXERCISE 2 Run the fingers up and down as if typing or playing the piano to loosen the finger joints.

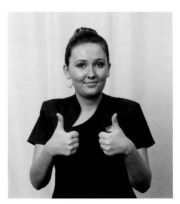

EXERCISE 3 Thumb circling: rotate one way, then the other.

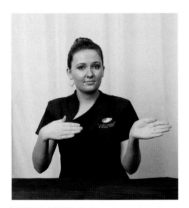

EXERCISE 4 Rotate wrists in a circle, and then rotate in the opposite direction to loosen them up.

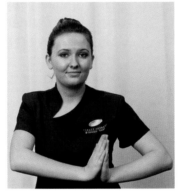

EXERCISE 5 Place hands flat together and draw a figure of eight; go clockwise and then anticlockwise to loosen up the wrists.

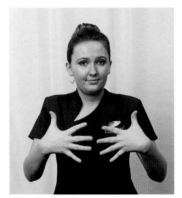

EXERCISE 6 Shake out the hands.

Preparation of the treatment area

The treatment area should be fully prepared before the client arrives. You should make sure that all work surfaces have been cleaned and are tidy and organised. Clean and disinfect any equipment you will need to use, such as the couch and trolley, before you begin. Make sure that any equipment or products you may need are ready and easily accessible before you start, so that you do not have to break contact during the massage and interrupt the flow of your treatment to go and get anything. Check that any equipment you require is plugged in and is in working order.

The treatment environment

The client needs to be comfortable during their treatment. The following should all be checked and adjusted if necessary.

INDUSTRY TIP

If you are aiming to attract the male market you should make sure that the reception area is neutral and includes male-oriented displays. Include current magazines for both male and female clients.

INDUSTRY TIP

Choose shoes that will enable you to move around quietly, for example with rubber soles. This will help you avoid disturbing clients or other colleagues.

Environmental condition	How to make the client comfortable
Lighting	■ Use subtle lighting. ■ Make sure to avoid glare in the client's eyes.
Ventilation	■ Maintain good air circulation to avoid stale air building up. ■ Avoid draughts.
Sound/music	■ Choose soft, gentle, relaxing music. ■ Check that having music is okay with the client – some clients may actually prefer to have their treatment in silence. ■ Avoid any unnecessary noise during your treatment, or sounds that might disturb the client.
Client privacy	■ The client will be removing their clothes and parts of their body will be exposed during a massage treatment, so it's important to make sure they have privacy. Modesty should be protected with careful towel management during treatment.
Hazards	■ Check your work area for hazards such as trailing wires. ■ Reduce any risks to you and your client.
Warmth	■ You will be exposing parts of the client's body as you carry out the massage routine, so keep the area warm and free from draughts.
Aroma	■ Make sure the room has a pleasing aroma – avoid the build-up of stale odours and pay attention to personal hygiene.

HANDY HINT

Never pour unused products down the sink, especially oils – these will build up on the inside of the pipe and cause bad odours. Eventually the pipe may become blocked. Blot or soak up any products with couch roll or tissue and then place into a refuse bin.

HANDY HINT

You don't have to use towels – a large sheet or lightweight duvet cover works well, as long as it is managed well during treatment.

INDUSTRY TIP

Clean up oil from work surfaces such as trolleys. Oil residue becomes sticky and is a breeding ground for bacteria.

HANDY HINT

Avoid using any more towels than you need to, as these can be bulky and get in the way. A large bath sheet and a small hand towel are often all that you need.

INDUSTRY TIP

As a guideline, to check you are working at the correct height, stand sideways on to the couch and place a clenched fist on the surface. Your knuckles should just touch the couch.

HANDY HINT

Spirit-based product is essential for removing any oil from equipment to avoid any sticky residue.

Disposal of waste

You should have a pedal bin, lined with a new bin liner. To ensure hygiene and avoid cross-infection, make sure that you do not touch the bin directly with your hand(s) once sanitised. During the treatment, dispose of your waste as you work and do not let it collect on a trolley or work surface. Do not let the bin overflow.

Equipment

- seating
- treatment chair
- clean towels/blankets/sheets
- steps
- bowls/containers
- gowns/slippers
- infrared lamp (if using).

Complete a safety check on any equipment you plan to use to make sure it is ready, then switch it on, ready for use. If using infrared, check that the bulb is working and that there is no damage to the lighting case. Make sure that both the bulb and protector are secure.

Treatment couch

The treatment couch is the main piece of equipment needed to carry out a massage. It should be sturdy, well cushioned and padded. It is preferable to have a face hole (not all clients like to use one, but it is useful to keep the neck straight when working on the back). The couch should be adjustable to allow for different therapists to work at it. It should be cleaned regularly with a suitable cleaner for hygiene reasons and to remove any oil residue, and then covered with a couch cover.

The couch should be neat, tidy and ready for the client. Towels should be freshly laundered and washed after every client to maintain hygiene standards.

There should be a small pillow or towel for the client to put their head on to support the neck. An additional towel or blanket may be required for warmth. If the client is very tall, you can place a hand towel on the couch and fold it over the client's feet to keep them covered and warm.

Trolley

Position your trolley so it is within easy reach. The trolley should contain all the products that you will require during the massage.

Products

- base oil: apricot kernel oil, grapeseed oil, coconut oil, evening primrose oil, jojoba oil, almond oil, olive oil
- cream
- powder (to include liquid talc and cornflour)
- gel

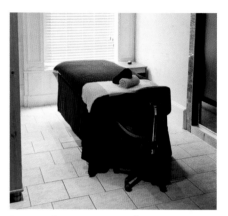
Prepared treatment couch

VALUES & BEHAVIOURS
Effective, hygienic and safe working methods

- pre-blended oils (relaxation and sense of well-being, joint and muscle pain, invigoration and uplifting, improvement of skin and body conditions)
- product to cleanse the feet.

Skincare products

If the client is having their face treated, make sure you remove any make-up, cleanse and tone their skin before you start your treatment. A suitable product should also be available for use to cleanse the client's feet before beginning a full body massage.

Consumables

You will also require some consumables:

- cotton wool to remove cleanser
- tissues
- couch roll to protect towels and maintain hygiene
- spatulas to decant products hygienically.

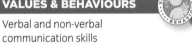

The consultation

A detailed consultation to establish the client's priorities and needs must take place before every treatment. Further information on the consultation process can be found in the Values and behaviours chapter.

Communication and behaviour

It is important to behave in a professional manner at all times. For more information on appropriate behaviour, communicating with the client and providing a professional consultation, please see the Values and behaviours chapter.

The consultation process

Carry out the massage consultation somewhere quiet and private. Greet your client by name and introduce yourself, then lead your client to the consultation or treatment area. You should sit beside your client so that you do not have any physical barrier, such as the couch, to communication – you should be able to maintain eye contact. You should confirm the treatment the client is booked in for before proceeding.

The aim of a consultation is to find out what treatment objectives the client has. It is an opportunity to discuss treatment options or to upgrade the treatment you are giving, if this is possible. To make sure your client leaves satisfied, it is important to listen to the client carefully and match the treatment objectives to their needs.

It is vital to agree the treatment objectives with the client during the consultation so you can make the correct choice of oils, massage

VALUES & BEHAVIOURS

Verbal and non-verbal communication skills

Communicating with clients

Identifying and confirming the client's expectations

Being courteous and helpful

Communicating appropriately

Checking the client's expectations

Promptly and positively responding to questions and comments

Providing information about services and products

Explaining why client expectations cannot be met

VALUES & BEHAVIOURS

Personal and professional ethics

Adhering to instructions

Meeting your salon's standards of behaviour

Greeting the client respectfully and in a friendly manner

VALUES & BEHAVIOURS

Providing information about services and products

techniques and consider any adaptations you might have to make. The client's expectations may not always be realistic or what you are expecting – if so, you need to be tactful and provide the client with a realistic treatment plan. If you feel that the client's expectations are unrealistic you should politely explain this and suggest alternative treatments that can be supported with appropriate recommendations. Allow the client plenty of time to ask questions.

Remember that as part of a thorough consultation you should include postural analysis. This will help you to be aware of where you may need to apply different techniques to work on tight or over-stretched muscles. Also remember to check for contra-indications.

Contra-indications

One of the purposes of the consultation is to check for contra-indications. A contra-indication is a reason why a treatment cannot be carried out. It may prevent the treatment or restrict it. If there is a reason why you cannot carry out the treatment you should tactfully explain why to the client. If possible, offer the client an alternative treatment. If you think that the client should seek medical advice, suggest this, but remember that you are not a medical practitioner and you are not qualified to make any form of diagnosis.

If the client speaks to their medical practitioner and they have agreed that there is no reason why the massage cannot go ahead, you should record this on the client's record card and get the client to sign to agree to the treatment going ahead.

In some cases the contra-indication will just restrict the treatment in some way. An example of this would be a bruise or an open wound that must be avoided. It may be that the treatment will need to be adapted, for example if there is a contra-indication involving a large part of a limb. You should always explain to the client if you are going to have to avoid an area or adapt a treatment – the client must agree to this before you start. It may be advisable for the client to rebook to benefit from the full treatment at a later date rather than be disappointed with only part of a treatment now.

You will need to review the following contra-indications and make sure that you are familiar with each condition before offering a massage treatment.

Contra-indications to massage

The main contra-indications to massage are as follows:

- Prevent treatment: contagious skin diseases (fungal, bacterial, viral, infestations), severe eczema, severe psoriasis, severe skin conditions, deep vein thrombosis, during chemotherapy, during radiotherapy.

 Watch a video of a body massage consultation on SmartScreen (unit 303).

■ Restrict treatment: broken bones, recent fractures and sprains, cuts and abrasions, recent scar tissue, skin disorders, skin allergies, product allergies, epilepsy, uncontrolled diabetes, high/low blood pressure, metal pins or plates, recent piercings, pregnancy, some medications, varicose veins, undiagnosed lumps and swellings.

Thermal testing

Infrared uses heat and it is therefore an important part of the consultation prior to this treatment to carry out thermal sensitivity testing.

To carry out thermal (hot and cold) testing, you will need one hot item and one cold item. You can use special tubes designed for this function, or you can use small bottles to carry out this test. Place the two items randomly over the treatment area and ask the client to tell you whether they feel hot or cold. If the client cannot feel the difference between hot and cold, they cannot have the treatment, as they will not be able to tell you if something is too hot and may sustain burns as a result.

Product sensitivity

Pre-blended oils contain ingredients that a client may be sensitive to – for this reason there may be occasions when it will be necessary to carry out a test patch.

First cleanse the skin with warm water, then apply a small amount of the product to be tested. If this is a single product, do this in the small dip behind the ear, as this area is hidden. If more products are being tested it may be preferable to use the inside of the forearm. Be careful to remember where you place each product and make sure there is no overlap. Carefully document this information.

The client should be asked to monitor the area for at least 24 hours, or according to the manufacturer's instructions, for any redness, irritation, itching or inflammation, any of which would be a contra-indication.

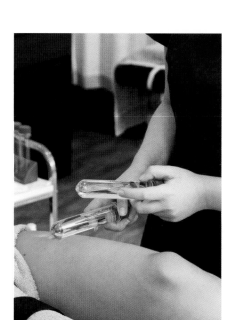

Thermal testing

Client analysis

As part of your consultation process you should visually observe the client, considering each of the following general characteristics. These will influence your decision about which products and techniques to use. They may also influence the treatment objectives.

Age

A client's age will affect their skin condition. A young client will generally have good skin tone and elasticity. As skin ages, it becomes thinner and less elastic, causing a loss of body contour. If the skin is very thin it should be treated gently to avoid damage. You should avoid movements that drag the skin.

Maintaining muscle tone becomes harder as we age, and muscle tone can become weaker as a result. Poor muscle tone is also associated with a lack of physical activity and is often not related to age. (See chapter 302, Anatomy and physiology.)

Another factor associated with women as they get older is a loss of bone mass, which can lead to osteoporosis. Elderly clients who are thin and frail should always be treated with care. Avoid using tapotement techniques.

Skin type

General skin types are detailed in chapter 302, Anatomy and physiology. You should also be aware of the general differences in skin between the different genders and ethnic groups. It is important to look at the client's skin, even on the body, and choose an appropriate treatment oil. You should consider whether the skin is dry, oily, mature, sensitive, dehydrated or moist, and consider the elasticity and thinness of the skin.

> **INDUSTRY TIP**
>
> Some clients have naturally moist skin. This is usually due to overactive sweat glands, but can also be caused by anxiety.

Male clients

Treating a male client will be different from treating a female client. Consider the following:

- Body hair – if the client is very hairy, this will influence your choice of massage media and technique, to avoid pulling the hair or generating unnecessary friction.

- Muscle bulk – there is a tendency for male clients to have more muscle definition or bulk, though this does depend on the level of fitness. Where muscle bulk is more defined, you can use the definition to help apply your techniques more effectively into the muscle tissue, especially when applying petrissage techniques.

- Fat distribution – fat is distributed differently around the body, particularly when there is excess weight. It is more difficult to get to the muscle tissue and working on a client with lots of excess **adipose tissue** can be hard work. Using more tapotement will be beneficial to help stimulate the tissue. Some clients with very hard, firm adipose tissue have quite sensitive skin, so make sure you check your technique with the client.

- Treatment considerations – the lower abdomen below the navel and inner upper thighs (also referred to as the 'femoral triangle') are **erogenous zones**. Therapists are advised to avoid massaging this area on a male client to avoid causing any embarrassment to the client or therapist.

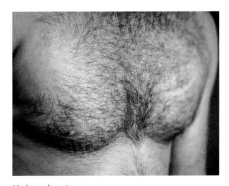
Hairy chest

> **Adipose tissue**
>
> Body fat.

> **Erogenous zone**
>
> Area of the body that has increased sexual sensitivity (eg the inner thighs).

Body fat

Body fat is called adipose tissue, and is a type of connective tissue. This tissue is made up of special cells called adipocytes. Eighty per cent of adipose fat is subcutaneous and is stored under the skin (the rest surrounds organs). Different genders and ethnic groups store fat in different areas. There are three types of body fat in the context of beauty therapy:

- Soft fat – adipocytes are loosely packed and have some room for movement, making the tissue soft to the touch and easily shifted using a 'wringing' movement.

- Hard fat – this tissue has tightly packed adipocytes with no room for movement, giving a firm, hard surface that is difficult to manipulate.

- Cellulite – fat cells are housed in clusters in free-standing chambers separated by vertical walls of connective tissue. When the fat cells expand these walls collapse under the pressure. This change in structure allows fluid to collect around the cells, resulting in a dimpled appearance of the skin and is commonly referred to as cellulite. This condition is commonly observed around the thigh and buttock areas but can also be found on the abdomen and upper arms. Loose cellulite is more obvious than compacted cellulite, which can be seen by gently squeezing the skin or clenching the muscles in the area exaggerating the dimpled appearance.

INDUSTRY TIP

Males tend to store excess fat around their middle, whereas women commonly store it on their hips, thighs, buttocks and bust.

HANDY HINT

When measuring a client's height and weight, always take the measurements on a hard floor – never carpet. The client should remove bulky clothes and shoes first.

Somatotype

Body type or physique.

Postural analysis

A postural analysis is used to:

- assess client treatment needs

- recognise any problems that may require medical referral

- plan an effective treatment.

Where there are figure faults or other areas of concern the massage can be adapted to take these into account. For example, work can be carried out on tight muscles if there is a postural fault, or an appropriate massage medium can be chosen if the skin is very dry.

You should also consider the following:

- weight

- height

- body frame

- **somatotype**

- posture and postural weaknesses.

Activity

Some of your clients will still work in imperial measurements rather than metric. It is useful to be able to covert one to the other.

Weight

Pound = lb, kilogram = kg

   1lb = 0.45kg

   1kg = 2lb 3oz

   1kg = 1000g

   1lb = 16oz

To convert kilograms to pounds, multiply by 2.2.

To convert pounds to kilograms, multiply by 0.045, or divide by 2.2.

Calculate the following:

   Work out how many pounds are in 65 kilograms.

   Work out how many kilograms are in 132 pounds.

Height

Centimetre = cm, metre = m, inches = in, feet = ft

   1cm = 0.4in

   1in = 2.5cm

   12in = 1ft

   100cm = 1m

To convert centimetres to inches, multiply by 0.39.

To convert inches to centimetres, multiply by 2.54.

Calculate the following:

   Client is 5ft 5in. Convert this to centimetres.

   Client is 182cm. Convert this to feet and inches.

Postural considerations

When the client comes into the salon, observe them closely and make a mental note of the following:

- how they move
- how they carry themselves
- their overall posture.

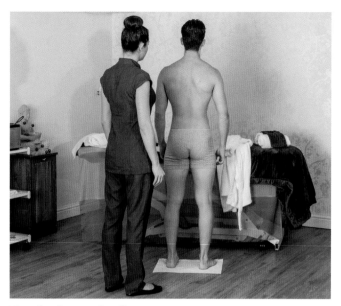 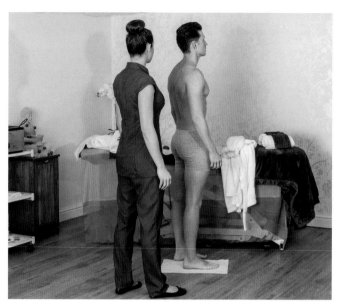

Visually observe the client

By assessing each of the above, you can find out a lot about your client before you ask any questions. If the client is moving very slowly or awkwardly this might indicate a problem that is restricting their movement. If they carry their body so that they are not symmetrical, eg leaning more to one side, this could indicate a possible joint problem that has led to a change in posture. Postural change is usually the result of avoiding discomfort or pain from a change in the underlying structures. Over a period of time, muscles will lengthen and shorten to accommodate the change in posture, further distorting alignment. This impacts the affected muscles, placing them under stress and strain, altering their structure over time. By considering these factors you can look to where your treatment might need to be adapted during massage to help alleviate symptoms, including feelings of muscular tension, tightness and discomfort.

Consider the following when analysing the client's posture:

- Posture of head and neck – head should be mid-line, not forward of the shoulders. Ears and eyes should be level.

- Shoulders – do they roll inwards? Note the level of the scapulae. Winged scapulae, rounded or very square shoulders, dowager's hump?

- Breasts – is there good or poor tone? Is ligament attachment good? Under- or over-developed? Stretch marks?

- Ribs – the rib cage should be symmetrical, as should the clavicles. Is the rib cage very defined or expanded? Pigeon or hollow chest?

- Arms – solid, muscular, in proportion? Thin or loose crêpey skin? Poor circulation on the backs of upper arms giving a rough texture to skin?

- Abdomen – good or poor muscle tone, giving a flat or protruding stomach? Waist high or low? Any excess fat below waist? Excess skin or stretch marks?

- Thighs – consider general distribution of fat, including cellulite. Consider proportion – are legs heavy or too thin? Muscular? Stretch marks?

- Legs – bow legs, hyper-extended knees, knock knees, varicose veins, broken capillaries?

- Feet – swollen ankles, fallen arches, hallux valgus (bunions), hammer toes, calluses, corns? Note the position of the feet and any abnormalities which may affect posture, such as poor circulation or athlete's foot.

- Back – curvature of spine, kyphosis, lordosis, scoliosis, flat back, round back, excess fat over latissimus dorsi muscle? Note the proportion of the upper back to trunk.

- Pelvic tilt – dimples on pelvis, if evident, should be level. Does the pelvis tilt forwards, backwards or to the side?

- Buttocks – **gluteal folds** should be level. Protruding buttocks may indicate anterior pelvic tilt, excess fat or cellulite. Note the level of gluteal drop – is the gluteal fold in line with the pubis?

Somatotypes

Somatotypes are names given to the most common body types. Most of us are a combination of more than one. The three somatotypes are:

Gluteal folds

The horizontal folds at the base of the buttocks.

Activity

Find three images from magazines to represent each of the different somatotypes.

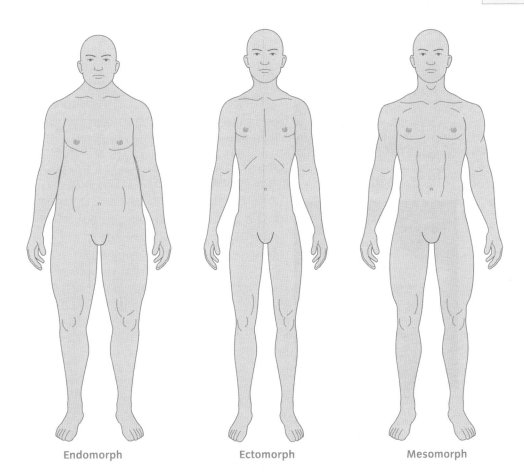

| Endomorph | Ectomorph | Mesomorph |

Endomorph	Ectomorph	Mesomorph
Tendency to gain weight.	Narrow shoulders and hips.	Inverted triangular shape – shoulders are wider than the hips.
Hips are wider than the shoulders and shorter limbs.	Long, thin trunk.	Boyish physique.
Heavy build.	Long bones, giving long limbs.	Athletic build; potential for well-toned muscles while active.
Higher percentage of fat to muscle bulk.	Lacks muscle bulk.	
	Low percentage of fat.	Sturdy, straight shoulders.
Tendency towards padded contours.	Often underweight with a lack of curves.	Low percentage of fat.
Hands may be small and delicate.		

Postural problems

For more about kyphosis, lordosis and scoliosis, see page 182.

Postural problem	Description and cause
Dowager's hump	A true Dowager's hump is usually associated with older people. It can be observed as a kyphotic curve of the upper thoracic vertebra causing the shoulders to become rounded and the chin to poke forward. The condition is caused by osteoporosis which causes the bone structure at the front of the vertebrae to collapse. There is often a pad of fat overlying the vertebra which further exaggerates the curve.
Winged scapula	This condition affects the serratus anterior muscles and causes the lower angle of the scapula to stand out prominently, giving a winged appearance. Weak or abnormal function of the serratus anterior.

Postural problem	Description and cause
Pigeon chest 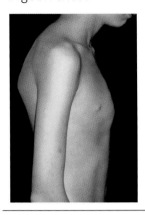	The chest becomes pushed out, as in taking a very deep breath, and the sternum bone raised. It is caused by excessive growth of the rib cartilage, some spinal conditions such as scoliosis or a genetic disorder.
Pelvic tilt 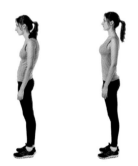	The pelvis can be tilted in a range of directions: forward (anterior), backward (posterior), lateral or rotated. The postural fault and the muscles that are affected will depend on the direction of the tilt. Anterior tilt causes the bottom to stick out, lordosis or flat back. Posterior tilt causes kyphosis and lateral or rotated pelvic scoliosis.
Bow legs 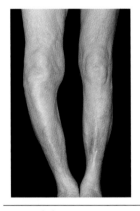	When standing with the feet together, there is a defined arched gap between the legs. It can be caused by nutritional deficiency (lack of vitamin D), leading to rickets.
Knock knees 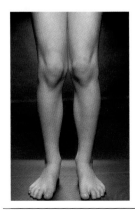	The knees rotate inwards so that they brush together. This condition is caused by slack tendons around the knee joint or an abnormal curvature of the bones of the lower legs.

Postural problem	Description and cause
Flat feet or fallen arches 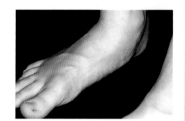	Collapse of one or both of the arches of the feet. This condition can be caused by weak muscles, injury, being overweight or ill-fitting shoes. It may also be hereditary.
Flat back 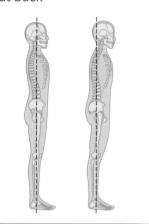	Increased posterior pelvic tilt, loss of natural lumbar and thoracic spinal curves giving the appearance of a flat back, with the head angled forwards.
Sway back 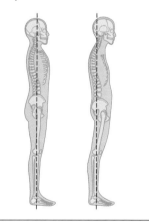	Increased anterior tilt of pelvis causing exaggerated lumbar arch, protruding stomach and shoulders extended back.
High arches 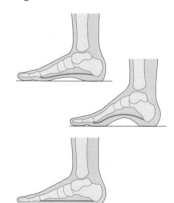	Increased foot arch, toes may also be flexed as if clawing. Condition may be hereditary or due to a neuromuscular disease.

Preparation of the client

To encourage the client to have confidence in you, always give them clear instructions about what to do, how to prepare and what treatment you are going to perform. Remember that this massage might be different from other treatments they have had, or it may even be their first massage treatment.

Ask the client to:

- remove their jewellery, watch, piercings (including from the face and abdomen) and contact lenses; make sure these items are stored safely

- undress down to their briefs (if the client prefers you can provide them with disposable paper briefs); you should leave the client while they do this to protect their modesty and give them clear instructions about where to leave their clothes

- get on to the couch once they are ready, and lie on their back, covering their body with a towel (leave this ready for them to use).

INDUSTRY TIP

Suggest to the client that they might like to use the toilet prior to the treatment so they are comfortable and to avoid them having to get up partway through.

VALUES & BEHAVIOURS

Maintaining customer care

Communicating with clients

Keeping the client informed

HANDY HINT

When the client is lying prone (face down) and you are carrying out a back massage, look up the back at the spinal alignment. This position will also exaggerate any pronounced curves or flattening in the natural curves of the spine.

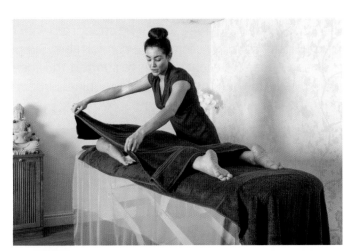

Covering the client with towels helps to maintain client modesty

HANDY HINT

A headband may be applied if the client requests one to protect their hair from oil.

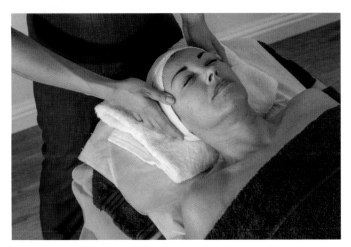

Secure a headband on the client's head to protect their hair from massage products

You should:

- check for contra-indications
- check the skin of each area before you apply oil
- always check the feet and sanitise the client's feet using an antiseptic wipe or spray
- if the face is being included in the treatment, cleanse it to remove any make-up.

Before the client gets on the couch, you may be required to carry out a postural assessment (see pages 265-266).

Once the client is on the couch, you can make them comfortable. Make sure their head is supported on a small pillow, bolster or folded towel if you are starting with the client in a **supine** position. Check that you can still get your hands around the back of their neck and shoulders for when you massage this area so that you don't have to disturb your client later by adjusting the head support. Ask the client if they want their arms tucked under the cover or out.

It is very unnatural to lie completely flat – this puts strain on the natural curves of the body. Natural curves should be supported with towels or similar props to help make the client more comfortable. Supports should be placed under the client's knees to support the knee joints and prevent any strain when the client is lying supine. Supports are placed under the ankles when lying **prone**.

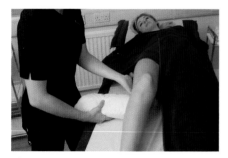

Placing support under the client's knees will make them more comfortable

Supine

Lying on one's back or spine (think of the 'S' to help you remember).

Prone

Lying on one's front.

INDUSTRY TIP

An unsupported neck can put pressure on the blood vessels that run up the side of the neck and curve around the vertebrae and can cause some clients to feel unwell.

INDUSTRY TIP

You can make a support by rolling up a small hand towel. Alternatively many manufacturers have pre-shaped supports which can be purchased.

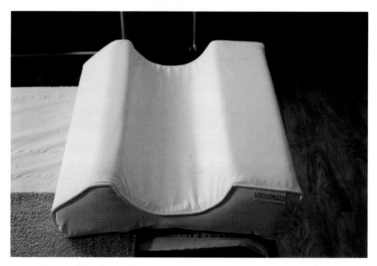

For a client with a large bust, a massage pillow can be used to aid their comfort

Provide body massage treatments

Your posture

Maintaining good posture is essential to enable you to use your body efficiently and to avoid becoming tired or straining ligaments and muscles. During treatment avoid locking your joints such as elbows, wrists, thumbs and fingers, as this puts a lot of strain through the joint. Remain relaxed, bend at the knees and keep the abdomen tucked in. Keep your back straight and your shoulders loose (check to make sure you are not tensing them, making them rise up). Avoid twisting as much as possible.

There are two specific stances that are used when providing a massage treatment:

■ Walk standing – used when working down the length of the body, for example effleuraging the leg. Stand at the side of the couch with your hip next to the couch, as if about to take a long stride. Weight is transferred from one foot to the other, almost in a rocking motion. This stance is important when applying forearm massage to allow a long following movement without breaking contact with the skin.

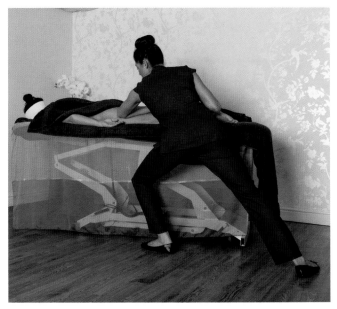
Walk standing

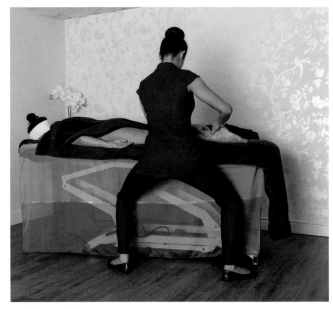
Stride standing

■ Stride standing – used when working crossways across the body, for example hacking. Stand facing the couch with feet hip-width apart, and bend at the knees to lower yourself so that your back stays straight.

The effects and benefits of massage therapy on the body

The effect is the result of your treatment and the benefit is how the client will feel as a result.

There are two types of effects that can be achieved with any treatment:

- psychological – this is how the treatment makes you feel mentally (eg uplifted)
- physiological – this is the effect the treatment has on the body (eg producing an erythema).

Psychological effects

Body massage has many possible effects on the client, including:

- mental relaxation
- feelings of well-being (eg contentment, calm)
- uplifting effects
- motivational effects – these can be used as a pleasurable incentive to help the client achieve targets such as weight loss
- emotional effects (eg crying).

Desquamation

The removal of dead skin cells from the surface of the skin.

Physiological effects on systems of the body

Body system	Effects and benefits
Skin	Improves the circulation – bringing oxygen and nutrients to the tissues and improving the general appearance and condition of the skin.
	Sweat and sebaceous glands are stimulated, producing more sebum and making the skin soft and supple.
	Aids **desquamation** as the dead skin cells are rubbed off the surface during massage. This leaves the skin feeling much softer than before.
	Improved circulation gives the skin a healthy glow.
	Oil or cream used nourishes and softens the skin.
Lymphatic	The action on the tissues helps pump the tissue fluid, making it more responsive, especially when directed towards the nearest lymph nodes.
	Stimulates the removal of waste products from the intercellular tissues.
	Excess tissue fluid is directed towards the lymph nodes for filtration.
Skeletal	Increased circulation encourages nutrients into the skeletal system and removes waste products.
	Passive joint movement helps to improve joint mobility by encouraging the movement of synovial fluid within the joint.

Body system	Effects and benefits
Muscular	Stimulating the circulation increases uptake of nutrients in the muscle cells and removes waste products, such as lactic acid, from within the muscles.
	The stretching and kneading of the muscle tissue helps to improve elasticity.
	Relieves muscular aches and pains.
	The movement of the muscle fibres during massage helps to keep them more mobile, increasing the circulation and reducing tension.
Respiratory	Circulation to the bronchioles is improved, which brings nutrients to the tissues.
	Mucus may be dislodged.
	Gaseous exchange is improved due to the increased circulation to lung tissue (replenishing oxygen and removing carbon dioxide).
Digestive	Direct massage to the abdominal area increases **peristalsis**, which in turn stimulates digestive enzymes.
Urinary	Aids the removal of waste products and toxins.
	The general increase in cellular activity stimulates urine production to aid removal of waste products.
Endocrine	Release of certain hormones helps maintain homeostasis and a sense of well-being.
Nervous	Stimulates, invigorates or soothes the nerve endings dependent upon the massage technique used.
	Endorphins are released, which help to suppress pain. Being relaxed will help to improve sleep patterns. Clients often experience a great night's sleep following a massage.

Massage techniques

The massage techniques you choose will enable you to achieve your client's treatment objective.

Effleurage

The word 'effleurage' comes from a French word meaning 'to skim over', and includes stroking movements. During effleurage the whole of your palm and fingers are used. Keep your hands and fingers relaxed so that they can mould to the client's body and maintain maximum contact.

Peristalsis

Involuntary muscular movements in the walls of the digestive system that move food through the system.

Endorphins

'Feel good' chemicals released by the pituitary endocrine gland.

HANDY HINT

Endorphins transmit electrical signals within the nervous system. When endorphin levels are high we feel less pain and fewer negative effects of stress.

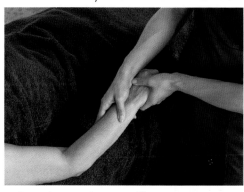

A therapist carrying out effleurage movement

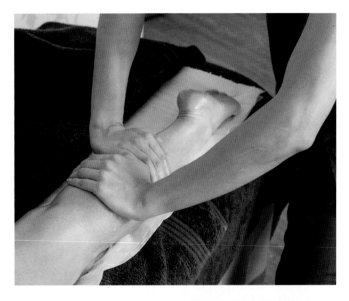
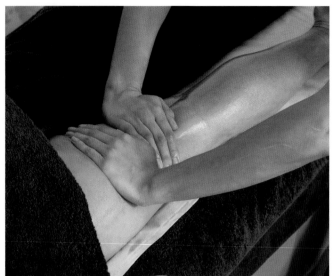
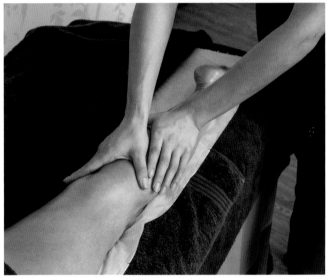
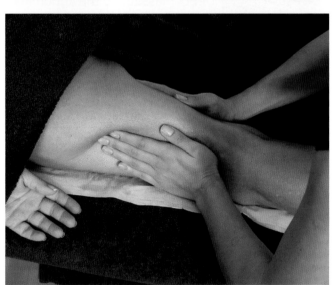

Effleurage movements carried out on the leg

Application of effleurage

- It is used to apply massage mediums to the skin.
- It is used for the first contact and last touch of a massage.
- The movements allow the client to become accustomed to the therapist's touch.
- It links different movements together so that the treatment remains flowing and continuous.
- It assists lymphatic and venous drainage.
- It increases micro-circulation, warms the skin and produces erythema.
- It increases cellular activity and metabolic rate.
- It can be applied in different ways for different effects. If applied slowly and lightly it will induce relaxation; if applied at a brisk pace it will stimulate and uplift.

HANDY HINT

Double-handed effleurage can be used as a soothing movement over the abdomen.

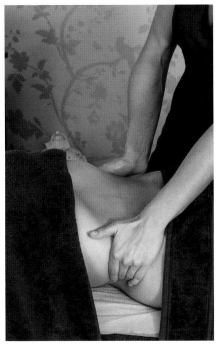

Effleurage movement being carried out on the abdomen

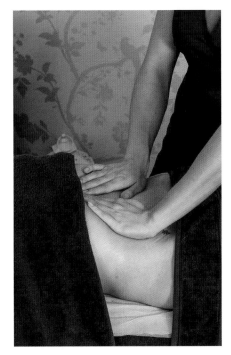

Effleurage movement being carried out on the back

Petrissage

This movement involves lifting and squeezing muscles and tissues, and is often referred to as kneading. Any pressure applied below the heart should always be applied in the direction of the heart. There are several different ways in which petrissage can be applied.

Technique	Parts of the hands and arms used	Method
Kneading	Palms of the hand Heels of the hands Forearms Thumbs Fingers	Work in a circular motion. Hands can work singularly or in pairs – the circular motion may be applied in opposite directions for a deeper effect.

Technique	Parts of the hands and arms used	Method
Picking up	Fingers Thumbs	Pick up tissue with one hand and pass it to the other while gently lifting and squeezing it.
Wringing	Palms of the hands Forearms	Use hands in opposite directions, lifting the tissue up, sliding the hands against each other and releasing the tissue again. Use this over larger areas of tissue (eg thighs and abdomen) to prevent discomfort.
Rolling	Fingertips Thumbs	Lift the body tissue up with the fingers and then push down towards the fingers using the thumbs.

Technique	Parts of the hands and arms used	Method
Ironing (reinforced kneading) 	Palms of the hands Heels of the hands Forearms	Place one hand on top of the other and place the palm and fingers on to the body tissue. Apply firm pressure, working in a circular motion.
Knuckling 	Using the knuckles of the hand	Work in circular movements; this is a deep technique.

Application of petrissage

◾ It can assist lymphatic drainage.

◾ The squeezing action of the muscles stimulates arteriole circulation, including in the skin, muscles and bones, causing vasodilation and erythema.

◾ It loosens tight tissue.

◾ It increases cellular metabolism.

◾ It stimulates peristalsis when used over the abdominal area.

◾ Wringing improves muscle elasticity by stretching movements along the length of the muscle tissue, and softens hard subcutaneous fatty tissue.

◾ Rolling improves skin elasticity, and softens subcutaneous tissue.

INDUSTRY TIP

When muscles become over-worked they produce too much waste. This causes the muscle fibres to become sticky and immobile and the circulation does not flow easily. We can feel this as an area of hardness or tightness within a muscle as we massage over it. Massage helps to encourage the circulation in this sluggish area, to remove the waste and encourage the muscle fibres to move more freely again.

Frictions

These are small movements, made either in a circular motion or with a backwards and forwards (transverse) movement, with constant pressure applied. They are often classified as petrissage movements. The palms of the hand or the fingers or thumbs are used to rub the skin and underlying tissue briskly. This action can be done in circles or backwards and forwards in a criss-cross movement.

Application of frictions

- They loosen muscle adhesions.
- They help with rapid increase of the circulation, causing vasodilation and erythema.
- They assist with lymphatic circulation in the area.
- They soften scar tissue by stretching and softening collagen fibres.
- They stimulate nerve endings.

INDUSTRY TIP

When applying massage techniques, don't waste energy using muscles you don't need – keep your hips still and just let the upper body do the work.

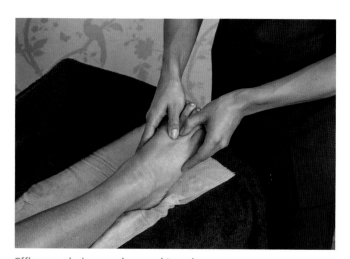

Effleurage being used around tarsals

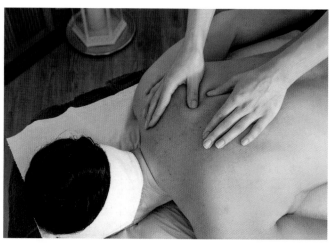

Frictions being used around erector spinae muscles

Vibrations

The vibrations technique involves shaking the skin tissue and muscle. It can be applied with the fingers or palms of the hands. Vibrations can be static and applied in one area by trembling the fingertips, forming a vibration on the skin. They can also be applied with the hand moving (which is often easier to do), creating running vibrations over a larger area.

Vibrations are also very effective lymph drainage techniques, but they do need to be light.

Application of vibrations

- They soothe and clear nerve pathways.
- They relax muscle fibres.
- They stimulate lymphatic activity in an area.

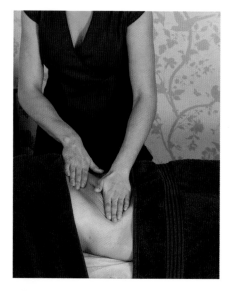

Vibrations on the body

Tapotements

Tapotements are quick, brisk movements that are carried out rhythmically, which is why they are often referred to as percussion movements. They are very beneficial when used appropriately and are no more tiring than other techniques when carried out correctly. Tapotement techniques are not usually used with pre-blended massage oils to avoid over-stimulation that could be caused by the combination of the product and technique.

Technique	Parts of the hands and arms used	Method
Cupping	Cupped hands	With cupped hands and elbows slightly bent, flex and extend the wrist – quickly moving alternate hands up and down on the area. A hollow, clapping noise should be heard as the hands create a vacuum effect between the flesh and the hands. If you hear slapping, review your technique.
Hacking	Ulna border of both hands	Have your fingers held loosely together and relaxed. The little finger and ring finger gently strike the area. Keep your hands working alternately in a brisk rhythm.
Pincement	Fingertips and thumb	Fingertips pick up loose tissue in an alternating action. (This is excellent on areas of poor circulation such as the backs of the arms and the toes.)

Technique	Parts of the hands and arms used	Method
Pounding	Ulna border of loose fists	Think of pounding on a door – hands pound in an alternating action over the area. This movement is only used over areas that are well padded, such as the upper thighs and gluteals.
Beating	Ulna border of loose fists	Keep your thumbs relaxed and tucked into loosely clenched fists, and elbows slightly bent. Alternately press the fists lightly on to the body, developing a brisk, stimulating rhythm. Think of beating batter in a bowl – your hands rotate around each other towards your body, striking the flesh using the ulna border. The circular movement lifts the tissues. This movement is only used over areas that are well padded, such as the upper thighs and gluteals.

Application of tapotements

- They give a rapid increase in circulation, leading to vasodilation and erythema.
- They stimulate nerve endings in the muscles, causing minute muscle contractions as a reflexive response.
- They increase cellular metabolism.
- They are great over the upper back to help loosen chest mucus.
- They can be applied gently towards the end of a treatment to gently wake the client up.

Additional techniques

Passive joint movements

These are used to take a joint such as the ankle or wrist through a range of movements unaided by the client – they just relax. This helps to improve and maintain joint mobility and flexibility. When using this technique the joints should never be forced or over-extended.

Lymphatic massage

These are light movements that work just below the skin to stimulate the drainage of lymph within the body tissues. Lymph, or tissue fluid,

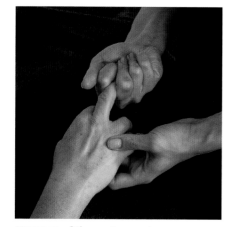
Massage of the metacarpals

vibrates rather than flows like the blood, and moves very slowly – about 1cm per minute. There are two main types of lymphatic drainage movements:

- slow stroking or fanning movements, performed in the direction of the nearest lymph nodes and in the direction of the heart
- pumping or light repetitive pressure using the fingertips.

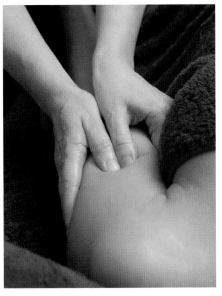
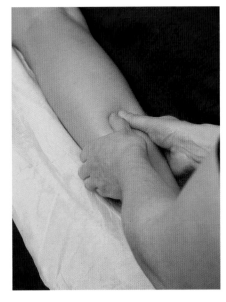
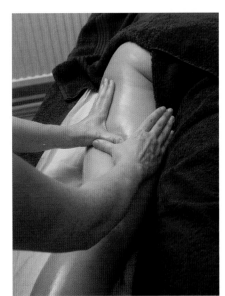

Pressure point movement

Neuromuscular massage technique

This technique has an effect on both the nerves and muscular tissues. Static pressure is applied to points in a muscle using either the thumbs, knuckles or elbows. These points are usually the tender spots where nodules and areas of dense tissue are found in the muscles. The client takes a deep breath and pressure is then applied as the client breathes out. This pressure is maintained for up to 30 seconds. When the pressure is released, circulation rushes into the tissues and helps to alleviate the symptoms of muscular aches and pains.

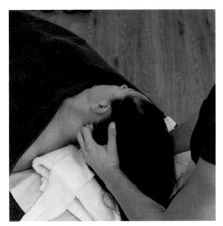

Neuromuscular massage

Massage mediums

There are a variety of massage mediums available to use. When choosing one, consider the following:

- skin type
- skin condition
- client preference
- allergies
- amount of hair in the area
- 'slip' required
- whether massage is to be combined with another treatment.

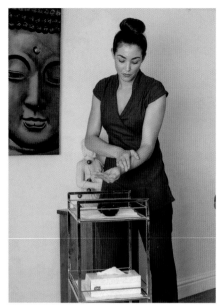

Massage oil being applied to the therapist's hands

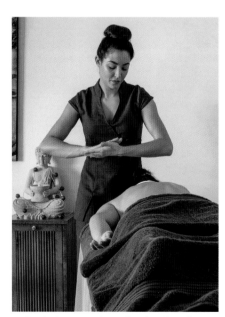

A therapist warming oil in her hands

Familiarise yourself with the different skin types and conditions before selecting your massage medium, to ensure you are using the most beneficial product for the client.

Massage oils

Massage oil is the most popular choice of medium for body massage, as it gives the best slip, allowing the hands to glide easily across the skin's surface.

The most beneficial oils are natural vegetable, fruit or seed oils. The skin readily absorbs natural oils, and they can help to soften and nourish the skin, keeping it supple. Different oils are suitable for different skin types and give different effects.

Mineral oils are the main ingredient in many massage oils and leave the skin feeling soft and supple. Mineral oils are not absorbed as easily as base oils, because they are made up of large hydrocarbon molecules, by-products of the oil refining process. This kind of oil stays on the surface of the skin for longer and is a popular ingredient in perfumed body lotions and creams.

Massage creams

Massage cream can be very effective on dry skin and is ideal to use on clients who do not like the feel of oil. Creams are easily absorbed into the skin – but it is only necessary to use a small amount as cream spreads widely once warm.

Pre-blended massage oils, creams and balms

Many companies produce a range of massage products to use for massage treatments. Often these are developed for a signature treatment that will follow a set routine.

Pre-blended massage products are formulated for specific treatment objectives. Familiarise yourself with the products and their ingredients so that you can be sure they are suitable for use on particular clients.

Pre-blended oils can:

■ enhance relaxation

■ provide a sense of well-being

■ ease joint and muscle pain

■ be invigorating and uplifting

■ improve skin and body conditions.

The benefits of using pre-blended products are that no measuring of essential oils and carrier oils is required, and they are easy to select according to the client's needs. They are often marketed under a brand name, which will give the client confidence in the treatment. The disadvantage of using pre-blended products is that the client may not like the smell of the blend most suited to their needs.

Powders

Choose the finest, unperfumed powders for use with massage. Powder will permit a firmer massage because it does not provide slip, as an oil or cream would. It is rarely used in the industry today, but it is a suitable alternative for use on a client with oily skin or if the client has a perspiration problem. If the skin is dry, powder will dry the skin further because it will absorb any oil and moisture on the skin's surface. The skin will need to be cleansed following treatment to remove the residue.

Powder your hands rather than pouring the product directly on to the client's skin. Keep powder use to a minimum, and avoid shaking it, as it creates a dusty atmosphere and will get in the eyes and nose of the client. Powder has also been found to aggravate respiratory conditions such as asthma.

INDUSTRY TIP
Refresh your product knowledge regularly so that you know what ingredients the oils contain.

INDUSTRY TIP
Powder is sometimes used on a hairy male client to avoid friction.

Activity

The amount of oil you use will depend on several factors including the client's skin type (texture, and condition) and the size of the client. Some oils are more viscous and absorb less easily, while other are less viscous and absorb more easily than others.

A typical full body massage will use about 20–40ml of oil. (As a rough guide, 10ml for the back, 5ml for the scalp and 5ml for the face.)

If a bottle contains 473ml, how many full body treatments will you get out of the bottle? How many back massage treatments (10ml each)?

What percentage of the bottle will you use per treatment?

HANDY HINT
Soy and jojoba are often used to make candles that, once lit, melt the wax so that it can used warm to massage with. These make great retail lines in the salon. Always test the temperature to prevent any risk of burning before applying.

Safety precautions

All products should be used according to health and safety guidelines. There are some further safety considerations when using base or carrier oils and pre-blended products.

Correct storage

As with all products, correct storage of massage mediums is important. Carrier oils and blended essential oils need to be stored in dark bottles. Check the manufacturer's instructions for correct storage methods.

Toxicity

If a product is toxic, it means it is poisonous. In some cases, it might even be fatal in large quantities (for example, large amounts of essential oils).

INDUSTRY TIP
The average shelf life once a container is open will vary and you should check for the symbol on the product container to guide you. (This is usually a small picture of a container with a number in it.)

Phototoxicity

This means that a product is sensitive to sunlight, and may cause a skin reaction when exposed to ultraviolet rays. If the skin is exposed to the sun after having oil applied, the mixture of the essential oil and the ultraviolet rays may result in itching, redness or burning, or an increase in skin pigmentation in the area. The main phototoxic oils are citrus oils.

Irritants

The skin may become irritated when an essential oil is applied to it. The skin cells may produce a histamine reaction and the area may become red, itchy and inflamed. The severity of the irritation will depend on the strength of the blend used.

Over-exposure

Over-exposure to products can cause irritation, sensitivity or result in toxic levels being used.

Disposal of massage mediums

It is a good idea to measure out what you need or to use a container that has a pump dispenser to avoid waste. If there is any product left over after the massage, it should be soaked up with a tissue and placed in a lined bin ready for disposal.

Activity

To see how loss in profit can add up, calculate how much it would cost to dispose of 5ml of massage cream. The bottle costs £3.99 and contains 150ml.

Treatment timings

A full body massage or massage using pre-blended oils should take one hour. If the face and scalp are included, it will take 75 minutes. A back treatment on its own should take 30 minutes. If you need to adapt or modify your treatment, it should still last for the expected duration – you will need to extend the treatment in an appropriate area to achieve this.

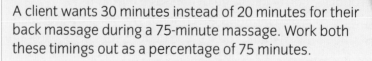

Activity

A client wants 30 minutes instead of 20 minutes for their back massage during a 75-minute massage. Work both these timings out as a percentage of 75 minutes.

How much would 7 minutes be as a percentage of a 60-minute massage?

Massage sequence

Massages can follow different routines and orders of work. They should be modified to suit each client, and each therapist will perfect their own routines. The exception is when you are performing a signature treatment, where the routine will be set to suit specific products. Each training centre will have a specific routine which will be used for training until you are confident enough to adapt it and work on your own routine.

As a general rule, effleurage is always used first, followed by petrissage. Other techniques may then follow. Frictions are excellent for increasing the circulation quickly. Tapotement is often used last before finishing the treatment area with further effleurage to drain and soothe.

Select a massage medium suitable for the client's skin type and condition. Apply it to your hands and lower arms up to the elbows. Then apply the medium to the client's skin with light effleurage movements, starting across the décolleté and moving up the neck and face.

A simple massage routine is given below to demonstrate the logical sequence of a treatment. You will be given a more detailed routine to follow by your tutors.

Effleurage should be applied at the start of each treatment area to apply your oil and between each technique to maintain the flow and continuity of the massage.

VALUES & BEHAVIOURS

Creativity skills

 Watch a video of this body massage treatment on SmartScreen (unit 303).

Consultation

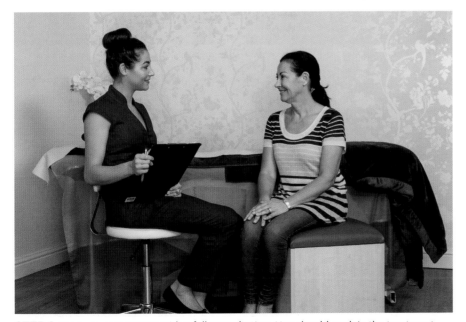

STEP 1 Start your treatment with a full consultation. You should explain the treatment process in full and agree your client's treatment objectives and a treatment plan. The client should give you verbal and signed consent. You can then leave your client to get undressed and position themselves on the couch.

Supine

Legs

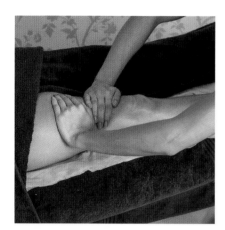

STEP 2 Start with the left leg. Apply your medium using effleurage.

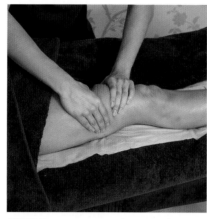

STEP 3 Petrissage to the upper leg, including kneading.

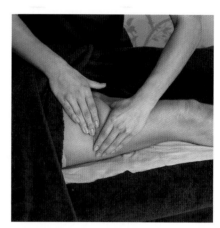

STEP 4 Pick up and squeeze.

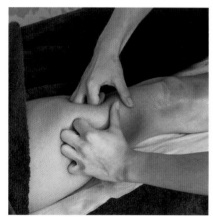

STEP 5 Knuckling.

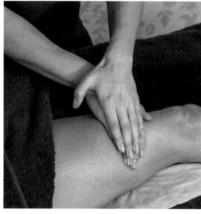

STEP 6 Reinforced kneading and tapotement to upper thigh – hacking cupping interspaced with effleurage.

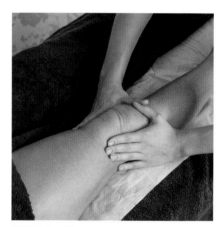

STEP 7 Effleurage around patella.

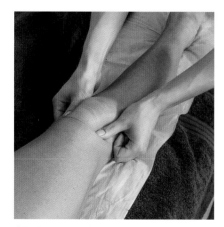

STEP 8 Kneading around patella.

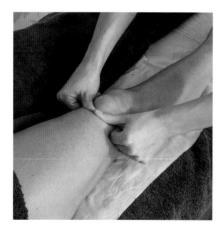

STEP 9 Frictions around patella.

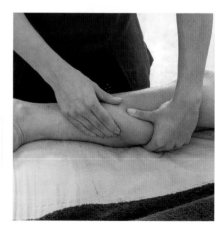

STEP 10 Petrissage to lower leg.

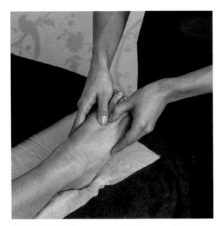

STEP 11 Effleurage, petrissage, friction to foot. Effleurage whole leg to finish. Repeat on right leg.

HANDY HINT

You can put a rolled up hand towel under the client's knee to offer extra support.

Arms

Massage the left arm and then the right so that you work around the body anticlockwise. Support the arm well during the treatment to make sure the client is relaxed as it can often feel an awkward area to work on. Make sure you continue to monitor and maintain good posture.

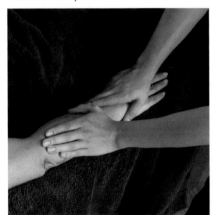

STEP 12 Effleurage to apply oil and warm up tissues.

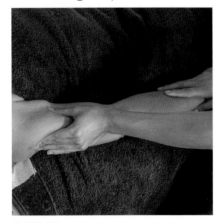

STEP 13 Petrissage to upper arm kneading, make sure you include the deltoid around the shoulder.

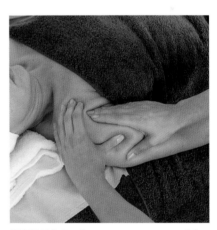

STEP 14 Petrissage to upper arm pick and squeeze.

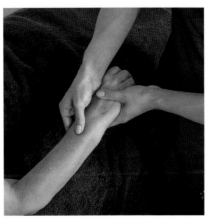

STEP 15 Effleurage the lower arm.

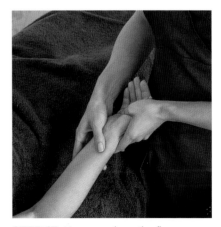

STEP 16 Petrissage to lower arm. Particularly along the extensor muscle which is often very tight.

STEP 17 Massage along the flexors.

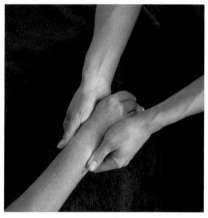

STEP 18 Massage around the wrist with petrissage; frictions can also be used here.

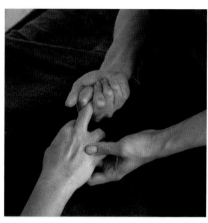

STEP 19 Onto the hand, massage each finger in turn. Effleurage whole arm to finish.

Abdomen

To avoid disturbing the client, check before you start whether the client wishes to have this area included.

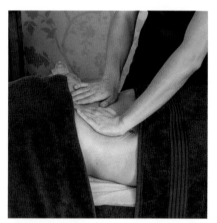

STEP 20 Effleurage up and around the abdomen.

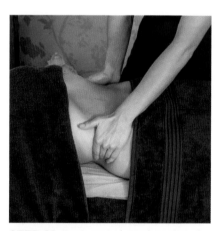

STEP 21 Petrissage along the sides of the abdomen, including kneading; pick up and squeeze.

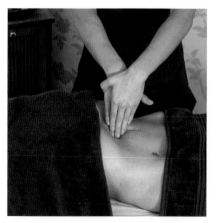

STEP 22 Using reinforced kneading massage clockwise around the abdomen. This is a good move for anyone with a sluggish digestion.

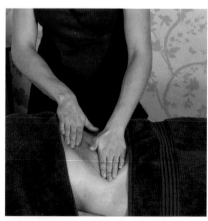

STEP 23 Vibrations across the abdomen will help stimulate the digestion. Finish with more effleurage.

Neck and shoulders (décolleté)

Lying supine the neck is in a more relaxed position than when the client is lying prone and a good opportunity to relieve stress and tension in the muscles. You can also work down the top of the arms in a more relaxed position.

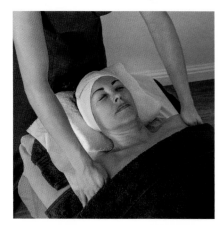

STEP 24 Effleurage around the chest, shoulders and neck.

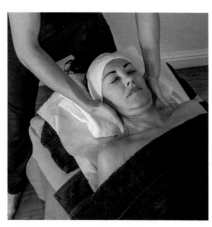

STEP 25 Effleurage up the neck and stretch the muscle well.

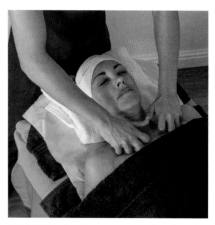

STEP 26 Petrissage across the chest using kneading and knuckling.

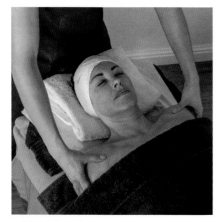

STEP 27 Make sure you include the shoulders and upper arms.

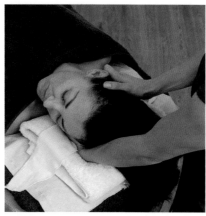

STEP 28 Slowly turn the neck to one side and knead around the neck and behind the ear.

Face

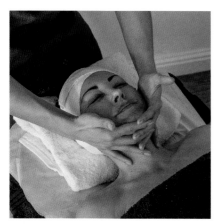

STEP 29 Effleurage up the neck and across the mandible.

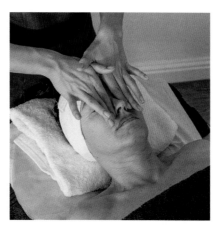

STEP 30 Effleurage up the sides of the nose.

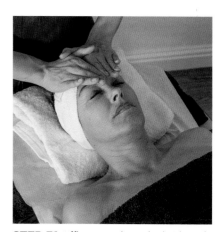

STEP 31 Effleurage along the bridge of the nose.

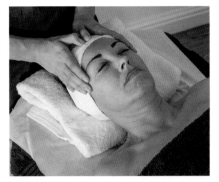

STEP 32 Effleurage across the forehead and circle the temples.

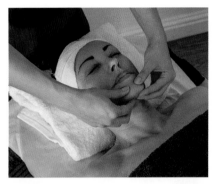

STEP 33 Pressure point massage to the chin.

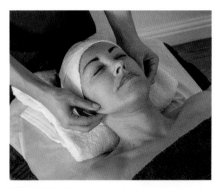

STEP 34 Pressure point massage along the mandible.

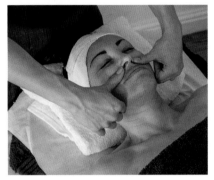

STEP 35 Pressure point massage along the maxillae (upper jaw).

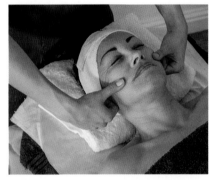

STEP 36 Pressure points below the zygomatic bone.

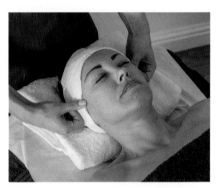

STEP 37 Pressure points along the zygomatic bone.

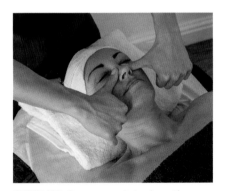

STEP 38 Pressure points along the eye socket.

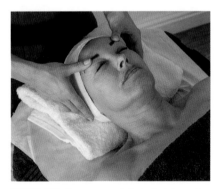

STEP 39 Pressure points to bridge of nose.

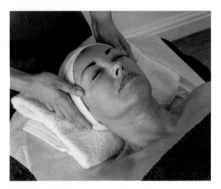

STEP 40 Pressure points along eyebrow line.

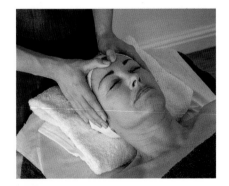

STEP 41 Pressure points across forehead.

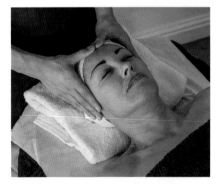

STEP 42 Slowly work up forehead continuing to apply pressure points moving out across the forehead. The last line of pressure points will be in the hairline.

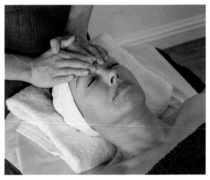

STEP 43 Smoothe along the forehead with effleurage.

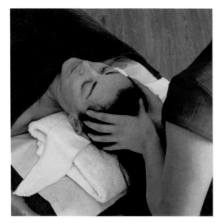

STEP 44 Massage into the hairline with finger petrissage (shampooing).

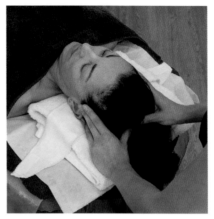

STEP 45 Apply pressure points along the scalp.

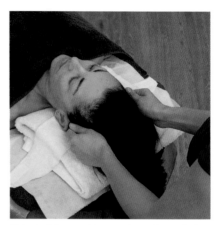

STEP 46 Finish by stroking through the hair.

Prone

Help the client to turn over, carefully managing the towels to maintain modesty.

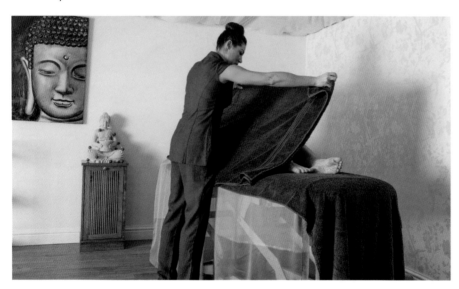

Legs

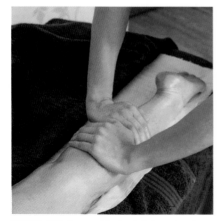

STEP 47 Start with the left leg. Apply your massage medium.

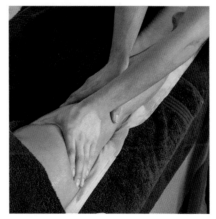

STEP 48 Effleurage the whole leg.

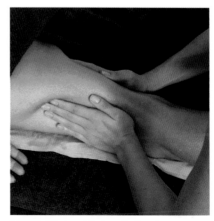

STEP 49 Double-handed pick-up to thigh.

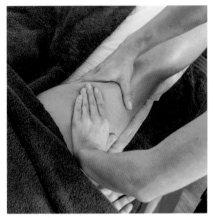

STEP 50 Petrissage, kneading.

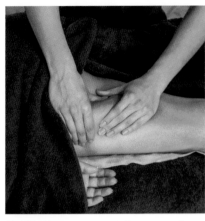

STEP 51 Petrissage, picking up and squeezing.

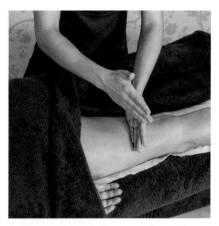

STEP 52a Finish the upper leg with tapotement, first hacking.

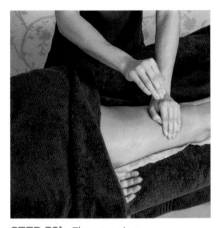

STEP 52b Then cupping.

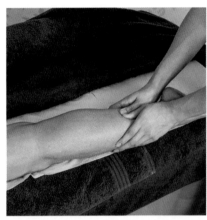

STEP 53 Effleurage down the leg to the calf. Many people find that deep work on the back of the calf can be quite uncomfortable, so monitor the client's body language.

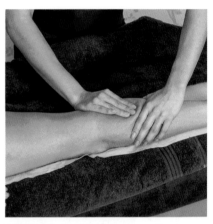

STEP 54 Petrissage to the calf using kneading and pick up and squeeze.

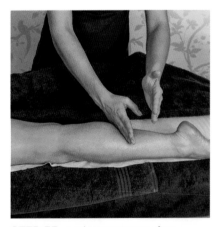

STEP 55 Apply tapotement, first hacking.

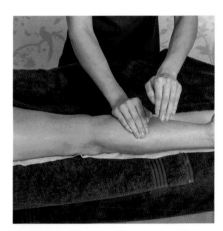

STEP 56 Then cupping. Finish with effleurage. Cover the leg and repeat to the other leg.

Back

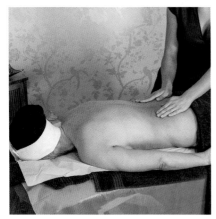

STEP 57 Effleurage the back.

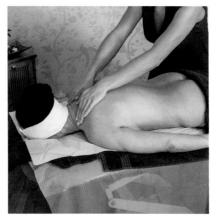

STEP 58 Ensure you massage over the tops of the shoulders.

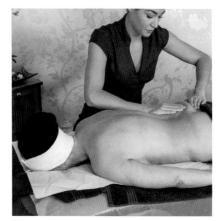

STEP 59a Petrissage using a range of movements including kneading.

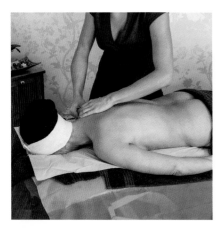

STEP 59b Finger kneading.

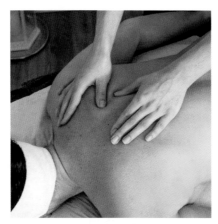

STEP 59c Thumb kneading, in particular around the edge of the scapula.

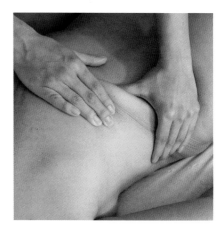

STEP 59d Wringing.

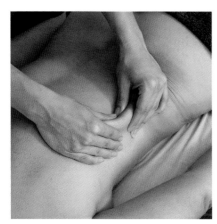

STEP 59e Skin rolling along sides of back and across shoulder.

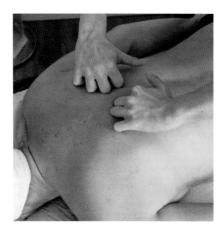

STEP 59f Knuckling.

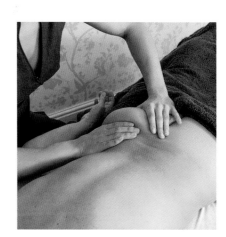

STEP 60a Include the top of the gluteal with your petrissage. Kneading.

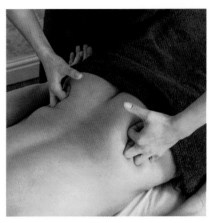

STEP 60b Knuckling.

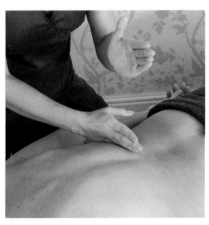

STEP 61a Finally some petrissage to stimulate. These movements will also help to wake the client up as you come towards the end of your massage. Hacking.

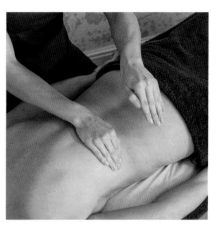

STEP 61b Cupping.

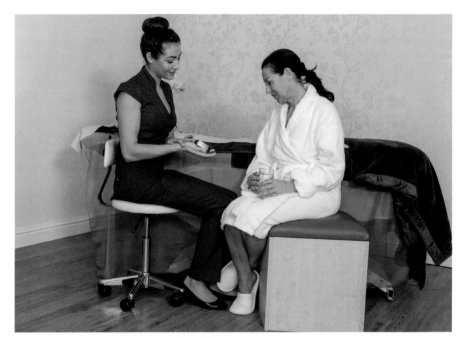

STEP 62 Complete your massage with some slow effleurage. Give the client a few minutes to relax and then help them up from the couch onto a chair. Offer the client advice and recommendations while they drink a glass of water.

Massage using the forearms and elbows

Massage isn't just about the hands – other parts of the arm can be used to help take the pressure off the joints of the hands and prevent repetitive strain injuries.

With any massage it is important to try to use the pressure of your body weight rather than push into the joint as this will over-stretch and strain the tendons.

Massage without using the hands predominantly uses the forearm or the elbow to achieve a similar soft tissue massage effect as the hands.

These strokes cover a larger area and can feel much deeper than normal massage techniques to a client. They are usually applied with slower, more sweeping movements to enhance relaxation.

The forearm

The forearm is excellent for covering a large area while applying even pressure. When applying this technique it is important that the hand is loose so that the flexor and extensor muscles of the forearm are in a relaxed state. The soft muscles of mainly the flexor groups are used to massage the skin. Occasional the ulna and border and the extensor muscles can be used. If the muscles are tense it changes the feel of the technique and it will feel hard and uncomfortable both to perform and receive.

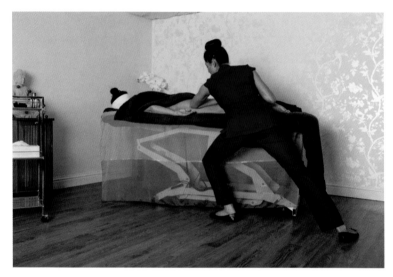

Massage using the forearm

The elbow

The proximal end of the ulna (olecranon) is used to replace the pressure often used by the thumb to get deep into the tissue. It is often used with the other hand to support the area around it and to guide the elbow. This helps to prevent the elbow slipping and causing discomfort.

Posture

When applying techniques without the hands, the therapist will need to give their posture different considerations. These techniques involve more movement from the therapist than in traditional Swedish massage, as there are often long strokes requiring more bending and stretching. The recommended posture is to stand with the knees bent, back straight and to rock through the legs to shift the weight from side to side. The therapist will need to develop strong leg and back muscles to support their posture as they work, and a supple body to enable it to move freely during treatment while maintaining good posture. The techniques mean

INDUSTRY TIP

In some Eastern massage techniques, the feet are used – this might be something you might like to try.

HEALTH & SAFETY

Continually applying pressure and over-extending damaged tendons will cause permanent damage. The tendons need time to begin normal repair and then have pressure gently increased as healing progresses.

INDUSTRY TIP

Attend a tai chi class – this will help you to understand both the flow of movement and working with the breath during movement.

that the therapist will be working much closer to the client's body and so will need to be more aware of personal space and body contact.

Techniques using the forearm

These can be applied in a stroking effleurage style. The forearm can be used so that it glides along the length of the legs or back.

On the legs a version of this technique is used. One hand slides the length of the leg while the other supports the hand by holding the wrist.

Both hands can be used together to sweep up using the ulna and inner forearm across the area; the arms slide down the sides of the back or leg to glide down.

The forearm can also be used to apply petrissage and knead the tissues. Care must be taken to keep the arm soft and relaxed during this technique. The arm sweeps over the area forming small circular movements, while gently rotating the wrist. This can be applied to the limbs, back and abdomen.

Take the forearms across the body in alternating sweeps. Tissue can be lifted between the forearms, lifting and compressing it.

The strokes can also be applied taking the hands down the body on the back and then sweeping the hands out. From this position you can apply some deeper work using the elbows as the arms sweep out.

The ulna border can be used in a pivoting movement, with the elbow resting on the plinth. This is a great movement when applied to the shoulders, pushing down to relax them and sweeping out towards the arm.

The upper inner arms can also be used for scooping, as if embracing the client's upper arm into the therapist arms; the client's arm can be gently compressed and stretched as the therapist draws their own arms down towards the hand. A similar technique can be used on the legs.

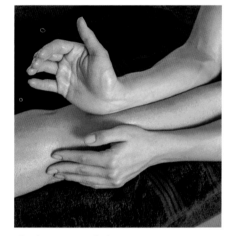

The forearm technique

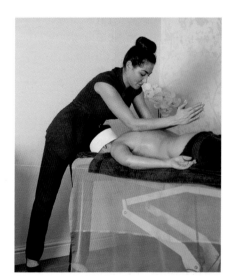
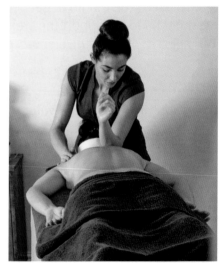

The ulna border of the forearm can be used to push into a muscle and hold a stretch

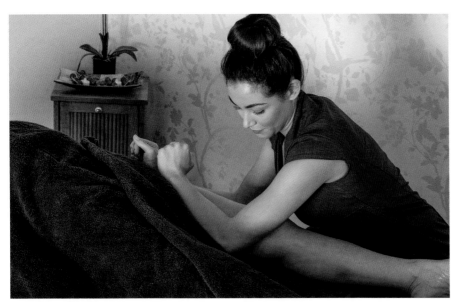

Scooping technique on the legs

Techniques using the elbow

These are used for deeper tissue work to help improve specific areas of tension within a muscle. The elbow is usually used when working on the back or gluteal. Care should be taken to check the pressure when applying this technique with the client and to use the other hand to guide the elbow as you work, especially when working close to the centre of the spinal column.

Apply forearm massage techniques

A simple forearm massage routine is given below to demonstrate the logical sequence of a treatment. You will be given a more detailed routine to follow by your tutor.

Effleurage should be applied at the start of each treatment area to apply your oil and between each technique to maintain the flow and continuity of the massage. You can also use traditional massage techniques to personalise your massage routine.

Watch a video of this forearm massage treatment on SmartScreen (unit 303).

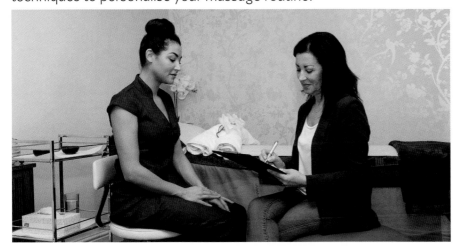

STEP 1 Start your treatment with a full consultation. You should explain the treatment process in full and agree your client's treatment objectives and a treatment plan. The client should give you verbal and signed consent. You can then leave your client to get undressed and position themselves on the couch.

Prone

Back

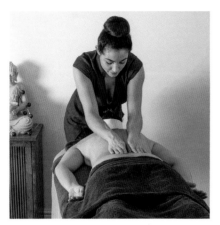

STEP 2 Apply your massage medium. Effleurage the back.

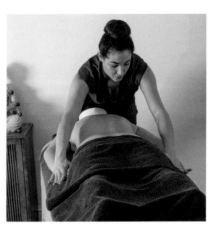

STEP 3 Sweep right down to the hands.

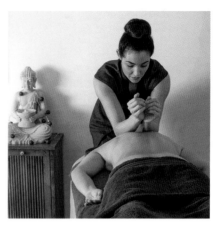

STEP 4 Sweep forearms using the elbows to gently apply deeper pressure.

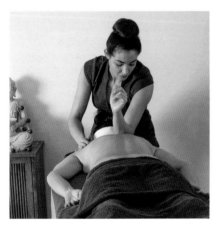

STEP 5 Knead using forearm and slight elbow rotations around scapula and neck.

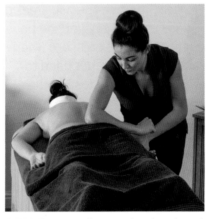

STEP 6 Scoop down to the gluteals and knead, maintaining a slight stretch in the muscle.

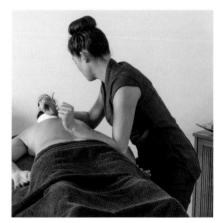

STEP 7 Stretch along the muscles and hold.

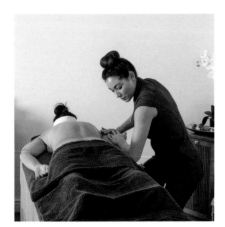

STEP 8 Work down the arms, supporting with one hand and sliding down with the forearm of the other. Keep the movement continuous.

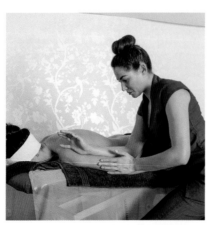

STEP 9 Supporting the limb with one hand, slide with the forearm and knead over the arm.

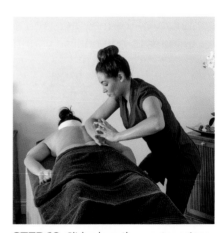

STEP 10 Slide along the erector spinae, applying deeper pressure, working up and down with a continuous movement.

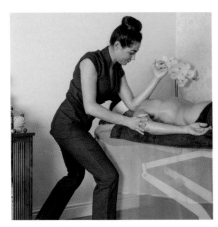

STEP 11 Slide the forearm in to sit in the groove between the neck and shoulder. Push down and hold the stretch. You can also knead in the same position using the forearm.

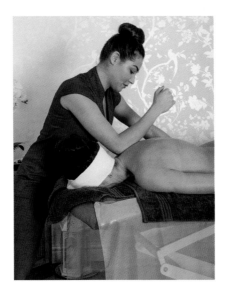

STEP 12 Knead across the top of the shoulders, keeping the movement fluid.

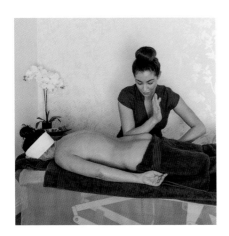

STEP 13 Knead along the edge of the back with the forearm.

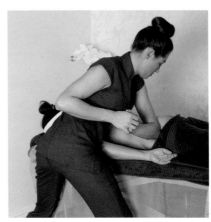

STEP 14 Pressure points can be applied using the elbow. Working into the sciatic point is shown here.

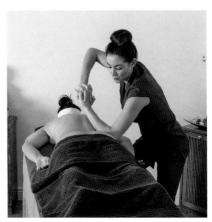

STEP 15 With your hands linked, perform a 'rocking boat' movement up the side of the spine.

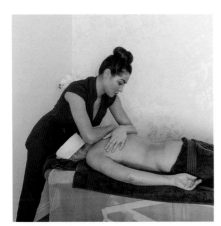

STEP 16 Lean into the arms and apply pressure to work down the back and stretch the muscles.

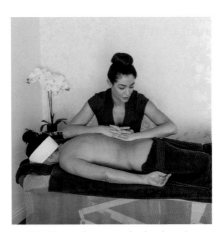

STEP 17 Work across the back and stretch using the large surface of both forearms. Knead around the gluteals.

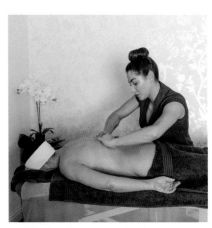

STEP 18 Effleurage to finish.

Back of the legs

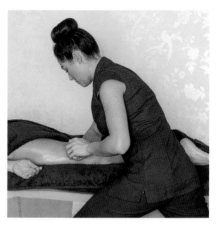

STEP 19 Mould the client's leg between your hands, support the ankle with one hand while sliding up the leg with the other forearm, keeping the hand moulded to the shape of the leg.

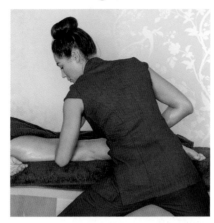

STEP 20 Support the leg with the right arm. Using the ulna side of the forearm, apply deep pressure by leaning into the movement and effleurage up the leg, using the hand to mould to the leg to return.

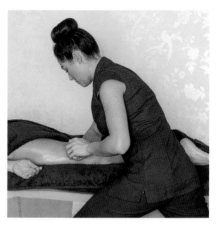

STEP 21 Support the right hand with the left to keep control. Apply deep pressure with the right forearm by leaning into the client's body as you effleurage up the thigh.

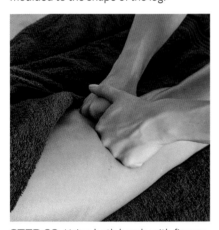

STEP 22 Using both hands with fingers flexed, lean into the hands to apply deep pressure, slowly effleuraging up the leg. Mould the open hands to the thigh to return.

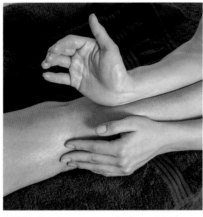

STEP 23 Supporting the leg with the left hand to keep it stable, and using the forearm of the right arm, knead along the gastrocnemius.

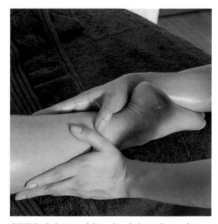

STEP 24 Moulding both hands to the leg to keep it stable, start at the ankle and effleurage up the leg using the forearms.

Supine

Front of the legs

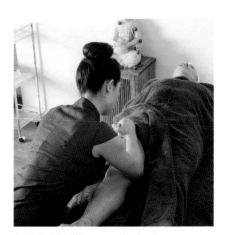

STEP 25 Effleurage the leg.

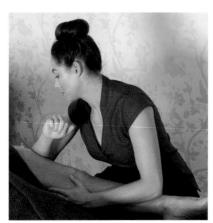

STEP 26 Knead, using the right arm and supporting the leg with the left.

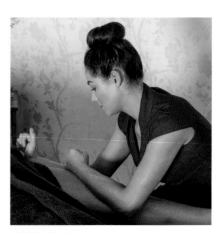

STEP 27 Knead, using both arms in a continuous flow.

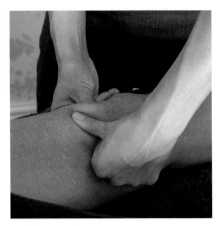

STEP 28 Work with the thumbs to knead around the patella.

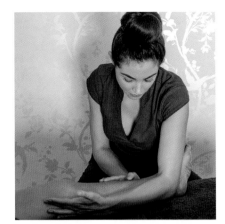

STEP 29 Slide with one hand, supporting with the other, to massage the inner calf.

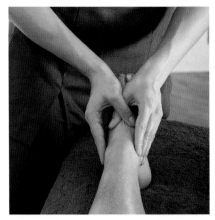

STEP 30 Massage across the top of the foot using the thumbs. Effleurage to whole leg.

Arms

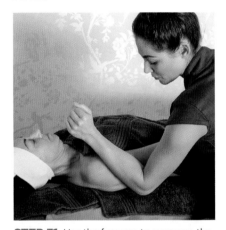

STEP 31 Use the forearm to massage the upper arm, supporting with the other hand.

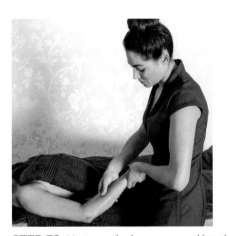

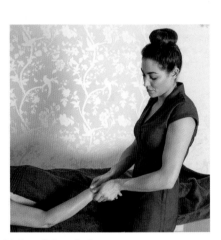

STEP 32 Massage the lower arm and hand with Swedish techniques.

Abdomen

To avoid disturbing the client, check before you start whether the client wishes to have this area included. Abdominal massage is more pleasant than clients often expect it to be, so it is worth encouraging clients to have the experience.

INDUSTRY TIP

It is very important to avoid bone-on-bone contact when performing forearm massage, as this will be very uncomfortable for both the therapist and the client.

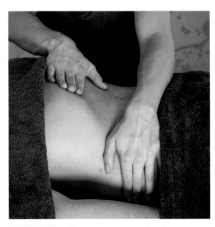

STEP 33 Effleurage using the forearms.

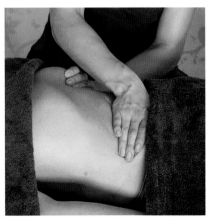

STEP 34 Knead across the abdomen.

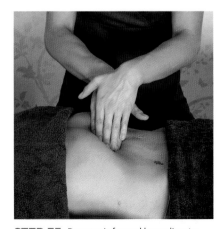

STEP 35 Deep reinforced kneading to stimulate digestion. Effleurage to finish.

Décolleté

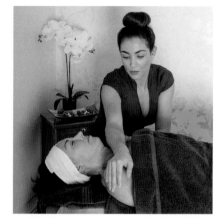

STEP 36 Effleurage around décolleté.

STEP 37 Using the forearm, effleurage the over chest.

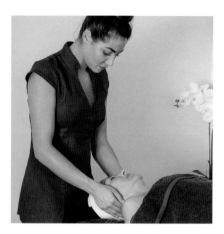

STEP 38 Effleurage the neck and stretch the neck muscles.

Finish

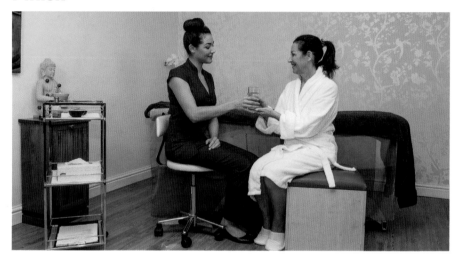

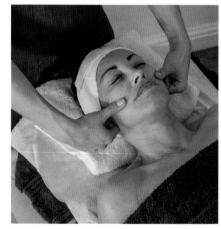

A therapist massaging a client's face from the front position

Adapt massage techniques to achieve treatment objectives

The selection and use of techniques will depend on the client's requirements. The massage should be adapted to suit the client's treatment objectives, unless it is a signature treatment following a set routine.

The treatment objectives for massage therapy include the following:

- Relaxation – use preheat before treatment to help relaxation (unless using pre-blended oils, when heat should be avoided as it may result in intensified contra-actions). To achieve a relaxation treatment, keep effleurage and petrissage movements slow and light, keep techniques rhythmic and use a relaxation blend. Tapotement should be omitted for massage using pre-blended oils but may be useful towards the end of a body massage to wake the client up.

- Sense of well-being – the aim of this treatment is to make the client feel happy and content. A pre-blended oil tailored to this objective could be used.

- Stimulation – use brisk, deep techniques and increase petrissage. Frictions are particularly good for stimulation, and incorporate tapotement techniques when carrying out a body massage.

- Invigorating or uplifting – use techniques that will not sedate the client. Keep up a good pace throughout the treatment and use an uplifting pre-blend such as citrus.

- Sedation – keep techniques light and very slow. Make effleurage slow and long. Using quite repetitive movements, particularly effleurage, as a stroking, soothing movement can be quite hypnotic and calming.

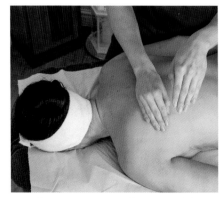

Avoid slow, repetitive effleurage if the client needs stimulation

- Invigoration – use deep, brisk techniques such as vibrations and tapotement.

- Assistance with the improvement of the appearance of cellulite – work predominantly on the problem areas where fat is stored, such as the buttocks and upper thighs. It is also useful to work over the abdomen. Use slow, deep movements and concentrate on petrissage and tapotement.

- Improvement of skin and body conditions – all massage techniques help to assist the natural desquamation of the skin. Using the most appropriate oil for the client's skin type and condition will help to nourish and moisturise the skin leaving it feeling soft, smooth and supple.

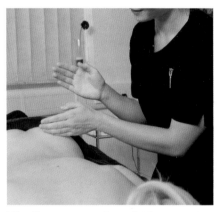

Vibration movements assist in invigoration

Massage modifications

When performing a massage treatment the therapist may have to modify (alter) the treatment in order for it to be effective, for example if the client is obese, very muscular or requires a relaxing or stimulating massage.

Obese client

- Deeper movements are necessary.
- The skin may be sensitive.
- Deep petrissage techniques and, when performing a body massage, hacking, cupping, beating and pounding should be used on areas of excess adipose tissue.

Muscular client

- Use deep, firm effleurage.
- Use slow, deep kneading over tense areas to relax muscles.
- Avoid deep petrissage movements on short contracted muscles, as this may be painful. Use stretching instead.
- Use infrared to preheat before body massage to warm the muscles.

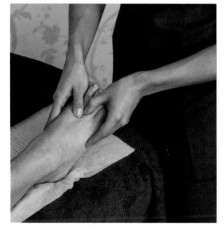

Adapt your treatment depending on your client. Treatment areas like toes in older clients, for instance might be fragile

Elderly client

■ Avoid tapotement over bony areas.

■ Use gentle pressure throughout as the skeletal system may be more fragile.

■ Use infrared to preheat (body massage only).

■ Apply extra frictions around joint areas to stimulate synovial fluid and increase joint mobility.

■ Use passive joint movement to increase mobility.

■ Use lighter effleurage and stroking, to avoid dragging delicate, thinner skin.

Infrared treatment

An infrared (IR) lamp provides a deep heat using infrared rays from a bulb (these rays are part of the electromagnetic spectrum). Infrared is a heat radiation treatment, and the lamp is also known as a 'non-luminous lamp' as the heat can be felt but the rays cannot be seen.

The rays emitted from the lamp vary in intensity depending on how close the lamp is to the skin and the duration of the treatment. The inverse square law says that the light intensity decreases with the distance from the light source. So the further away the lamp is from the subject, the bigger the area it covers and the longer it can be left on.

Where IR travels through air (ie with nothing absorbing the rays), each time you double the distance from the source of the infrared you will halve the original intensity.

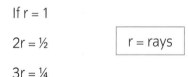

If r = 1

2r = ½   r = rays

3r = ¼

For example, if the lamp is at a distance of 40cm, it can be left on for five minutes. If the distance of the lamp is doubled to 80cm, the time it can be left on for is quadrupled to 20 minutes. So if the distance is doubled, the time is multiplied by four. It is much kinder to the skin to have the lamp further away but to leave it on for a longer length of time. The figure below shows moving the lamp further away from the client reduces the intensity of the rays.

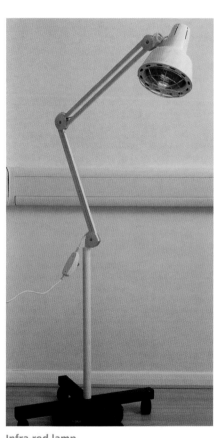

Infra-red lamp

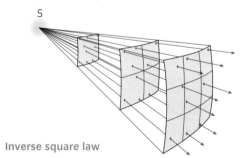

Inverse square law

Infrared enhances the treatment:

- It encourages vasodilation – it increases the body temperature slightly.
- It softens the muscle tissues and relaxes the muscles.
- It stimulates the sebaceous glands and lubricates the skin.
- Its mild heat has a soothing and calming effect on sensory nerve endings.

Application of infrared treatment

Following consultation and preparation of the client:

 Watch a video of infrared treatment on SmartScreen (unit 305).

1 The most common area treated in this way is the back, so position the client prone, with pillows for support that tilt the body slightly towards the lamp.

2 Ensure the eyes are protected by sunbed goggles if the client if having a treatment lying supine, or by draping a towel so that it shields the eyes.

3 Position the lamp so the light rays hit the area at a 90° angle – never put the lamp directly over the client.

4 Follow the manufacturer's instructions on distance and time. Use a tape measure to ensure that the distance is correct. As a guide, lamps are usually left on for 5–20 minutes at a distance of 45–90cm.

5 Observe the skin's reaction throughout, by looking and touching. You should also ask the client how they feel. For safety reasons, never leave the client alone during an IR treatment.

6 At the end of the treatment, switch off the lamp and place it in a safe area to cool down. Place a towel on the lamp so that you can move it. This also acts as a warning to others that the lamp may be hot.

7 Continue with further treatment, such as a back massage.

Provide advice, recommendations and treatment evaluation

Following the treatment you should give the client suitable advice and recommendations. This will help to maximise the benefits of the massage.

General advice

INDUSTRY TIP

For safety and insurance reasons you must never recommend the use of individual aromatherapy oils unless you have been trained as an aromatherapist.

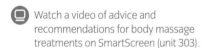 Watch a video of advice and recommendations for body massage treatments on SmartScreen (unit 303).

The client should be advised to do the following after their treatment, ideally until the following day:

- Relax and avoid any strenuous activity – this will give the body time to heal, cleanse and eliminate toxins while benefiting from the relaxed mental and physical state.

- Avoid physical exercise.

- Ensure that food intake following the treatment is light – avoid spicy foods and heavy meals, as these are more difficult to digest.

- Avoid alcohol, which will put toxins back into the body.

- Increase water intake, or drink fruit/herb infusions to keep the body hydrated and flush waste products out of the body.

- Avoid stimulants such as caffeine in coffee, tea, fizzy drinks and energy drinks to maximise the relaxation effect.

- Avoid ultraviolet light and sunbathing – the skin will be more sensitive and pre-blended aromatherapy oils may be phototoxic.

- Drive with extra care if calming or relaxing pre-blends have been used – suggest the client keep the windows slightly open to ensure they remain alert.

- Leave products on the skin and hair to allow them to penetrate – where pre-blended products have been used, the essences need time to change chemically for a longer-lasting effect; oil left on the hair will leave it glossy and hydrated after it has been washed out.

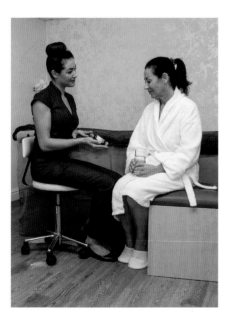

Suggest products for a long-term skincare routine as part of the advice and recommendations

Client-specific advice

There is also longer-term advice to consider:

- Suggest that the client follows a home skincare routine to maintain treatment results and objectives.

- Link-sell and encourage the clients to use any pre-blended products you have used when they go home – there may also be supporting products such as bath, body products and candles.

- Recommend products for your client to use that they will personally benefit from.

- Suggest further treatments to maximise results and reduce the effects of stress. Let the client know how often they should return for repeat treatments.
- Where appropriate, recommend lifestyle changes the client could make to improve their physical well-being. Be tactful and only discuss issues that the client has raised. Suggestions might include:
  - ways to increase physical activity
  - healthy eating advice
  - tips on finding time to relax and de-stress
  - help with reducing or giving up smoking
  - reducing caffeine and alcohol intake.
- Advise on postural awareness according to the client's needs.
- Advise the client what to do if they have a reaction or contra-action.

> **Activity**
>
> Think of some lifestyle changes that you might discuss with a client. Make a list of the benefits to the client from following the advice you give.

Contra-actions

Sometimes a contra-action is referred to as a 'healing reaction'. They are less likely to happen with a body massage when using a carrier oil, but may occur if pre-blended products have been used, as the essential oils they contain can have a more dynamic effect on the systems of the body.

Severe erythema/skin irritation

This might be due to over-stimulation of the skin or to excessive heat being applied (infrared or overuse of gyratory massage). It could also be a sign that the skin is reacting to a product. Stop and review what you are doing. If you are applying massage, are you using appropriate techniques? Cool compresses (or cold stones if you have them) should be applied to the skin to reduce the circulation.

Allergic reaction to a product

The skin will feel hot and the client will feel irritation, tingling or itching. Remove the product completely with lukewarm water. Apply a cool compress and discontinue treatment. Refer the client to a medical practitioner if the irritation does not subside. Sometimes the reaction can be delayed and it may reoccur once the client has returned home. In this case, advise the client to bathe the skin with lukewarm water and apply a cool compress. They should seek medical advice immediately if the symptoms worsen.

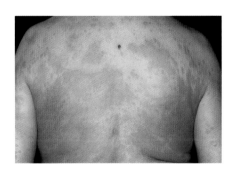

A client with an allergic reaction to a product

Fatigue

Following a good relaxation treatment it is not unusual to feel very sleepy and relaxed. Sometimes this can go on for longer than desired and this is a sign that the body needs to rest and heal. The client should be advised to follow their body's signals and rest and relax for as long as possible. An early night is always a good remedy.

Headache

During a massage treatment the body begins to get rid of waste products from cellular activity. These flood into the circulatory system and to the liver and kidneys to be filtered out and removed. If the waste products build up to a higher level than can be eliminated quickly, the client may experience a headache. Advise the client to sip water to keep the body hydrated, and to rest until the headache goes away.

Nausea

During massage the circulation is redirected to the area being treated. If a client has had a meal before their treatment, the blood will be directed away from the digestive system, and this may cause the client to feel nauseous. Ideally the client should not have a massage for at least an hour after eating. If the client has eaten recently, always avoid massaging the abdomen. Sometimes the experience of the body getting back into a more balanced state can make the client feel nauseous. Advise the client to sip water and rest until the feeling subsides.

Over-application of infrared to the back of the neck can also make some clients feel nauseous – if this occurs, stop the treatment.

Heightened emotions

When the body is in a relaxed state, it 'lets go'. Emotions that have been held in are suddenly released and a client may get very emotional – possibly tearful and weepy. The best remedy is to have a box of tissues handy and listen to the client if they want to talk. Offer the client reassurance that the feeling will pass. Avoid hugging the client or becoming emotional yourself, as this will not help. Sit with the client and place a hand on the forearm or shoulder. Offer them a drink to sip and take them somewhere quiet to rest if possible until they are feeling calmer. On rare occasions the client may become very chatty and excited, sometimes laughing out of character. Again, allow the client to chat and rest somewhere quiet until they feel more balanced.

VALUES & BEHAVIOURS

Maintaining customer care

Verbal and non-verbal communication skills

Communicating with clients

Responding to different client behaviours

Communicating appropriately

Excessive thirst

The body will require additional fluids to help support the kidneys while they remove any toxins and waste products generated as a result of the massage treatment. If the client feels excessively thirsty, encourage them to sip water frequently, rather than drink a large glass straight down, as the body adjusts.

Increased urination

During a massage treatment the body begins to get rid of waste products from cellular activity. This is transported by the circulatory system to the liver and kidneys. The body needs plenty of fluids (water) to help eliminate the waste products from the kidneys, which will result in increased urination.

Muscle aches

It is important to use effleurage and other techniques which help to stretch out the muscles at the end of a massage or mechanical treatment. This is to prevent a rapid increase in circulation to an area, which is then suddenly stopped. This would prevent the drainage of waste products from the area, leaving the muscles feeling tight again rather than helping to remove any tension. Over-treating an area can also cause this.

HANDY HINT

For skin irritation or an allergy, it is often advisable to suggest a client speaks to a pharmacist. This will be quicker than making an appointment to see a GP and the pharmacist will usually have something that can be purchased over the counter without the need for a prescription.

HANDY HINT

It is not unusual for clients to feel tender following a deep or firm massage. This is because massage creates some changes in the tissues; the increased circulation initiates a natural anti-inflammatory response which in turn stimulates the nerve endings. Lots of stretching will help to alleviate these symptoms.

Evaluation and feedback

It is important to gain feedback from the client. This will help you to reflect on your treatment application and form a plan for further professional development. If you carried out an effective consultation and met your client's objectives, your feedback should be positive. It is also good to receive constructive feedback to include areas which you could develop further. When you have completed the treatment, you should seek confirmation from the client that they are satisfied with the results, and make a note of this on the client record card along with any other constructive comments from the treatment.

INDUSTRY TIP

If you want objective feedback, get someone else to carry out a questionnaire. Clients are more likely to complete one if they feel it is being organised by someone impartial.

Answers at the back of the book.

1 Which one of the following is a petrissage technique?

a Pounding

b Hacking

c Ironing

d Beating

2 Which one of the following is the main reason why ultra-violet should be avoided following a massage with pre-blended oil?

a Uneven tanning

b Burning

c Allergic reaction

d Urticaria

3 If a client wants an uplifting, stimulating massage, which two techniques should be increased?

a Effleurage and vibrations

b Friction and petrissage

c Petrissage and effleurage

d Friction and vibrations

4 Which one of the following massage techniques produces rapid erythema?

a Effleurage

b Vibrations

c Compression

d Friction

5 What must you avoid during a forearm massage?

a Movements towards the heart

b Movements away from the heart

c Working over bony areas

d Pressure over the spine

6 Which one of the following is a contra-indication to a body massage treatment?

a Eczema

b Psoriasis

c Broken skin

d Urticaria

7 Which one of the following is a characteristic of an endomorph?

a Narrow shoulders and hips

b Tendency to gain weight

c Low percentage of body fat

d Sturdy straight shoulders

8 What is the type of movement used when you transfer from one massage movement to another?

a Rolling movement

b Transfer of movement

c Linking movement

d Rotating movement

9 What is the correct therapist posture for providing massage?

a Knees bent, back straight, both feet on the floor

b Knees bent and rock between the legs

c Back straight, keeping one foot in contact with the floor

d Back straight and apply pressure with your arms

10 Which one of the following is a contra-indication to abdominal massage?

a Excessively hairy skin

b Loose crêpey skin

c Very thin clients

d Menstruation

304
PROVIDE FACIAL ELECTROTHERAPY TREATMENTS

As the term suggests, electrotherapy treatments use an electrical current.

Electrotherapy treatments:

- improve the skin's condition
- improve muscle tone
- aid lymphatic drainage.

Often a client will need a course of treatments to be able to see the results. It is not always possible to see a result after only one treatment.

In this chapter you will learn how to:

- prepare for facial treatments using electrotherapy
- provide facial treatments using electrotherapy
- provide advice, recommendations and treatment evaluation.

Facial electrotherapy treatments

In this chapter, you will cover the following facial electrotherapy treatments:

- high-frequency treatment
- galvanic treatment
- vacuum suction (also known as lymphatic drainage)
- microcurrent treatment
- microdermabrasion.

It is essential that you understand fully:

- the effects and benefits of these treatments
- how the equipment works
- some basic electrical terminology
- the correct products to use with the equipment
- the length of treatments and how often the client should have them
- any noises or sensations associated with the treatments (so that you can explain them fully to the client).

Prepare for facial electrotherapy treatments

In this part of the chapter you will learn about:

- preparing yourself, your client and your work area for a facial electrotherapy treatment
- consultation
- contra-indications to electrotherapy treatments
- selecting equipment and products for electrotherapy treatments
- preparing your client for a facial electrotherapy treatment.

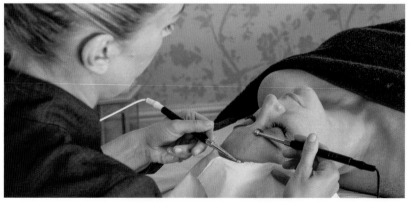

Facial electrical treatment

Prepare yourself, your work area and your client

You should be fully prepared prior to a client arriving for their treatment. You need to make sure that:

- all the equipment and products are to hand and that once the treatment begins you will not need to leave your client unattended
- the trolley and couch are clean and prepared
- the treatment environment (ie lighting, sound, heating and ventilation) is suitable and makes the treatment experience pleasant for the client; requirements may vary from client to client so check that they are comfortable before you begin
- you are fully prepared to meet, greet and treat your client.

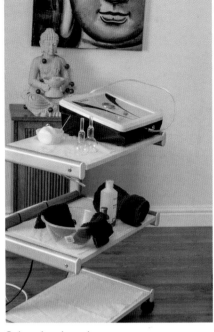

Set up treatment area

Consultation

Consultation is a vital process during which you should assess the client's needs and objectives and their suitability for the treatment.

During the consultation you will need to:

- discuss what the client hopes to achieve from the treatment
- find out about a client's needs/objectives
- agree a treatment plan
- give the client a full explanation of the treatment (ie what is going to happen – sensations, sounds)
- explain realistic achievements associated with the treatment
- carry out a skin analysis and figure diagnosis
- record details of the client's medical history and previous treatments (to make sure you are using the correct procedure for them).

Allow the client plenty of time to ask questions as they may be nervous, especially if they have not had an electrotherapy treatment before.

 Watch videos of consultation for electrotherapy treatments on SmartScreen (unit 304).

VALUES & BEHAVIOURS

More detailed information on the consultation process and communication techniques can be found in the Values and behaviours chapter.

Contra-indications to electrotherapy treatments

In addition to the general contra-indications listed in the Values and behaviours chapter (pages 30–31), there are a number of contra-indications that are specific to facial electrotherapy treatments.

Contra-indication	Treatment	Restricts/ prevents treatment	Reason
Pacemaker	All facial electrotherapy treatments	Prevents	Could affect the rhythm of the heart.
Metal plates or pins Piercings Excessive metal in a particular area (eg dental fillings, bridge work)	All facial electrotherapy treatments	Restricts	Might increase electrical current through the body and make the treatment uncomfortable.
Sunburn	Any electrotherapy treatment of the sunburnt areas	Restricts	Erythema could develop.
Acne rosacea	All facial electrotherapy treatments	Restricts	Treatment will be painful. High risk of cross-infection.
Migraines	All facial electrotherapy treatments	Restricts	May cause a migraine.
Recent Botox injections	Facial microcurrent treatments	Prevents	Risk of interference with Botox treatment.
Collagen/dermal fillers	Facial microcurrent treatments	Prevents	Risk of interference with collagen/dermal filler treatment. Could displace collagen or fillers and have a negative effect on cosmetic procedures.
Loose crêpe-like skin	Vacuum suction treatments	Restricts	Suction will cause capillary and tissue damage.

Once you have completed the consultation with your client and have decided on the programme or treatment that meets their objectives, you can begin treatment.

Select equipment and products for electrotherapy treatments

To achieve the best results, clients will need a course or series of treatments. Throughout the course of treatments you might need to change the equipment you are using to meet the client's needs. You might also need to use more than one piece of equipment to achieve

HANDY HINT

The best results are achieved when clients:
- have a course of treatments
- follow a healthy eating plan – nutrition has an effect on the skin.

the treatment objectives. It is therefore important that you understand which pieces of equipment work well together and the course of treatments that will suit your clients.

To select the correct piece of equipment you also need to understand:

- what it is used for
- how the equipment works
- the electrical current it uses
- specific contra-indications and contra-actions
- how application to the face and body differs
- how to prepare for the treatment (yourself, your client and your work area).

Prepare the client for a facial electrotherapy treatment

The specific techniques you use during treatments will vary. However, the preparation for the client will be similar. The following steps outline the preparation of the client for facial electrotherapy treatments.

HANDY HINT

If you need to, refer back to your Level 2 beauty therapy textbook to remind yourself of the products, tools and equipment for carrying out a facial (see chapter 204/224, Provide facial skin care/Facial care for men).

INDUSTRY TIP

In addition to the electrotherapy equipment you will need:

- any accessories that are to be used alongside the machine
- products, tools and equipment for carrying out a facial.

HANDY HINT

Before the client arrives, check that the machine is working so that, if it isn't, a replacement can be used or the client can be notified that the treatment they have booked is not available on that day. If this is the case, the client could be offered another treatment or the appointment could be rebooked.

INDUSTRY TIP

Some facial procedures include a facial massage, which can be adapted to suit the needs of the client and the treatment.

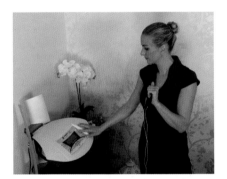

STEP 1 Prepare the treatment room including all equipment.

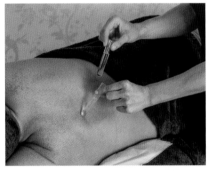

STEP 2 Perform a consultation and tactile and thermal sensitivity tests on the area to be treated. Ask the client to remove all jewellery from the area to be treated. If it cannot be removed, cover it with insulating tape.

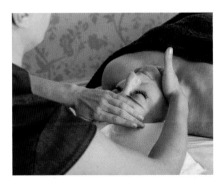

STEP 3 Cover the client with towels/blankets and protect the client's hair with a net or towel.

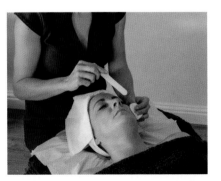

STEP 4 Cleanse, tone and exfoliate the skin. Make sure the toner doesn't contain any alcohol, as alcohol is **flammable**.

Flammable

Easily set alight.

Carry out facial electrotherapy treatments

In this part of the chapter you will learn about:

- high-frequency treatment
- galvanic treatment
- vacuum suction
- microcurrent treatment
- microdermabrasion
- general contra-actions to electrotherapy treatments
- general home-care advice and recommendations for facial electrotherapy treatments.

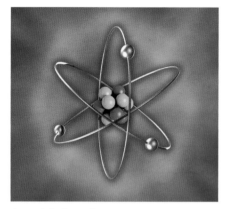

A model of an atom

| **Atom** |
| The smallest part of a chemical element that can exist. |

| **Nucleus** |
| The centre of an atom. |

| **Neutron** |
| Uncharged particle. |

| **Proton** |
| Positively charged particle. |

| **Electron** |
| Negatively charged particle. |

| **Anion** |
| A negatively charged atom that has more electrons than protons. |

| **Cation** |
| A positively charged atom that has more protons that electrons. |

| **Ion** |
| An atom that has lost or gained some electrons. |

| **Electrical current** |
| A flow of electrical charge. |

Electricity

Electricity is a form of energy that is made from electrons which are part of an atom. Everything on the planet is made from **atoms**. Each atom is made up of:

- a **nucleus**
- **neutrons**
- **protons**
- **electrons**.

If an atom contains the same number of protons and electrons it has no charge because it is balanced.

If the atom has more electrons than protons it is negatively charged (–ve) (technically known as an **anion**).

If it has more protons than electrons it is positively charged (+ve) (technically known as a **cation**).

When the balance between the protons and electrons is upset, an atom may gain or lose an electron (an **ion**). The loss of electrons from atoms is what creates an **electrical current**.

Electrical currents

The electrical current for electrotherapy equipment can come from two sources:

- mains electrical supply: equipment is plugged into a wall socket. This type of current is called alternating current (or ac current)
- battery power: equipment runs on a battery that produces electricity from a chemical reaction. This type of current is called direct current (or dc current).

Alternating current (ac)

An alternating current changes direction – it flows one way and then in the opposite direction. It continually repeats this forwards and backwards cycle. This cycle happens many times per second and is measured in hertz (Hz). This is the **frequency** of the current. UK mains' electrical supply is 50Hz, which means the direction of the current changes 50 times every second. The pressure needed to make the current work is measured in **volts** (V). UK mains electrical supply is 240V.

When you apply an electrical pulse (during electrotherapy treatments) you can vary the width of the pulse, the depth of the pulse and the frequency (rate of pulses) to have different effects.

1 For example, the current may flow at 2 milliamps (mA) in one direction and then 2mA in the opposite direction – on a graph, the wave would look square.

Square wave

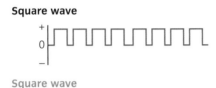

Square wave

2 If the current starts at 0mA and builds up to 2mA, then returns to 0mA before changing direction, it will look like a wave.

Wave flow (sine)

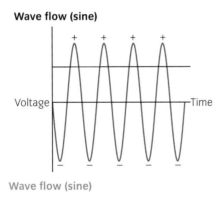

Wave flow (sine)

Direct current (dc)

Direct current flows from positive (+ve) to negative (–ve). Electrodes are needed to complete this circuit from positive to negative. An electrode is a device that **conducts** electricity (a conductor) and helps current to flow from positive to negative. Positively charged electrodes are called anodes and negatively charged electrodes are called cathodes. Both of these electrodes are needed to make the circuit complete so that it works. The current passes through an **electrolyte** solution to get from positive to negative.

Currents used within electrotherapy treatments

A direct current is used in galvanic treatments and a modified direct current is used in microcurrent treatments.

Frequency

The number of times per second that the current changes direction. It is measured in hertz (Hz) (eg 250,000Hz means that it changes direction 250,000 times per second).

Volt

The force needed to push energy around an electrical circuit (a pathway through which electrical current flows from its source through a conductor (a material that is a good transmitter of electricity, eg most metals) and back to its source).

Conducts

Transmits energy (here electricity).

Electrolyte

A substance that produces an electrically conducting solution when dissolved in a polar solution, such as water.

WHY DON'T YOU...
Look at a battery. There will be a +ve symbol on one end and a –ve symbol at the other. The battery has an electrolyte solution inside it which helps the current flow from +ve to –ve.

Treatment	Current	Wave form
Galvanic	Direct current – constant direct flow.	**Galvanic wave** Voltage ⟶ ⟶ ⟶ ⟶ Time on off
Microcurrent	Modified direct current: ■ alters depending upon the machine programme selected ■ current usually builds up like a wave.	**Microcurrent wave 1** + 0 − A basic interrupted direct current shows as a square wave **Microcurrent wave 2** + 0 − Gradual attack

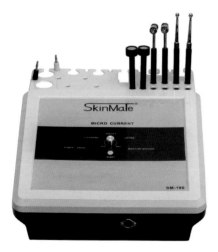

High-frequency machine

Electrode

A device that conducts electricity (a conductor) and helps current to flow from positive to negative.

Saturator

A device which is normally made from glass; this is used on the skin to conduct the electrical current to the client.

Oscillating

Moving backwards and forwards rhythmically.

High-frequency treatment

High frequency can be used on the face or the body (usually the back) to improve the skin's condition.

There are two kinds of high-frequency treatment:

■ Direct high frequency – a glass **electrode** is applied directly to the skin in the treatment area.

■ Indirect high frequency – during an indirect high frequency treatment, the client holds the **saturator** electrode to channel the current. The client may experience a mild tingling sensation. The therapist may also feel this in their fingertips. The lighter the therapist's pressure, the more stimulation occurs.

How high-frequency machines work

The high-frequency machine uses an **oscillating** alternating current. The frequency of the machine (ie the number of times per second that the current changes direction) is very fast – up to 250,000Hz. As the pulses of current are very quick, rather than causing the muscles to contract, the high-frequency machine creates a gentle heat which increases circulation and warms and relaxes the treatment area. This high-frequency current also causes a buzzing noise.

Tools and equipment used in high-frequency treatment

Electrodes

There is a selection of glass electrodes that can be used for high-frequency treatments. They vary in size and shape and are selected according to the area of the face or body that is being treated.

Inside the glass electrode is a gas. The current passing through the electrode causes the gas to **ionise**. The type of gas will determine the colour that the electrode glows.

Gas	Colour that the electrode glows
Argon	Violet
Mercury vapour	Blue
Neon	Orange

Different types of high-frequency electrodes

Electrode	Use
Mushroom electrode	Available in a variety of sizes – the smaller the electrode the more stimulating the effect. Can be used on the face or the body.
Horseshoe electrode	Curved. Used over contours of the body and neck.
Roller electrode	Used on large flat areas (eg the back).
Fulgurator	Used for a technique called **sparking**, which is used on papules and pustules.

HEALTH & SAFETY

Being made from glass, the electrodes are very delicate and need to be treated with care. If you drop them they will smash and break.

Ionise

To convert into ions by removing one or more electrons.

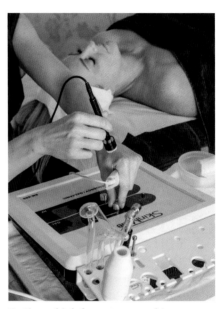

Testing a high-frequency machine

INDUSTRY TIP

Be sure to make your client aware of the noise of the machine prior to starting treatment.

Sparking

The electrode can be used to create a spark by lifting the apparatus away from the skin; this creates a break in electrical flow. Then, by adding the electrode back to the skin's surface this reconnects the current. This process should be used with caution as it can damage the skin.

Electrode	Use
Glass saturator	Either a metal bar or a glass tube containing a metal spiral.
Metal saturator	Used for indirect high frequency.
Rake saturator	Specifically designed for hair and scalp treatment.

Products used in high-frequency treatment

Product	Use
Powder (talc free)	Applied to the body during direct high frequency.
	Also applied to the hand the client is going to hold the saturator with.
	Absorbs any moisture.
Oxygenating cream	Recommended by some manufacturers when using direct high frequency.
	Has a soft creamy feel.
	Should be used with face gauze to stop the electrode sliding over the area too quickly.
Gauze	Used alongside oxygenating cream.
	A piece of gauze is applied to the face.
	May be necessary to cut a hole in the gauze for the eyes, mouth and nose.
	Gauze face masks with eye and mouth holes already cut out are available from some suppliers.

Effects and benefits of high-frequency treatment

The following list shows the benefits and effects of a high-frequency treatment:

- Causes vasodilation of blood vessels, resulting in improved colour to the skin.
- Stimulates sebaceous gland when applied for short amount of time (about five minutes), which is beneficial to dry skin.
- Stimulates cellular metabolism.
- Improves condition of blemished skin (by leaving a **germicidal** layer of **ozone** on the skin that destroys bacteria).
- Stimulates **superficial** sensory nerve endings.
- Tightens the pores.
- Destroys bacteria and heals pustules.
- Dries out oily skin.
- Increases lymph circulation, which helps with removal of waste products.

Germicidal

Destroying germs.

Ozone

A colourless gas made up of oxygen atoms formed by electrical discharge in the air. It is created when a high-frequency current mixes with air. Too much ozone is damaging to the skin.

Superficial

Near the surface.

Contra-indications to high-frequency treatment

Please refer to general contra-indications to electrotherapy treatments on page 315.

 Watch the video of this direct high-frequency facial treatment on SmartScreen (unit 304).

Application of direct high-frequency treatment to the face

Carry out steps 1–4 from facial electrotherapy preparation (see page 317).

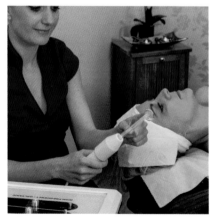

STEP 1 Explain the buzzing noise to the client before you begin the treatment.

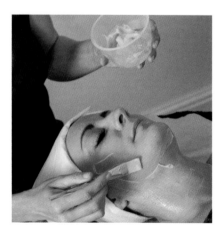

STEP 2 Apply oxygenating cream and gauze or powder to the treatment area.

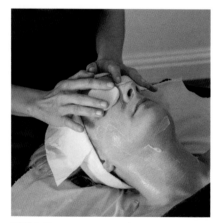

STEP 3 Secure eye pads to the client's face.

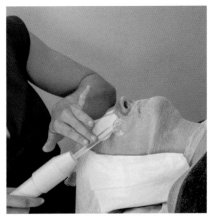

STEP 4 Starting with the mushroom electrode, place the electrode in contact with the client's skin before switching on the current. Turn up the intensity according to manufacturer's instructions.

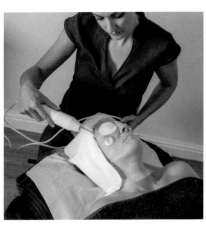

STEP 5 In a small circling motion, work the electrode across the treatment area.

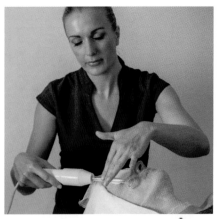

HEALTH & SAFETY ⚠

Sparking occurs when the electrode is lifted from the skin

Application of indirect high-frequency treatment to the face

Carry out steps 1–4 from facial electrotherapy preparation (see page 317).

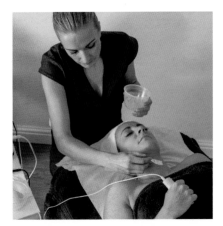

STEP 1 Apply powder to the client's hands and double-check that any jewellery has been removed. Place a sanitised saturator into the client's hand, ensuring they have a firm grip on it.

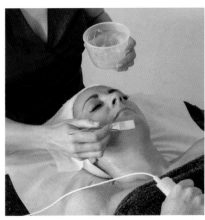

STEP 2 Apply a medium (eg massage cream) to the treatment area.

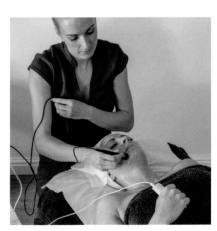

STEP 3 Put one hand on the area to be treated and make small circular movements. Switch the machine on and turn up the intensity. The client will feel warmth in the area. Check the intensity is comfortable for them and place both hands on the area to be treated.

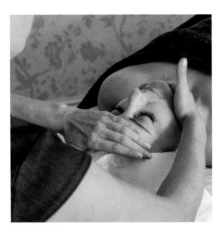

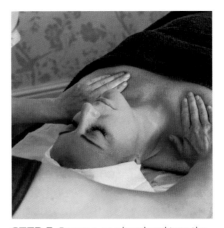

STEP 4 Massage the area to be treated, avoiding tapotement, as lifting away from the client's skin may cause sparking. Do not lose contact with the skin.

STEP 5 Remove one hand and turn the intensity back to zero. Continue to massage for a few minutes to allow the current to disperse before removing the hands completely from the skin.

Activity

Carry out some research into the use of direct high frequency alongside galvanism. How many skincare companies use both direct high frequency and galvanism together as one of their signature treatments? You could visit a trade show to try to find out this information as well as seeing it in action.

Contra-actions to high frequency treatments

Refer to page 315 for general contra-actions to electrotherapy treatments.

Home-care advice and recommendations for high frequency treatments

Refer to page 356 for general advice and recommendations for electrotherapy treatments.

Galvanic treatment

Galvanic treatment improves the skin in two ways:

- **desincrustation**: removal of surface blockages and thorough cleansing of the skin – it literally means to remove a covering crust
- **iontophoresis**: the introduction of water-soluble substances into the skin – this technique is used to push products into the skin.

On the face, it helps improve the skin's texture through **desquamation**. It cleanses the skin and helps to introduce beneficial ingredients into the skin to improve its condition.

HANDY HINT

Observe the client's skin reaction throughout the treatment. Application time is 8–12 minutes in line with the manufacturer's instructions.

INDUSTRY TIP

Facial direct high frequency is a highly effective treatment when used in conjunction with facial galvanism. Together they contribute to improved skin condition.

Desincrustation

A deep cleansing treatment that softens sebum.

Iontophoresis

A technique of introducing ionic medicinal compounds into the body through the skin by applying a local electric current.

Desquamation

The shedding of the outermost membrane or layer of a tissue.

HANDY HINT

Losing contact with the client can cause discomfort to them through sparking.

How galvanic machines work

A galvanic current is a low-voltage, direct current that flows in one direction. It works on the basic laws of **polarity**:

- +ve attracts –ve
- +ve repels +ve
- –ve repels –ve.

The galvanic machine has a polarity switch for selecting and changing polarity. The machine also has sockets for connecting electrodes. An anode (an electrode with positive polarity) and a cathode (an electrode with negative polarity) are needed for the system to work because opposite poles attract. Products containing positively or negatively charged ions are used during galvanic treatments.

Example of how a galvanic facial treatment works:

1 A gel containing anions (negatively charged ions) is applied to the skin.
2 The client holds an **indifferent electrode** (a metal bar electrode) in their hand, which has a positive polarity (ie an anode).
3 The roller electrodes (the **active electrodes**) that are negatively charged (ie a cathode) are applied to the face.
4 This creates a circuit (from positive to negative) allowing the current to flow.
5 As the polarity of the roller electrodes is the same as the polarity of the gel, they are repelled and the ions in the product are attracted through the skin to the positive electrode in the client's hand.

Effects of the electrodes used in galvanic treatment

Anode (+ve polarity)	Cathode (–ve polarity)
Acid reaction (hydrochloric acid)	Alkaline reaction (sodium hydroxide)
Vasoconstriction	Vasodilation
Pores are tightened	Pores are relaxed
Decreases erythema	Sebum is softened and broken down (**saponification**)
Soothes nerve endings	Stimulates nerve endings
Decreases lymph	Increases lymph
Skin tightening	Skin softening

Polarity

Like poles repel each other but opposite poles attract each other.

INDUSTRY TIP

Facial galvanic treatment and direct high frequency treatment should be used together to help deep cleanse problematic skin.

Indifferent electrode

The electrode held by the client that completes the circuit.

Active electrode

The electrode that comes into contact with the client's skin.

HANDY HINT

The active electrode (eg rollers) must be of the same polarity as the galvanic solution/gel so that products are pushed into the skin.

HANDY HINT

The active ingredients in galvanic solutions are marked with a plus (+) or a minus (–) to show whether they are positive or negative. Always check that the correct polarity of cosmetic products is used to make sure that an effective treatment is achieved.

HANDY HINT

The polarity of the products and the machine setting will have an effect on the treatment. It is important to remember that like poles repel, so:

- negative (–ve) to negative and positive (+ve) to positive would push away from each other
- positive to negative and negative to positive would be attracted to each other as opposites attract.

Saponification

The breaking down of fat by an alkali to form soap.

Equipment used in galvanic treatment

Equipment	Use
Indifferent metal bar electrode	Held by the client. Wrapped in a sponge envelope. Completes the electrical circuit.
Indifferent metal plate electrode	Placed under the client's shoulder. Wrapped in a sponge envelope. Completes the circuit.
Ball electrode	Ideal for treating the sides of the nose, the chin and around the eyes.
Roller electrode	Two rollers are used on the face and neck area in a slow rhythmic rolling motion.
Tweezer electrode	Lint soaked in desincrustation fluid is wrapped around the points. Used to target problematic areas.

HANDY HINT

A therapist would choose whether to use the bar or plate electrode but they would not use both at the same time.

Products used in galvanic treatment

Product	Use/benefits
Cleanser and toner	For preparing the skin for treatment.
Mask	Enhances the treatment, has properties such as anti-ageing, firming and nourishing.
Moisturiser, eye gel and lip balm	Protect and nourish the skin, eyes and lips.
Disinfectant	For disinfecting the equipment before and after use.

Effects and benefits of galvanic facial treatments

The following list shows the benefits and effects of galvanic treatment:

- improvement of skin type and condition by pushing beneficial products (eg moisturisers) into the skin
- deep cleansing
- desquamation (ie improves skin texture).

Precautions

It is important to perform all the following safety checks before carrying out galvanic treatments to avoid the risk of galvanic burns:

- Make sure all jewellery (both client's and therapist's) is removed.
- Cover cuts/blemishes with petroleum jelly.
- Make sure that the sponge pockets are not split or ripped.
- Make sure that wires are not split or damaged.
- Check that the machine has been PAT tested and that it is still valid.
- Make sure that the client does not have any contra-indications that prevent treatment.
- Do not exceed 2–3mA on the galvanic unit (as per manufacturer's instructions).

Contra-indications to galvanic treatment

In addition to the general contra-indications listed in the values and behaviour chapter on pages 30–31, it is important that you are aware of these contra-indications to treatment:

- pregnancy (and post-pregnancy until the postnatal check or GP's advice)
- epilepsy
- diabetes
- cuts or abrasions in the treatment area
- varicose veins
- kidney disorders due to the diuretic effect of the treatment.

Application of galvanic treatment to the face – desincrustation

The cathode is the active electrode.

Carry out steps 1–4 from facial electrotherapy preparation (see page 317).

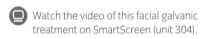

Watch the video of this facial galvanic treatment on SmartScreen (unit 304).

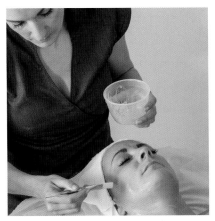

STEP 1 Check the equipment prior to use. Apply the negatively charged desincrustation product (eg cream, gel, contents of ampoule) to the client's skin.

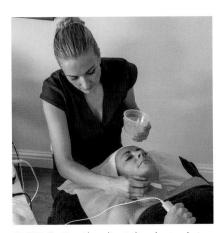

STEP 2 Give the client the electrode to hold or place one under their shoulder, making sure it is not touching any metal (such as a bra clip) and that the electrode is covered with either dampened lint or a sponge pocket.

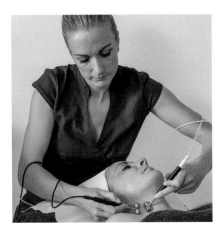

STEP 3 In small circling motions, work the electrode across the treatment area for between three and five minutes for general cleansing and eight to ten minutes for oily areas.

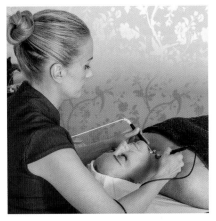

STEP 4 Carry out the roller sequence starting on the jawline.

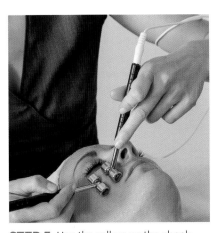

STEP 5 Use the rollers on the cheek area.

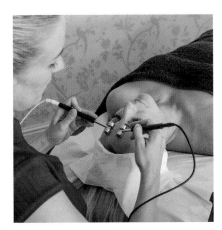

STEP 6 Use the rollers across the forehead.

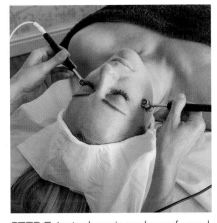

STEP 7 Iontophoresis can be performed at this point. If you aren't applying iontophoresis then reverse the polarity for two to three minutes to tighten the pores and restore the pH balance of the skin, before applying a mask.

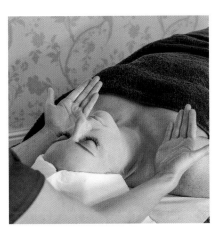

STEP 8 Remove the mask and apply toner and moisturiser.

> **HANDY HINT**
>
> Select the negative polarity as this softens the sebum and relaxes the pores.

> **HANDY HINT**
>
> Observe the client's skin reaction throughout the treatment and reduce the intensity over bony areas.

> **HANDY HINT**
>
> There is a milliamp meter on a galvanic machine that should not exceed 1.5mA during treatment as the skin's resistance breaks down above this level. It is therefore important to monitor the milliamps throughout the treatment.

> **INDUSTRY TIP**
>
> If the client has an oily congested skin you can apply direct high frequency for five to eight minutes after extraction and before reversing the polarity. Remember to apply over oxygenating cream and gauze. This will have a healing, drying and germicidal effect.

Application of galvanic treatment to the face – iontophoresis

The anode (+ve) is the active electrode).

Carry out steps 1–4 from facial electrotherapy preparation (see page 317) and give the indifferent electrode to the client as per the instructions above.

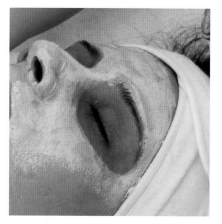

STEP 1 Apply iontophoresis products to the face and throat area using a mask brush.

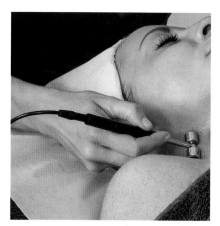

STEP 2 Pick up one of the rollers and start on the neck. Slowly turn up the intensity and wait for 30 seconds to allow any resistance to be broken down. Then turn up the intensity again until the client feels a tingling sensation. As with desincrustation, the current should not exceed 1.5mA.

> **HANDY HINT**
>
> Reduce the current slowly. Once the current has reached zero, keep the rollers moving for a moment or two to allow any left-over current to disperse.

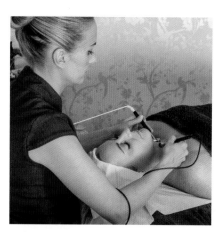

STEP 3 Pick up the other roller so that two rollers are used in sequence. Start at the neck and work in a sequence up the face to the forehead. Make sure that the two rollers do not clash. Work in a slow, smooth rhythmic manner for five to seven minutes.

> **HANDY HINT**
>
> During a galvanic treatment tissue fluid is drawn toward the negative electrode (cathode/black). This is known as electro-osmosis and can help to improve the appearance of lumpy tissue/cellulite.

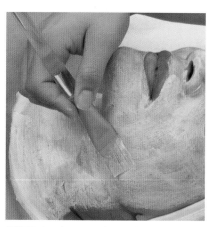

STEP 4 After switching off the machine and removing the indifferent electrode from the client's hand, remove the iontophoresis product from the skin unless the instructions recommend you apply a mask over them.

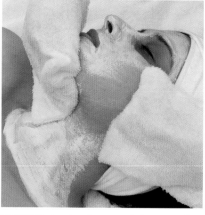

STEP 5 Apply a face mask, leave on for the recommended time and remove with warm water or a hot towel.

Contra-actions to galvanic treatment

You need to be aware of general contra-actions such as product allergies. However, there are also some contra-actions that are specific to galvanic treatments.

Contra-action	Description	Action to be taken
Sensitisation due to intensity of the treatment or products	Severe erythema.	Apply a cool compress. If it happens during treatment, reverse the polarity for two to three minutes, then apply a cooling soothing gel.
Galvanic burn	Usually the result of poor practice (eg not applying enough product or over-treating the area). A chemical burn results from a concentration of alkali on the skin. Skin is dark, split and surrounded by an inflamed red ring.	Flush the area with lots of cool water. Apply a dry sterile dressing. Advise client to seek medical advice immediately.
Metallic taste	If the client has fillings or bridge work they may taste metal in their mouth.	Use rubber gum shields to help prevent this.

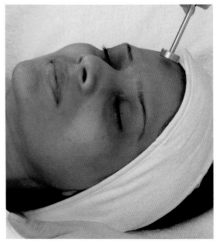

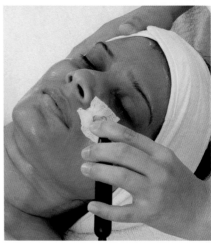

An alternative method of application is using electrodes. Refer to the manufacturer's instructions as to how to use these

Home-care advice and recommendations for galvanic treatment

Please see page 356 for general advice and recommendations for electrotherapy treatments.

Vacuum suction

Vacuum suction is a **mechanical method** of lymphatic drainage treatment.

How vacuum suction works

It is performed using a **ventouse**, which is applied to the skin with a straight and light gliding manner towards the **lymph nodes**. This encourages drainage of lymph fluid from within the lymph spaces. Although the unit operates by using an electrical current, no current passes through the body or face.

Mechanical method

A method using a machine (ie does not involve passing an electrical current through the body).

Ventouse

Glass cup used in vacuum suction.

Lymph nodes (or lymph glands)

These filter and clean lymph fluid before it is returned to the bloodstream. Help to prevent infection.

Equipment used in vacuum suction

Equipment	Use
Vacuum suction unit	Creates a vacuum that causes skin tissue to be sucked into a ventouse.
	Simple to use.
	Has an on/off switch and intensity control for the amount of suction needed.
Facial cup	For lymph drainage on the face.
	Also for deep cleansing.
Body cups	For stimulation of the circulation.
	Also for lymphatic drainage of the body.
Comedone ventouse	For extraction of comedones.
Flat-head ventouse	Desquamation along fine facial lines.
	For lymphatic drainage without over-stimulating the skin.
Pore blockage ventouse	For comedone or pore blockages when there is a group present.

Effects and benefits of vacuum suction

The following list shows the benefits and effects of a vacuum suction treatment:

- Aids with the flow of waste products and tissue fluids to the lymph nodes.
- Improves the appearance and tone of the skin.
- Can reduce fine lines.
- Improves fluid drainage and reduces fluid retention.
- Increases circulation.
- Mobilises fatty deposits.
- Helps prevent varicose veins (body).
- Assists with the removal of comedones and pore blockages.

- Increased blood supply will nourish bones.
- Has a soothing effect on nerve endings.
- Stimulates the lymphatic and circulatory system.

Contra-indications to vacuum suction

Please refer to page 315 for general contra-indications to electrotherapy treatments.

Application of vacuum suction to the face

Before performing vacuum suction, you need to know where the lymph nodes are positioned.

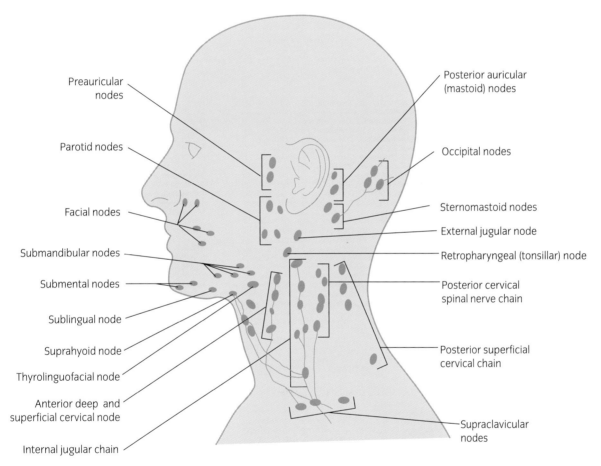

Preauricular nodes

Parotid nodes

Facial nodes

Submandibular nodes

Submental nodes

Sublingual node

Suprahyoid node

Thyrolinguofacial node

Anterior deep and superficial cervical node

Internal jugular chain

Posterior auricular (mastoid) nodes

Occipital nodes

Sternomastoid nodes

External jugular node

Retropharyngeal (tonsillar) node

Posterior cervical spinal nerve chain

Posterior superficial cervical chain

Supraclavicular nodes

Lymph nodes of the face and neck

Watch the video of this vacuum suction treatment on SmartScreen (unit 304).

Facial vacuum suction procedure

Carry out steps 1–4 from facial electrotherapy preparation (see page 317).

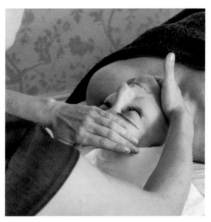

STEP 1 Prepare the client's skin for treatment with either massage oil or cream.

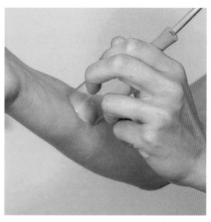

STEP 2 Select the correct cup for facial use. Test the vacuum suction machine on yourself.

HANDY HINT

To break suction, remove your finger from over the air hole on the ventouse. This will break the vacuum.

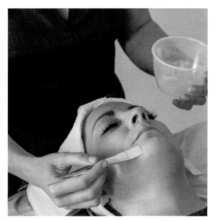

STEP 3 Explain to the client the sensation that they will experience. Apply the medium for the vacuum suction procedure.

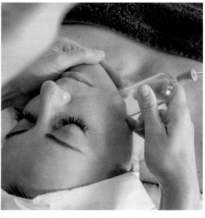

STEP 4 Start at the décolletage area and draw to the lymph nodes. Carry out the neck routine. Draw across the jawline. Work across the cheek area, and then across the forehead, remembering to reduce the suction when working on this area.

INDUSTRY TIP

Good practice tips

- Do not exceed 20% lift of skin.
- Ensure the skin is sufficiently lubricated to prevent dragging, which may result in bruising.
- Keep the skin taut throughout the treatment using your other hand.
- Always release the vacuum suction before removing the ventouse.
- Give advice and recommendations – advise the client about the importance of rehydration to help with lymphatic cleansing.

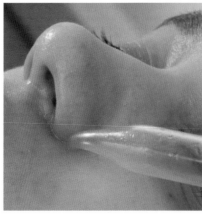

STEP 5 If you are working on a congested area, use the correct ventouse.

Microcurrent treatment

Microcurrent treatment is often referred to as a non-surgical lift, as it helps to lift and firm body and facial contours. Microcurrent treatment was originally used for the medical treatment of Bell's palsy, strokes, facial paralysis, pain control and scar healing, before becoming a beauty/spa treatment.

How microcurrent treatment works

It works by stimulating the muscles. Microcurrent stimulates the Golgi tendon organ (GTO) within the muscle rather than the motor point of the muscle.

The client feels very little sensation during a microcurrent treatment. The treatment uses a modified direct current with a frequency that is very similar to the body's own bioelectrical impulses. It therefore works in **synchronisation** with the body. Microcurrent is measured in **microamps**.

Synchronisation

Working at the same time.

Microamp

One millionth of an amp (symbol is μA).

Equipment used in microcurrent treatment

Microcurrent machines have advanced greatly over the years and the following types of machines are available.

Type of microcurrent machine	Use
Combination systems	Pads are applied to specific points. Probes are also used to stretch and re-educate the muscles.
Probe system	Microcurrent is applied through probes for the face and gloves for the body. This equipment varies between manufacturers.
Twin system	Can be used either with probes or pads.

The majority of programmes on the microcurrent machines are pre-set. Therefore all the therapist needs to do is apply the pads to the treatment area as recommended by the manufacturer, select the programme and press go.

Products used in microcurrent treatment

In addition to sanitising products and exfoliators, you will need positively (+ve) ionised gels, which contain ingredients such as collagen and act as a conductor to the current. Some equipment manufacturers will have their own ranges of products that they recommend for use alongside their machines.

Tools used in microcurrent treatment

In addition to the machine, have to hand:

- cotton buds cut to 1.5cm, which may be needed for facial probes
- adhesive tabs, which are needed to fix pads in place throughout the treatment.

Microcurrent also has positive and negative polarity, which is selected automatically on pre-set programmes and is easily recognised with probes as they have two leads, one of which plugs into the negative outlet and the other into the positive outlet.

Effects and benefits of microcurrent treatment

The following list shows the benefits and effects of microcurrent treatment:

- Improves the appearance of cellulite.
- Improves skin texture and colour.
- Tightens the skin.
- Reduces the appearance of dark circles and puffiness under the eyes.
- Increases fibroblast activity, which stimulates collagen production.
- Speeds up cellular metabolism.
- Effective on stretch marks as microcurrent tightens the collagen fibres that give the skin strength.
- Increases **ATP**, which increases the body's energy levels, reenergising muscles and producing a feeling of well-being.
- Tones and lifts sagging muscles, shortening them back to their original position.
- Softens scar tissue.

HANDY HINT

Gloves are not always used in the probe system. Some units have them and some don't. If the system doesn't have gloves, probes would be used on the body instead.

INDUSTRY TIP

If you are using the probe method, it might not be as simple as just applying the pads, selecting the programme and pressing go. There are different techniques to follow relating to each individual machine so you need to refer to the manufacturer's instructions.

INDUSTRY TIP

Increased fibroblast activity stimulates collagen product. This then rehydrates the skin and encourages moisture retention. Fine lines are plumped out and the appearance of wrinkles is reduced.

ATP

Adenosine triphosphate – a chemical substance found in all living tissue that provides energy for muscle contraction.

Contra-indications to microcurrent treatment

There are some specific contra-indications to facial microcurrent treatment. These are:

- Botox
- epilepsy
- phlebitis
- thrombosis
- cosmetic fillers.

Stages of microcurrent treatment

There are generally four sequential stages to a microcurrent treatment:

1 Increasing the circulation to the epidermis.
2 Drainage and relaxation; this aids the lymphatic system by removing toxins.
3 Muscle toning, lifting slack tissue and improving the pores.
4 Firming of muscles, reducing scar tissue, increasing circulation, second detoxification, improving skin texture, stimulating collagen production.

Application of microcurrent treatment to the face

Carry out steps 1–4 from facial electrotherapy preparation (see page 317).

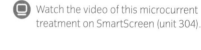 Watch the video of this microcurrent treatment on SmartScreen (unit 304).

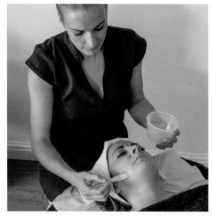

STEP 1 Apply a conductive cream, gel, serum or product ampoule to the client's face and neck in line with the manufacturer's instructions.

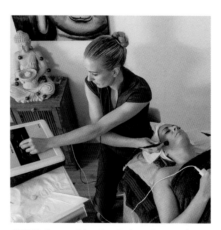

STEP 2 Double-check that the machine dials are all set to zero. If you are using probes on the face, place a cotton bud soaked in the conducting cream, gel or serum (often collagen gel) into the metal area on the probe. Select the required programme and then apply the pads or probes following the manufacturer's suggested sequence.

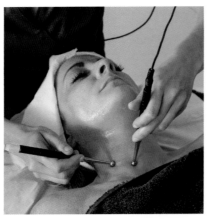

STEP 3 Explain the sensation to the client. Work in sequence across the face, starting with the neck.

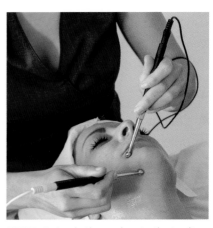

STEP 4 Apply the probes to the jawline.

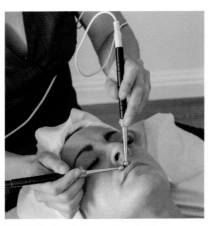

STEP 5 Apply the probes to the upper lip.

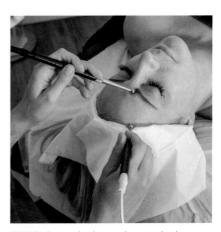

STEP 6 Apply the probes to the brow line.

HANDY HINT

Perform facial massage towards the lymph nodes for five minutes to remove the lymph waste that has been released during the muscle stimulation.

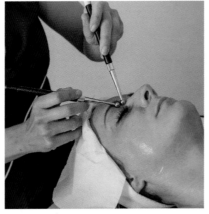

STEP 7 Apply the probes to the eye area.

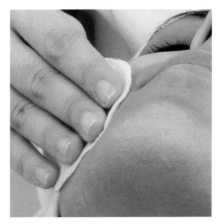

STEP 8 Remove products and apply toner and moisturiser.

General contra-actions to electrotherapy treatments

A contra-action is an undesirable effect that happens during or as the result of a treatment. It is essential that the therapist knows how to deal with a contra-action and that they can also advise the client on how to deal with one if it occurs once they have left the salon/spa. The most common contra-indications following a facial electrotherapy treatment are as follows.

Contra-action	Cause	Action to be taken
Excessive erythema (all electrical treatments)	Over-stimulation of the circulatory system.	Usually settles and disappears after a few hours. Apply a cool compress to reduce any further heat in the area. If it is still red and uncomfortable after 24 hours, the client should notify the salon and contact their doctor in case there is another cause.
Allergic reaction/ irritation (all electrical treatments)	Reaction to a product that has been applied to the skin.	Excessive erythema and inflammation. Might be accompanied by itchiness. Remove all products from the skin immediately using cool water and apply a cool compress to reduce any heat in the area. If the reaction is severe and has not disappeared after 24 hours, the client should contact their doctor and notify the salon of the results.
Galvanic burns (galvanic treatment)	Over-intensity used	Stop treatment and apply a cold compress to the affected area.

Microdermabrasion

Microdermabrasion exfoliates the skin. It is used for improving the appearance of the skin and treating various skin conditions. It is a very popular treatment because it has an immediate effect but it also has long-term effects due to the stimulation of the skin's repair functions.

Currently, there are two popular methods of microdermabrasion:

- Crystal microdermabrasion – very small crystals are sprayed onto the skin, at a variable pressure, to exfoliate the skin. The crystals and exfoliated skin cells are removed by a vacuum.

Micro

Very small.

Dermabrasion

Removal of layers of the skin by mechanical means.

- Diamond microdermabrasion – an abrasive substance is used to smooth out the top layers of the skin. Instead of using crystals to exfoliate the skin, a hand piece containing diamonds or other particles is passed over the skin. The diamond tip **abrades** the skin and, in a similar way to crystal microdermabrasion, the exfoliated particles are then removed by vacuum through the same hand piece. This is a newer procedure which is gaining popularity.

Most microdermabrasion machines will come with the option of using either crystals or diamond tips.

Abrades

Scrapes.

Preparation of the work area

There should be a high standard of cleanliness in the work area. Carry out the following preparation prior to a treatment being carried out:

- Disinfect all equipment in the work areas, such as the trolley, lamps, couch and electrical equipment.
- Check the temperature of the treatment area – it should be warm enough that the client feels comfortable but not too hot to cause flushing of the skin.
- Carry out all necessary electrical safety precautions and tests.

Prepare the client for microdermabrasion

Prepare the client by:

- asking them to remove their jewellery (eg earrings, necklace or any facial piercings) from the area to be treated
- positioning them on the treatment couch – making sure they are comfortable and that you can easily access the area to be treated
- checking that their expectations are realistic and that they are fully aware of the microdermabrasion process.

Equipment and tools

Crystals

Aluminium oxide

A natural metal compound found in the earth.

The most successful and most commonly used crystals for crystal microdermabrasion are **aluminium oxide** (corundum crystals). This is because in terms of hardness they are second only to diamonds which makes them excellent for abrading the skin.

Other types of crystals that are used include:

- magnesium oxide crystals
- sodium bicarbonate (baking soda) crystals

■ sodium chloride (salt) crystals

■ occasionally nut shells or fruit stones (generally labelled as organic grains).

Aluminium oxide crystals are the most commonly used in microdermabrasion because they are hard enough to provide the level of exfoliation needed and because they are the best crystals for use with the equipment. The other crystals listed above provide less effective exfoliation and may clog up the machine.

Diamonds/silicon carbide

Silicon carbide is often used in place of diamonds for diamond microdermabrasion.

Silicon carbide is a very hard manufactured **crystalline** material made from silicon and carbon. It comes as a powder.

Although silicon carbide is more commonly used than diamonds, the name diamond microdermabrasion is used because it sounds more attractive. Silicon carbide heads are less expensive than diamond heads so they can be disposed of and replaced more frequently.

Components of the different types of microdermabrasion machines

A microdermabrasion machine is made up of:

■ a crystal machine

■ a diamond machine.

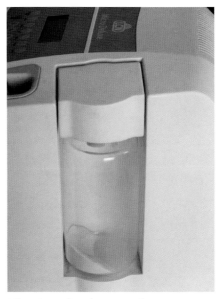
Microdermabrasion crystals

Crystalline
Having the structure of crystals.

HANDY HINT
Your work area should be well ventilated. The lighting should be bright enough to see the skin clearly but not too bright. Ensure the music isn't too loud and that the aromas are pleasant. You want to create a relaxing environment.

INDUSTRY TIP
Most modern crystal microdermabrasion machines do not spray crystals into the air. However, there is a small risk of inhaling stray crystals. It is therefore advisable to wear a face mask during treatment.

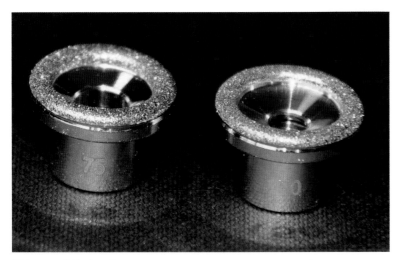
Silicon carbide heads

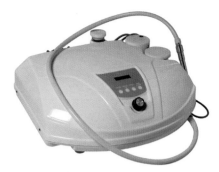

Crystal machine

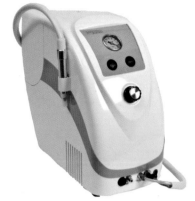

Diamond machine

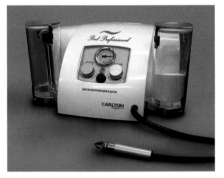

Microdermabrasion machine

Crystal machine	Diamond machine
Two tubes: ■ one for clean crystal spray ■ one for used crystal removal.	Single tube connected to machine and hand piece.
Operating buttons, eg: ■ on/off button ■ crystal settings ■ vacuum settings ■ anti-clog button.	Operating buttons, eg: ■ on/off button ■ vacuum settings.
Hand piece: ■ made from metal or glass ■ attached is a nozzle that targets the crystals onto the skin.	Hand piece: ■ made from metal or plastic ■ attached is the diamond head that is used on the client's skin.
Pressure gauge: ■ shows how much pressure is being applied to the skin from vacuum suction.	Pressure gauge: ■ shows how much pressure is being applied to the skin from vacuum suction.
Vacuum/air pump: ■ pulls and raises a small section of skin while pumping the crystals through the tube onto the skin ■ vacuums away the used crystals, skin and debris into the used crystal container.	Vacuum/air pump: ■ pulls and raises a small section of skin while pumping the crystals through the tube onto the skin.
Clean crystal container.	
Used crystal container.	

Vacuum operation

■ Vacuum settings button: by controlling the amount of vacuum suction, the vacuum settings button controls the amount of crystal flow. The higher the amount of suction, the higher the crystal flow.

■ Anti-clog button: the anti-clog button reverses the vacuum and sucks crystals away from the internal workings of the machine. Not all machines have an anti-clog button but the majority do.

INDUSTRY TIP

It is very important to be aware of the amount of pressure being applied to the skin by the **vacuum** operation of the machine. This is why an accurate pressure gauge is an important feature of a microdermabrasion machine.

Vacuum

To collect particles (eg crystals) by suction.

INDUSTRY TIP

The processes of pumping and vacuuming happen when the top of the hand piece is in contact with the skin. At this point the circuit of pumping and suction is closed, which is why this process is called closed or loop system microdermabrasion.

WHY DON'T YOU...

Use the internet to review the variety of microdermabrasion machines available. Compare the benefits and prices.

Advantages and disadvantages of the different types of microdermabrasion equipment

The advantages and disadvantages of the different types of microdermabrasion equipment are shown in the following table.

Type of microdermabrasion machine	Advantages	Disadvantages
Crystal microdermabrasion	More hygienic as crystals are used once only and can be disposed of. Crystals can penetrate into folds of the skin and wrinkles as they are fired under pressure.	Can be costly replacing crystals. Concerns about risks from inhalation of crystals.
Diamond microdermabrasion	Less expensive as diamond head replacement (ie consumables) is required less frequently than crystal replacement. No crystal residue to clear away after treatment.	Diamond heads can be more difficult to clean effectively. Longer treatment or more repeat movements are necessary to penetrate into the folds of the skin and wrinkles as the diamonds are **static** on the hand piece.

Static

Not moving; fixed.

Prepare products and equipment for microdermabrasion

1 Make sure you have all the necessary tools and equipment in place:

- microdermabrasion machine
- crystals or a selection of diamond heads
- disposable applicator heads (if using crystal microdermabrasion).

2 Prepare the machine according to the manufacturer's instructions, eg:

- the new crystal container is three-quarters full
- the container for the used crystals is empty
- the disposable nozzle cap on the applicator is clean.

3 Test the machine to make sure it is in good working order.

4 Cover the couch with a clean towel and/or disposable couch roll.

5 Ensure your trolley is stable and that it has enough shelves to put the equipment on the top and any products and water below to prevent any accidental spillage onto the machine.

6 Ensure you have a waste bin for general waste and a yellow waste bag for disposing of the crystals.

INDUSTRY TIP

A fully adjustable couch is advisable to suit the needs of different clients. A fully adjustable couch also helps prevent postural problems for the therapist.

Vinyl

A type of plastic that provides a reasonable resistance to oil and grease. It is not as strong or as resistant to tearing as nitrile.

Nitrile

A type of rubber with increased strength and resistance to oils and acids.

HANDY HINT

One towel should be available for the therapist to make sure that their hands are dry when touching the microdermabrasion machine.

HEALTH & SAFETY

It is important to wear disposable protective gloves (vinyl or nitrile) when performing a microdermabrasion treatment. (Powder-free gloves are recommended to reduce the risk of potential allergies.) During the treatment, you are removing the skin's protection so the client's skin is more vulnerable to bacteria. Wearing gloves helps to reduce the risk of cross-infection. As there is a small risk of breaking the skin and causing blood spotting, gloves also protect the therapist from infection.

INDUSTRY TIP

A stool with castors allows you to move freely during the treatment.

7 Make sure you have the following personal protective equipment (PPE):

- **vinyl** or **nitrile** disposable gloves for the therapist to prevent cross-infection (see health and safety tip below)
- a face mask for the therapist to avoid inhaling crystals (see industry tip on page 341)
- protective goggles for the client to prevent any loose crystals going into their eyes.

8 Prepare the trolley with the following equipment and products:

- tissues (for drying the client's skin)
- disposable sponges (for cleansing and mask removal)
- headband or bonnet (ideally disposable)
- cotton wool (used sparingly for eye make-up removal)
- selection of bowls (for water)
- spatulas
- mask brush
- skin cleanser
- serum
- ampoules of product
- mask (soothing and hydrating)
- moisturiser
- sun protection product.

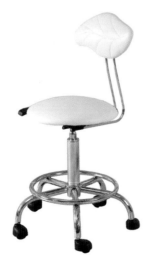

A therapist's stool

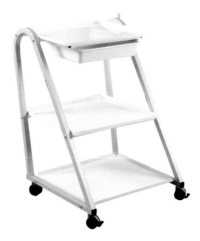

A stable trolley with enough shelves for storage

Consultation

Consultation is a vital process during which you should assess the client's needs and objectives and their suitability for the treatment. More detailed information on the consultation process and communication techniques can be found in the Values and behaviours chapter.

Skin analysis

It is important to carry out a skin analysis using visual and manual inspection techniques to assess the client's skin type, the pigmentation of the client's skin and any sun damage. This is because microdermabrasion can affect melanin. If the melanin in the skin is more active, there is a greater potential to cause unwanted pigmentation changes. Darker skins should be treated gently and gradually to avoid pigmentation problems.

A thorough skin analysis is important prior to any treatment. As microdermabrasion is an exfoliating treatment, when you are carrying out your skin analysis you need to assess whether the skin can withstand exfoliation and what adaptations should be made. You need to:

- assess the client's general skin type (ie dry, oily or combination)
- consider the client's skin's characteristics (ie dehydrated, mature skin, young skin, lacking in tone, wrinkles, blemishes (ie milia, pustules, comedones) and pigmentation variations)
- look at the client's skin tone (ie fair, medium or dark).

Manage clients' expectations

Microdermabrasion is a high-profile treatment, often used by and endorsed by celebrities. As a result, clients' expectations of the treatment might be unrealistic. It is therefore important to manage your clients' expectations. Microdermabrasion offers many benefits to many skin conditions but it can't miraculously turn back the clock.

Client treatment plan

During the consultation process, discuss and agree the treatment plan with the client in line with their needs and desired outcomes. Make recommendations to the client to get the best possible results from the treatment. Once you have discussed and agreed the treatment plan, summarise and confirm the client's objectives and the treatment process.

The thickness of the stratum corneum (outer layer of skin) will affect the level of exfoliation. Finer skins can't **tolerate** as much exfoliation.

INDUSTRY TIP

It is important to establish whether the client has any allergies to the products and equipment used in the treatment. It is also as important to find out whether the client has had an allergic reaction in the last two to four weeks even if the reaction is unrelated to the treatment. This is because the treatment also stimulates **histamine** production so any treatment may cause the skin to react.

Histamine

The chemical the body produces when having an allergic reaction. It causes blood vessels to dilate and an inflammatory response in the tissues.

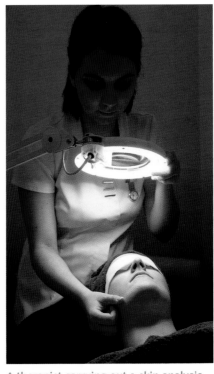

A therapist carrying out a skin analysis

INDUSTRY TIP

A mirror is a handy tool to use during a consultation. Allow the client to look in the mirror and point out to you exactly what they would like to improve.

Tolerate

Cope with.

The following table gives information on the type of microdermabrasion treatment you should provide based on the client's skin type or condition.

Skin type or condition	Treatment using the crystal method	Treatment using the diamond method	Products
Dry skin	▪ Light exfoliation only. ▪ Low pressure and low crystal flow. ▪ Use rapid movements with no repeat movements.	▪ Use a low-grade abrasion head and low pressure. ▪ Rapid movements with no repeat movements.	Nourishing and hydrating masks, serums and creams.
Oily skin	▪ Medium exfoliation. ▪ Medium pressure and medium crystal flow. ▪ Avoid any pustules. ▪ Repeat movements if necessary. ▪ Adapt speed of movement as required in each area. ▪ Rapid movements in areas with finer skin. ▪ Slower movements in areas of thickened skin.	▪ Use a medium-grade abrasion head and medium pressure. ▪ Avoid any pustules. ▪ Adapt speed of movement as required in each area. ▪ Rapid movements in areas with finer skin. ▪ Slower movements in areas of thickened skin.	Masks used to reduce sebum production.
Combination skin	▪ Light to medium exfoliation. ▪ Low to medium pressure and low to medium crystal flow. ▪ Adapt speed of movement as required in each area. ▪ Rapid movements in areas with finer or drier skin. ▪ Slower movements in areas of thickened skin.	▪ Use a low- to medium-grade abrasion head and low to medium pressure. ▪ Adapt speed of movement as required in each area. ▪ Rapid movements in areas with finer or drier skin. ▪ Slower movements in areas of thickened skin.	Hydrating, balancing and soothing masks, serums and creams.
Mature skin	▪ Light to medium exfoliation. ▪ Low to medium pressure and low to medium crystal flow. Always support the skin during treatment to avoid dragging. ▪ Adapt speed of movement as required in each area. ▪ Rapid movements in areas with finer skin. ▪ Slower movements in areas of thickened skin.	▪ Use a low- to medium-grade abrasion head and low to medium pressure. ▪ Always support the skin during treatment to avoid dragging. ▪ Adapt speed of movement as required in each area. ▪ Rapid movements in areas with finer skin, slower movements in areas of thickened skin.	Regenerating and hydrating masks, serums and creams.

Skin type or condition	Treatment using the crystal method	Treatment using the diamond method	Products
Dehydrated	■ Medium to deep exfoliation. ■ Medium to high pressure and medium to high crystal flow. ■ Adapt speed of movement as required in each area. ■ Rapid movements in areas with finer skin. ■ Slower movements in areas of thickened skin.	■ Use a medium- to high-grade abrasion head and medium to high pressure. ■ Adapt speed of movement as required in each area. ■ Rapid movements in areas with finer skin. ■ Slower movements in areas of thickened skin.	Hydrating and soothing masks, serums and creams.
Sensitive or fine skin	Not suitable for treatment.	Not suitable for treatment.	Masks, serums or creams for sensitive skin.
Pigmented skin	Initial treatment: ■ Light exfoliation only, low pressure, low crystal flow. ■ Use rapid movements with no repeat movements. Subsequent treatments: ■ If no contra-actions occur; medium to deep exfoliation. ■ Medium to high pressure and medium to high crystal flow. ■ Adapt speed of movement as required in each area. ■ Rapid movements in areas with finer skin. ■ Slower movements in areas of thickened skin.	Initial treatment: ■ Use a low-grade abrasion head and low pressure. ■ Rapid movements with no repeat movements. Subsequent treatments: ■ If no contra-actions occur; medium- to high-grade abrasion head and medium to high pressure. ■ Adapt speed of movement as required in each area. ■ Rapid movements in areas with finer skin. ■ Slower movements in areas of thickened skin.	Hydrating, brightening and pigment treatment masks, serums and creams.

Hyperpigmentation

Increase in pigmentation in the skin.

Hypopigmentation

Loss of pigmentation in the skin.

Haemophilia

A genetic condition in which blood clotting is reduced.

Sensitivity testing

It is recommended that you carry out a sensitivity test 24 hours prior to the treatment:

- Cleanse the area to be tested.
- All the products that will be used during the treatment (eg cleanser, crystals and aftercare products (eg serum, mask and moisturiser)) should be applied to an area just behind the ear approximately 2cm × 2cm.
- Carry out a second sensitivity test using only the crystals (ie no products). This is because the products (eg cleanser, etc) are the things most likely to cause a reaction.
- Ask the client to leave the area alone and return to the salon the next day for you to assess the reaction.
- Note any contra-actions that occur within 24 hours or any adverse reactions.

Contra-actions

Contra-actions include:

- mild erythema.
- slight flaking of the skin.

There is a risk of more serious adverse reactions, which can include:

- severe or prolonged erythema
- swelling (oedema)
- changes in pigmentation (**hyperpigmentation** or **hypopigmentation**).

If no adverse reactions are seen after 24 hours, a full treatment may take place. If any adverse reactions are observed, then the treatment should not go ahead. However, if adverse reactions are observed on the first test but not the second, treatment may go ahead using different products (after testing these).

Contra-indications to microdermabrasion

In addition to the general contra-indications listed in the Values and behaviours chapter (pages 30–31), there are a number of contra-indications that are specific to microdermabrasion:

Contra-indication	Restricts/prevents treatment	Reason
Vascular/fragile skin or acne rosacea	Prevents	■ The skin is very fragile and thin. ■ Cannot tolerate this type of exfoliation.
Cosmetic procedures (eg acid peels)	Prevents	■ The skin is already undergoing exfoliation. ■ It will be highly sensitised. ■ Cannot tolerate further exfoliation.
Roaccutane (medication for acne)	Prevents	■ Reduces sebum in the skin. ■ Skin is dry, thinned and highly sensitised skin during its use and for up to six months afterwards. ■ The skin cannot tolerate microdermabrasion.
Active viral lesions (eg herpes simplex or cold sores)	Prevents	■ High risk of cross-infection.
Cancer/chemotherapy and radiotherapy	Prevents	■ Microdermabrasion activates the circulation and lymphatic flow. ■ If cancerous cells are present there is a potential risk of mobilising them within the circulatory system.
Pregnancy	Restricts – some side effects of pregnancy may be worsened by treatment. For example, high or low blood pressure. It is also important to be mindful of the potential effects of an electric current passing through the skin.	■ Hormonal changes during pregnancy mean that the skin is more prone to hyperhypopigmentation.
Active acne lesions	Restricts if only a few are present but would prevent treatment if they are more widespread.	■ Treatment would spread the bacteria and cause cross-infection.
Moles	Restricts	■ If the nature of the mole is unknown, the client needs to seek medical advice prior to treatment.
Fine or young skins	Prevents	■ Skin cannot withstand this kind of abrasion. ■ Skin doesn't need this kind of abrasion.
Haemophilia	Prevents	■ Blood clotting is reduced. ■ As there is a potential to cause bleeding you should not carry out microdermabrasion.
Tattoo	Restricts – areas around the tattoo may be treated.	■ Deeper exfoliation over a tattoo may result in blurring and fading of the tattoo.

Skin cancer

Skin cancer is the most common type of cancer in the UK. A client may ask for a pigmentation mark to be removed. As a therapist, particularly one who provides microdermabrasion treatment, you are in a unique position to spot possible skin cancers. As a therapist you are not medically qualified to give a diagnosis of a skin condition. However, it is very important that you are aware of the key indicators of skin cancer and know how to direct the client to a medical expert without causing distress or alarm.

Effects and benefits of microdermabrasion

The following table shows the effects and benefits of microdermabrasion treatments.

Effects	Benefits
■ Stimulates cellular renewal and circulation. ■ Removes dark, keratinised cells and debris.	■ Improves skin's health and appearance (ie brightens dull skin). ■ Restores and revives mature skin. ■ Reduces fine lines and wrinkles. ■ Refines and reduces scar tissue.
■ Smoothes out uneven texture.	■ Smoothes and restores the skin's texture.
■ Removes the surface layer of the epidermis so that pigmented areas will appear lighter.	■ Reduces hyperpigmentation (eg age spots and sun damage).
Deep exfoliation: ■ removes debris from the surface of the skin ■ unblocks pores.	Deep facial cleansing.
■ Increases circulation and lymphatic flow, smoothing the skin.	■ Improves the appearance of cellulite.

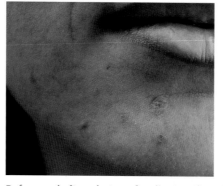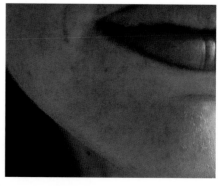

Before and after photos of a client undergoing a microdermabrasion treatment

Treatment times

The microdermabrasion process is relatively quick depending on the area to be treated. A session will usually last about 50–60 minutes; approximately 15–20 minutes of this time will be spent using the machine and the rest of the time will be for pre-cleansing and post-treatment care.

The number and interval of treatments will depend on:

- the required end result
- the skin's condition
- the skin's reaction to the treatment.

As a guide, clients are likely to have a course of between six and 12 treatments every seven to ten days in order to achieve the **optimum** results. Where deeper exfoliation has taken place, at least 10–14 days should be left between treatments to allow the skin time to heal and recover.

Carry out microdermabrasion treatments using the crystal and diamond methods

Once you have completed the consultation and the client profile, you can start the treatment. You also need to make sure that the response to the sensitivity test doesn't prevent treatment. Before you start, ask the client to remove their clothes and jewellery and put them somewhere for safekeeping.

A client's first treatment should always be carried out lightly (ie on a low pressure setting with rapid movements) to assess the skin's reaction. The depth of treatment can be increased at future sessions as long as there are no contra-actions.

INDUSTRY TIP

It is quite common for salons to offer a faster quick polish type microdermabrasion facial. This can be carried out in 30 minutes by excluding the lymphatic drainage prior to treatment and using cooling gel to finish the treatment rather than a treatment mask.

Optimum

The best possible; ideal.

INDUSTRY TIP

Do not apply any products to the skin while you are using the microdermabrasion machine unless the manufacturer's instructions say you can do so. Any products used on the skin will be sucked up into the machine and might stop it from working.

INDUSTRY TIP

Keep water and moisture well away from the machine and the crystals. Imagine you left a bowl of sugar or salt out in the open; any moisture in the air would cause the salt or sugar to clump together. This is exactly what will happen to the crystals if they are not kept in a sealed container away from moisture.

The same applies to the crystals in the machine. If you work on wet skin or keep a steamer near the microdermabrasion unit, the moisture will get inside the machine and form clumps of crystals.

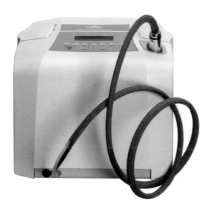

STEP 1 Set up the machine (check that it is in working order prior to use).

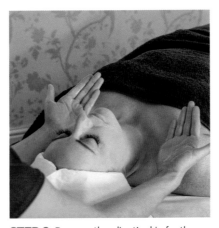

STEP 2 Prepare the client's skin for the treatment procedure by cleansing and toning with appropriate products for their skin type and check the skin for any issues such as broken capillaries.

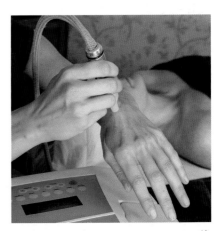

STEP 3 Test the equipment on yourself to make sure that everything is working correctly and that it is at the correct level.

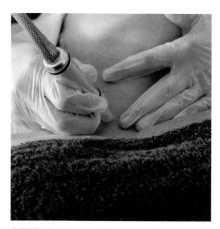

STEP 4 Carry out the procedure following the manufacturer's instructions. Start with the client's neck. Use tissue to collect debris from the treatment.

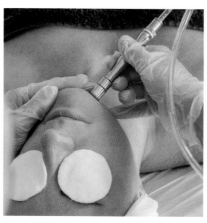

STEP 5 Next work across the client's jawline.

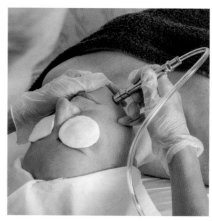

STEP 6 Work across the chin area in small movements.

HANDY HINT

If you are using the diamond method, after step 4 put the appropriate diamond head in place on the hand piece. Select the appropriate head according to the client's needs, the desired outcome and the manufacturer's instructions. Diamond heads are available with varying sizes of particles; bigger particles for deeper exfoliation and smaller particles for more superficial exfoliation.

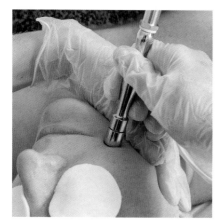

STEP 7 Work across the cheek area in a continuous motion.

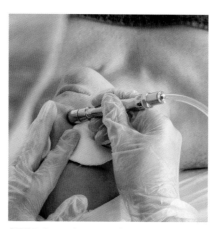

STEP 8 Work across the nose area in smaller steps.

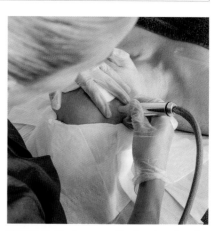

STEP 9 Work across the forehead and down the temples, looking at the skin reaction throughout.

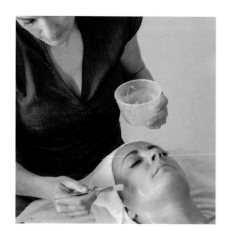

STEP 10 Using a soft brush, remove dead skin cells/debris from the client's face.

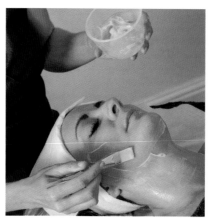

STEP 11 Apply facial mask evenly over the entire neck and face area, placing eye pads over the client's eyes for comfort. After the appropriate timing, remove the facial mask and tone the face.

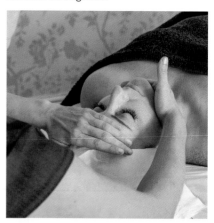

STEP 12 Moisturise the entire face, using the correct product for the client's skin type. Complete the client's record card and provide aftercare information.

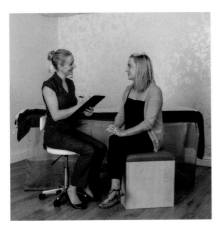

STEP 13 Clear and clean the machine after the treatment is complete. Complete the client's record card and provide advice and recommendations.

Watch videos of crystal and diamond microdermabrasion treatments on SmartScreen (unit 304).

At the end of the treatment you should evaluate the treatment by checking that visible treatment outcomes have been achieved (eg that the skin texture is refined and smooth). Give any advice and recommendations. Remind the client that certain outcomes (eg wrinkle reduction and pigmentation reduction) take time and might need further treatment.

Maintenance of the machine

It is important to maintain the machine so that it remains in good working order:

- Empty the used crystal container after each client. Try to prevent the used crystals and dead skin cells from entering the atmosphere.
- After every treatment, clean the filters and lids according to the manufacturer's instructions.
- Dispose of the diamond head or clean the nozzle on a crystal machine.

Activity

Practise your movements on friends and family. Remember to overlap your movements and keep them short and at a constant speed. Begin by working on the backs of hands until your technique improves.

Activity

For each skin type, suggest a list of post-care products (from the range at your college or another range you are familiar with) that would be suitable for use by a client following a microdermabrasion treatment.

INDUSTRY TIP

Clearly note on the client's record card the pressure settings or diamond heads used and the outcomes achieved.

HANDY HINT

Faster movements = lighter exfoliation.
Slow movements = deeper exfoliation.

INDUSTRY TIP

When carrying out exfoliation using microdermabrasion, use short movements from the centre of the face outwards. This will help you to make the speed and pressure more constant. Long sweeping movements often leave red lines on the client's skin.

HANDY HINT

Monitor the client's comfort and skin reaction throughout the treatment and adjust the level of exfoliation if needed.

INDUSTRY TIP

To keep the microdermabrasion machine in good working order, it is vital to follow the manufacturer's instructions on cleaning and maintenance. Filters will need replacing regularly.

INDUSTRY TIP

It is essential to use the correct pressure setting to get the best results. Your technique is equally as important. Practise as much as possible to improve your skills.

Adapt the treatment to suit client needs

- Wrinkles/scar tissue – work along the length of the wrinkle and from side to side within the borders of the wrinkle or scar. Continue to do this until red spots appear. This method works deeper and smoothes the area.

- Large areas (eg the back or tops of the arms) – treat the area in small sections. Take care to overlap each movement to avoid striping. Keep the movements fluid and in the same direction across the area.

- Cellulite – repeat the lymphatic stimulation stage at least three times over each area.

- Contra-indications – on most microdermabrasion machines the vacuum suction stage can be done as a **stand-alone** treatment. This can be very useful for brightening and reviving skin where exfoliation is contra-indicated.

Stand-alone

Able to be done on its own.

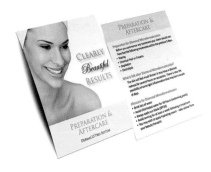

An advice leaflet

Contra-actions to treatment

A contra-action is an adverse reaction that can happen during or after a treatment. It is important to be aware of these reactions and provide advice to your client in case they do occur.

If contra-actions do occur during treatment, discontinue the treatment and provide appropriate action and advice.

Contra-action	Cause	Action to be taken
Erythema	<ul><li>Redness of the skin due to over-stimulation of the skin or an adverse reaction.</li><li>Usually occurs in first 24 hours but may be prolonged depending on the depth of treatment and skin sensitivity.</li></ul>	<ul><li>Avoid heat or further skin stimulation for at least 48 hours.</li><li>Protect skin from UV radiation.</li><li>Apply moisturising products.</li><li>Reduce pressure setting.</li><li>Increase speed of movements.</li><li>Avoid repeated movements over a specific area.</li><li>Avoid applying downward pressure on the hand piece.</li></ul>
Swelling (oedema)	<ul><li>Swelling due to fluid retention.</li></ul>	<ul><li>Make sure client has given you correct information about allergies.</li><li>Make sure that all products used in treatment were included in the sensitivity test.</li><li>Reduce pressure setting.</li><li>Increase speed of movements.</li><li>Avoid repeated movements over a specific area.</li><li>Avoid applying downward pressure on the hand piece.</li></ul>

Contra-action	Cause	Action to be taken
Flaking or peeling of the skin	■ A natural reaction. ■ Shows that the skin is renewing itself.	■ Apply moisturising products.
Excessive bleeding	■ Removal of the epidermis to expose the dermis. ■ Treatment too deep.	■ Reduce pressure setting. ■ Increase speed of movements. ■ Avoid repeated movements over a specific area. ■ Avoid applying downward pressure on the hand piece.
Changes in pigmentation (hyperpigmentation or hypopigmentation)	■ Dark patches on the skin (hyperpigmentation which is caused by an increase in melanin in the skin). ■ Light patches of skin where the pigmentation has been lost (hypopigmentation which is caused by a decrease in melanin in the skin).	■ Protect skin from UV radiation. ■ Apply moisturising products. ■ Reduce pressure setting. ■ Increase speed of movements. ■ Avoid repeated movements over a specific area. ■ Avoid applying downward pressure on the hand piece.
Red stripes on the skin	■ Too much downward pressure applied on hand piece. ■ Speed of hand piece was not constant.	■ Make sure speed of hand piece is constant. ■ Reduce pressure setting. ■ Increase speed of movements. ■ Avoid repeated movements over a specific area. ■ Avoid applying downward pressure on the hand piece.
Pin-point bruising	■ Flat, round red spots under the skin surface caused by bleeding between the epidermis and the dermis.	■ Reduce pressure setting. ■ Increase speed of movements. ■ Avoid repeated movements over a specific area. ■ Avoid applying downward pressure on the hand piece.

General causes of contra-actions

The following are general causes of contra-actions to microdermabrasion treatment:

■ speed of hand piece movement not constant

■ over-treatment

■ pressure setting on the machine too high

■ movements on the skin too slow

■ placing downward pressure on the hand piece

■ too many movements repeated over a specific area

■ allergic reaction

■ incorrect skin analysis.

Watch the video of electrotherapy advice and recommendation on SmartScreen (unit 304).

AHAs

Alphahydroxy acids.

HANDY HINT

Advise the client not to use 'dirty' moisturising creams (ie pots of cream into which they have put their fingers). These are likely to contain bacteria which can be transferred to their skin. Recommend that they purchase a new product and use a spatula for the duration of their microdermabrasion treatments.

HANDY HINT

It is important to be tidy in your salon. After the client has left, clean and sanitise the machine in line with the manufacturer's instructions and store away correctly. With the vacuum suction machine, wash the ventouses in hot soapy water, using an antibacterial soap, and leave them to dry before putting them away.

INDUSTRY TIP

If the client has a contra-action, write this up on their record card so the product/treatment can be avoided or altered in the future.

Home-care advice and recommendations

Following a microdermabrasion treatment, you should give your client suitable advice and recommendations to follow. This advice will help the client maximise the benefits of the treatment.

- Avoid alcohol, spicy foods, heat treatments and hard physical activity for 24 hours as these are stimulants and can contribute to the initial reddening of the skin.
- Do not use any products other than those recommended by your therapist. In particular, avoid perfumed products and those containing exfoliation ingredients such as **AHAs**.
- Avoid UV exposure and always use a sunscreen with an SPF 20 or above. Remember that you can't apply this for the first 24 hours.
- Avoid wearing make-up for 24 hours. If wearing make-up after this time, always use a clean applicator brush and try to use mineral make-up.
- Use a gentle cleansing lotion and apply plenty of moisturising cream (after the first 24 hours).
- Avoid further skin treatments to the area to let the skin settle down.
- Follow the therapist's advice if any contra-actions occur.

General home-care advice and recommendations for facial electrotherapy treatments

Following a facial electrotherapy treatment, you should give your client suitable advice and recommendations to follow. This advice will help the client maximise the benefits of the treatment.

- Provide recommendations for the correct skincare routine (eg products that will enhance their treatment).
- Encourage the client to:
  - drink plenty of water and reduce caffeine intake
  - quit smoking
  - follow a healthy eating plan
  - take regular exercise.
- Encourage the client to book a course of treatments:
  - muscle toning treatments (microcurrent): ten treatments with one to two a week and then monthly to maintain the effect
  - vacuum suction, high frequency and galvanic: up to twice a month.
- Explain how to deal with a contra-action if one occurs.

Answers at the back of the book.

1 What is the maximum percentage that the ventouse can be filled to during vacuum suction?

a 15%

b 18%

c 20%

d 23%

2 Petroleum jelly is used in electrical treatments to:

a Cover minor breaks in the skin

b Act as a medium for roller electrodes

c Cover the indifferent electrode

d Change the polarity

3 Where is the corrugator muscle situated?

a At the back of the head

b In between the eyes

c Around the lips

d Under the chin

4 What is the sensation created by a microcurrent treatment?

a Sharp shooting pains

b Sweeping and gliding

c Tingling

d Little to no sensation

5 What colour is a high-frequency glass saturator containing mercury vapour?

a Orange

b Green

c Violet

d Blue

6 Which one of the following needs to be replaced after every use of a microdermabrasion machine?

a Crystals

b Air pump

c Filters

d Nozzle

7 Which level of sun factor (SPF) should a client use following a microdermabrasion treatment?

a SPF 2

b SPF 4

c SPF 8

d SPF 20 or above

8 A conductor in electrotherapy is a device that is a:

a Poor transmitter of electricity

b Poor transmitter of energy

c Good transmitter of electricity

d Good transmitter of energy

9 What is the function of an electrode?

a Helps the current to flow from positive to negative

b Positively charges electrons

c Produces a chemical reaction on the skin's surface

d Negatively charged electrons

10 What causes the metallic taste in the mouth during facial electrotherapy?

a Amalgam fillings

b Tooth enamel

c Chemical reaction

d Ionisation

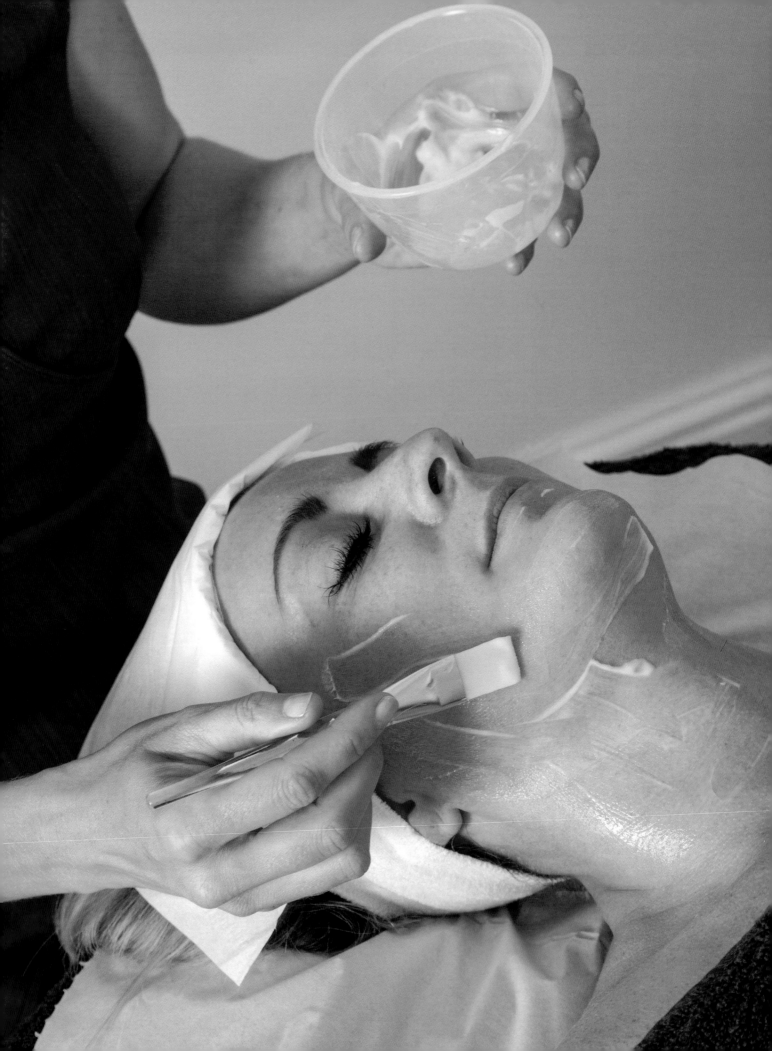

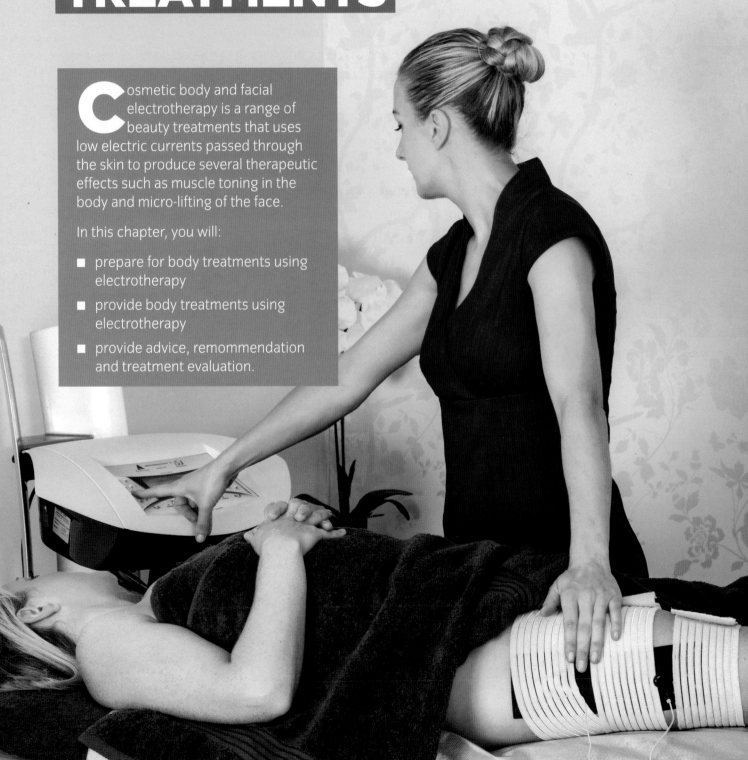

305
PROVIDE BODY ELECTROTHERAPY TREATMENTS

Cosmetic body and facial electrotherapy is a range of beauty treatments that uses low electric currents passed through the skin to produce several therapeutic effects such as muscle toning in the body and micro-lifting of the face.

In this chapter, you will:

- prepare for body treatments using electrotherapy

- provide body treatments using electrotherapy

- provide advice, remommendation and treatment evaluation.

Body electrotherapy treatments

The reasons for clients having body electrical treatments are to:

- re-educate muscles with poor tone, to condition and strengthen them
- re-shape the body contours through inch loss (eg after pregnancy or as part of a slimming programme)
- lift and firm body contours to maintain an attractive figure
- improve posture by stretching and toning shortened muscles, eg pectorals for a client with kyphosis
- improve poor circulation by stimulating the blood supply to an area, improving cell metabolism
- improve lymphatic circulation thus improving removal of toxins and waste products/detox
- improve the appearance of cellulite
- soften and aid dispersal of adipose tissue/aid weight loss
- reduce the appearance of and soften scar tissue
- reduce the appearance of stretch marks and hyperpigmentation
- improve skin texture and condition.

In this chapter you will learn about:

- consultation
- contra-indications to electrotherapy treatments
- selecting equipment and products for electrotherapy treatments
- preparation of a client for a facial electrotherapy treatment
- preparation of a client for a body electrotherapy treatment.

It is essential that you understand fully:

- the effects and benefits of these treatments
- how the equipment works
- terminology relating to body electrotherapy treatments
- the correct products to use with the equipment
- the recommended length and frequency of the treatments
- what the client can expect from the treatment, eg any noises or sensations associated with the treatment (so that you can explain this fully to the client).

Overview of body treatments

Galvanic treatment	Faradic treatment	Microcurrent treatment
• Improves cellulite conditions • Removal of toxins and waste • Increases circulation and metabolism • Improves skin colour and tone	• Tones, tightens and strengthens muscles • Improves body contours • Re-educates muscles • Increases circulation and metabolism	• Lifts, tightens sagging muscles • Stimulates muscle fibres/slows down ageing process • Improves skin conditions (eg cellulite/stretch marks) • Reduces oedema

Mechanical massage (G5) treatment

Lymphatic drainage treatment

Body treatments

Prepare for body electrotherapy treatments

It is vital to agree the client's treatment objectives during the consultation so that you can select the correct pieces of equipment to suit their needs. During the consultation you will need to take details of the client's medical history and former treatments to decide on the correct procedure to maximise the benefits of the treatment.

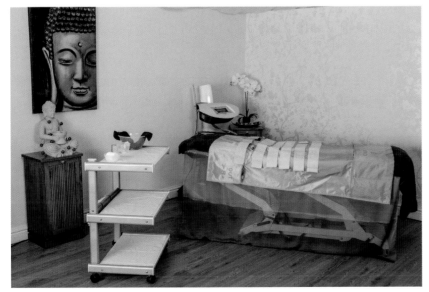

A prepared treatment couch

Prepare yourself, your work area and your client

You should be fully prepared prior to a client arriving for their treatment. You need to make sure that:

- all the equipment and products are to hand and that once the treatment begins you will not need to leave your client unattended

- the trolley and couch are clean and prepared

- the treatment environment (ie lighting, sound, heating and ventilation) is suitable and makes the treatment experience pleasant for the client (requirements may vary from client to client so check that they are comfortable before you begin)

- you are fully prepared to meet, greet and treat your client.

Consultation

Consultation is a vital process during which you should assess the client's needs and objectives and their suitability for the treatment. More detailed information on the consultation process and communication techniques can be found in the Values and behaviours chapter.

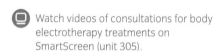
Watch videos of consultations for body electrotherapy treatments on SmartScreen (unit 305).

During the consultation you will need to:

- discuss what the client hopes to achieve from the treatment

- give the client a full explanation of the treatment (ie what is going to happen – sensations, sounds)

- explain realistic achievements associated with the treatment

- record details of the client's medical history and previous treatments (to make sure you are using the correct procedure for them)

- perform a figure diagnosis including checking the client's body type and condition.

Allow the client plenty of time to ask questions as they may be nervous or they may not have had an electrotherapy treatment before.

Contra-indications to body electrotherapy treatments

It is essential to establish any contra-indications prior to carrying out a massage treatment. The client can then be advised to have a different treatment or, where appropriate, to gain medical advice.

If the client has any of the following conditions, this would prevent the massage treatment from being carried out:

- any contagious disease, including skin diseases (bacterial, viral, fungal)
- treatment for cancer (chemotherapy or radiotherapy treatment)
- severe skin condition (eg severe psoriasis or eczema)
- infestation (scabies)
- dysfunction of the nervous system
- recent scar tissue
- undiagnosed lump or swelling.

Not all disorders are contra-indications; some may only restrict treatment. It is therefore vital that that the therapist is familiar with the diseases and disorders that they may encounter within the workplace that may restrict treatment:

- undergoing medical treatment/medication
- uncontrolled diabetes
- epilepsy
- varicose veins
- high or low blood pressure
- history of thrombosis or embolism
- pacemaker
- pregnancy
- metal pins or plates
- piercings
- product allergies
- cuts and abrasions
- heat rash or sunburn
- bruises
- anxiety
- micro-pigmentation (permanent make-up)
- IPL or **LASER** and epilation.

LASER

Light Amplification Simulated Emission of Radiation.

All therapists offering body treatments should be aware of the most common type of skin disorders and diseases that they may come across, and be able to make a decision as to whether the treatment is contra-indicated or not and therefore may or may be not be carried out.

When a client attends a body treatment you must ensure that you check visually (inspect the skin) as well as verbally for any contra-indications to the chosen treatment.

In addition to the general contra-indications listed above, there are a number of contra-indications that are specific to body electrotherapy treatments.

Contra-indication	Treatment	Restricts/ prevents treatment	Reason
Pacemaker	All body electrotherapy treatments.	Prevents	Could affect the rhythm of the heart.
Metal plate or pin Piercing Excessive metal in a particular area (eg dental fillings, bridge work)	All body electrotherapy treatments.	Restricts	Might increase electrical current through the body and therefore make the treatment uncomfortable.
Sunburn	Any electrotherapy treatment of the sunburnt areas.	Restricts	Erythema could develop.
Nervous client	All body electrotherapy treatments.	Restricts	Treatment will not be enjoyable for client.
Recent breast implants	Breast-lift microcurrent treatments.	Restricts	Risk of interference with implants. Could dislodge or affect the implants.
Muscular injury	Body electrotherapy treatments.	Restricts	Might make the condition worse.
Intrauterine device (IUD)	Body electrotherapy treatments.	Restricts	If IUD is copper avoid working over the abdominal area (ie over the uterus).
Very bony areas	Body electrotherapy treatments.	Restricts	Might be painful for client if treatment is applied over bony areas, which have little tissue.
Obesity	Body electrical muscle stimulation (EMS or faradic) treatments.	Restricts	Adipose tissue is an insulator. The muscles might not contract resulting in an ineffective treatment.
Loose crêpe-like skin	Vacuum suction treatments.	Restricts	Suction will cause capillary and tissue damage.
Excessive body hair	Vacuum suction treatments.	Restricts	Suction will drag on the hair. Will be uncomfortable for the client.
Recent stretch marks	Vacuum suction treatments.	Restricts	The skin tissue is already delicate. Vacuum suction could cause further trauma.

Once you have completed the consultation with your client and have decided on the programme or treatment that meets their objectives, you can begin your body analysis prior to starting the treatment.

General contra-actions to electrotherapy treatments

A contra-action is an undesirable effect which happens during or as the result of a treatment. It is essential that the therapist knows how to deal with a contra-action and that they can also advise the client on how to deal with one if it occurs once they have left the salon/spa. The following table shows the most common contra-actions following a facial or body electrotherapy treatment.

Contra-action	Cause	Action to be taken
Excessive erythema (all electrical treatments)	Over-stimulation of the circulatory system.	Usually settles and disappears after a few hours. Apply a cool compress to reduce any further heat in the area. If it is still red and uncomfortable after 24 hours, the client should notify the salon and contact their doctor in case there is another cause.
Allergic reaction/ irritation (all electrical treatments)	Reaction to a product that has been applied to the skin.	Excessive erythema and inflammation. Might be accompanied by itchiness. Remove all products from the skin immediately using cool water and apply a cool compress to reduce any heat in the area. If the reaction is severe and has not disappeared after 24 hours, the client should contact their doctor and notify the salon of the results.
Muscle fatigue (spasms or cramps) (faradic or microcurrent)	A lack of oxygen to the muscle and a build-up of waste products (eg lactic acid). Over-working the muscle.	Stop treatment and massage affected area to remove waste products and introduce fresh oxygen and nutrients to the area.
Galvanic burns (galvanic treatment)	Over-intensity used.	Stop treatment and apply a cold compress to the affected area.

Body analysis

When performing a body analysis the therapist should carry out a manual assessment alongside their postural analysis.

The manual assessment will help to identify the treatment objectives and influence your decision about which products, equipment and techniques to use.

The manual assessment should include:

- weight
- height
- calculating the BMI
- measuring the body or areas to be treated (as appropriate for inch loss, eg faradic, microcurrent and body wraps)
- body characteristics (fat distribution and type, muscle bulk)
- body condition (sluggish circulation, muscle tone)
- skin type and condition.

Weight

When assessing weight:

- always use the same scales – preferably calibrated digital scales
- make sure the scales are on a firm base
- always return the scales to zero prior to weighing
- the client should stand with their weight evenly distributed on both feet
- the client should wear minimal clothing
- check weight against height and frame size.

Height

When measuring height:

- ideally use a permanent fixed measurement on a wall
- client should have heels against the wall
- client should have their head held evenly and look straight ahead.

Calculate the client's frame size

It is useful to note the client's general frame size, as a person with a small frame will weigh less than someone of the same height with larger hands and feet. We can do this by looking at wrist circumference.

Wrist measurement in relation to frame size

	Women	Men
Large frame	6.5 or more inches	7.5 or more inches
Medium frame	5.5–6.5 inches	6.5–7.5 inches
Small frame	5.5 or less inches	6.5 or less inches

*2.5cm = 1 inch

The therapist should measure the body when the body treatments prescribed give inch-loss reduction, for example body wraps, EMS (faradic) and microcurrent toning and firming treatments. The client should be measured before and after the treatment or course of treatments, to determine the total inch loss achieved.

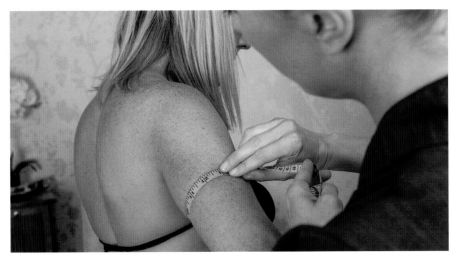

Watch a video of body analysis on SmartScreen (unit 305).

Measuring the bicep

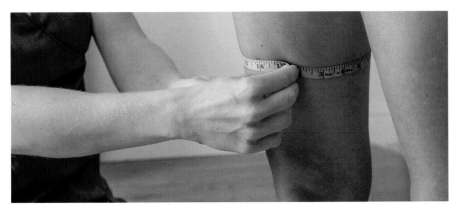

Measuring the thigh

Measure around the fullest part of the area of the body and ensure that the tape measure is:

- not too tight
- not twisted
- parallel with the ground
- placed in the same place each time.

HANDY HINT

If a client has booked a course of treatments with the aim of losing inches, record the size of the area at the start and at the end of the course of treatments.

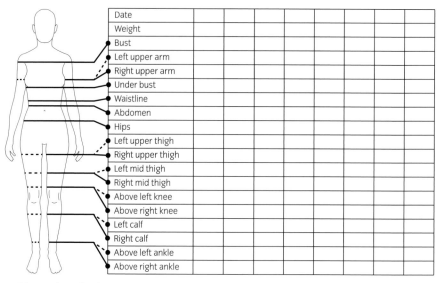

Date					
Weight					
Bust					
Left upper arm					
Right upper arm					
Under bust					
Waistline					
Abdomen					
Hips					
Left upper thigh					
Right upper thigh					
Left mid thigh					
Right mid thigh					
Above left knee					
Above right knee					
Left calf					
Right calf					
Above left ankle					
Above right ankle					

Measuring chart

Fat distribution and type

Assess the body's fat distribution and type:

- soft fat – loose packed adipocytes (fat cells), which are easy to grasp and have movement
- hard fat – tightly packed adipocytes; firm to touch and hard to grasp, difficult to manipulate
- cellulite – dimpled appearance to the skin; common around thighs, buttocks, abdomen and upper arms.

Muscle tone

Muscle tone is the slight but continuous tension or contraction in the muscles at all times while awake. This keeps the body upright. Without this the muscles would all relax at once and the body would collapse. Maintaining muscle tone becomes harder as we age, and muscle tone can become weaker as a result.

Good muscle tone:

- has a defined shape with good contours
- is firm to the touch
- is in a state of partial contraction
- contracts quickly to stimulation of the nerve.

Poor muscle tone is:

- little definition with slack contours
- soft to touch
- flabby and loose
- slow to contract.

Postural analysis

As a therapist you will need to have a basic understanding of the structure of the spine and how to identify postural and figure faults, along with body type, muscle tone, fat type and skin conditions.

A postural assessment is used to:

- assess any figure problems and faults
- recognise any areas of concern or that may require medical referral
- plan an effective treatment by selecting the most appropriate electrical or mechanical treatments and products for the conditions present.

Vertebrae/spinal column

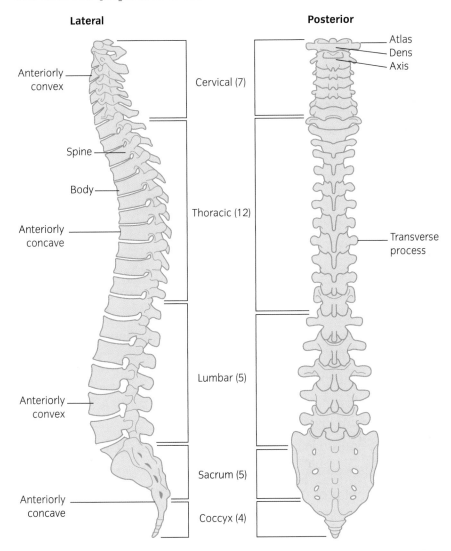

Lateral

Anteriorly convex

Spine

Body

Anteriorly concave

Anteriorly convex

Anteriorly concave

Cervical (7)

Thoracic (12)

Lumbar (5)

Sacrum (5)

Coccyx (4)

Posterior

Atlas

Dens

Axis

Transverse process

Lateral and posterior vertebrae

Good posture should include:

■ well-balanced position when standing

■ head held up, comfortable, with no protrusion of the jaw

■ body weight equally distributed

■ spine follows a natural curve

■ shoulders are even and not slouched; neither droop or over-extend

■ chest naturally elevated, arms loose at the sides of the body

■ abdomen pulled in flat and curves at the waist are even

■ pelvis balanced and without tilt

■ feet facing forward and slightly apart.

How to assess posture

When you first greet your client observe them closely and make note of the following:

■ how they move

■ how they carry themselves

■ their overall posture.

Postural considerations

1 Position of head and neck – head should be midline, not tilted or jaw forward; ears and eyes level.

2 Body weight evenly balanced.

3 Spine – follows a natural curve.

4 Shoulders – even, neither drooping nor rolled inwards. Check for dowager's hump.

5 Scapulae – blades should be even and equal distance from the spine without protrusion.

6 Arms – relaxed and at the sides.

7 Ribs – clavicles and rib cage should be symmetrical. Are the ribs over-extended? Pigeon or hollow chest?

8 Abdomen – pulled in flat and curves at the waist are even.

9 Pelvis – balanced and not tilted forward or backwards.

10 Buttocks – not protruding; gluteal folds level and in line with the pubis.

11 Legs – straight with knees facing forwards and level, not hyper-extended or bowed.

12 Feet – look at position of feet; do they turn in or out? Check for flat feet, high arches.

Postural faults

The following are types of postural conditions that a therapist may encounter.

Condition	Characteristics
Flat back	Pelvis tilted backwards, lumbar region of spine flat and hamstrings shortened.
	The client will tend to look erect with square shoulders.
Pelvic tilt – unbalanced pelvis	Tilts too far forward – the lumbar vertebrae become hyperextended.
	Tilts too far back – the lumbar region can become flattened.
Lordosis	Hollow back in the lumbar region.
	Pelvis tends to be inclined forwards, the abdominal and hamstring muscles become lengthened and stretched, lumbar muscles become shortened and the gluteals weakened.
Kyphosis	Exaggeration of the normal backward curve of the thoracic region in the spine.
	Poking chin, round shoulders, pectoral muscles tend to be tight, shortened and the upper back muscles overstretched and weak.
Scoliosis	This a sideways deviation (lateral) of the curve of the spine, forming either an 'S' or a 'C'. Commonly the thoracic vertebrae are rotated. The primary curve may vary in degree and a secondary curve develops below the primary curve to compensate and maintain posture.
	This condition can lead to other faults such as one leg being shorter than the other, one shoulder higher than the other, uneven scapulae or pelvic tilts.
Winged scapula	The medial border of the scapula vertebrae protrudes backwards away from the ribs. It is caused by a weakness in the serratus anterior muscle.
Knock knees (genu valgus)	There is an increased lateral angle of the tibia in relation to the femur causing the angle of the knee to move inwards from the hips. Women have a tendency to this postural fault due to the increased width of the female pelvis.
Bow legs (genu varus)	The lateral angle of the femur to the tibia is reduced causing the knees to become further apart.
Flat feet (pes planus)	Medial longitudinal arch is reduced giving reduced stability to the foot.
Dowager's hump	This condition generally develops over a period of time. The head becomes tilted forward and there is extreme kyphosis. The shoulders become rounded and movement is restricted in the area. There is often an accumulation of fatty deposits at the lower cervical and upper thoracic vertebrae.
Pigeon chest	The sternum protrudes forward.
Short limbs	Limbs are not in proportion to the body.

Postural faults of the spine

There are three main postural faults to be considered:

- kyphosis
- lordosis
- scoliosis.

Kyphosis

Also known as round shoulders. A kyphotic curve looks like the letter 'C' with the opening towards the chest, which causes an increase in the normal backward curve of the thoracic spine.

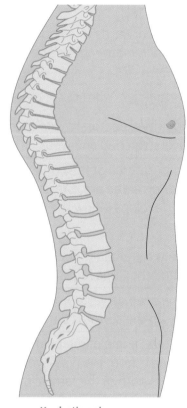

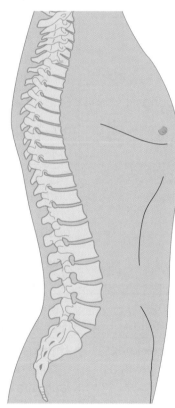

Kyphotic spine   Normal spine

Symptoms of kyphosis

These include:

- round shoulders, hunched back
- tight and shortened pectoral muscles, neck flexors, hamstrings and gluteals
- extensors of upper neck and back are lengthened/stretched and therefore weakened.

In kyphosis the ilium of the pelvis is tilted backward at a 45-degree angle and the pubis bone is tilted forward, which affects the hip flexors and hip extensors.

Causes of kyphosis

Kyphosis tends to start between the age of 10 and 20 years and its most common cause is habitual bad posture, eg faulty sitting position.

However, other causes include:

- congenital spinal problem (eg cerebral palsy)
- over-rapid growth rate in childhood
- lack of proper exercise
- trauma to the spine
- heavy breasts with lack of support.

Lordosis

Commonly referred to as hollow back or sway back. With this condition there is an abnormal and excessive inward curvature of the lumbar vertebrae. The angle of pelvic tilt is increased forward and the chest is elevated with the shoulders pulled back.

Symptoms of lordosis

These are:

- lower back pain
- buttocks/gluteals appear prominent due to excessive arching/ curving of the lumbar spine
- tightness of the hip flexors and hamstrings
- weakness in the abdominal and gluteal muscle groups.

Main causes of lordosis

These include:

- congenital defect
- pregnancy; pelvic tilt alters
- poor postural habits especially with people whose occupation requires long periods of standing (shop assistants, etc)
- being overweight, due to the angle of the pelvic tilt altering
- long-term practice of gymnastics, due to the posture frequently adopted
- may occur in childhood.

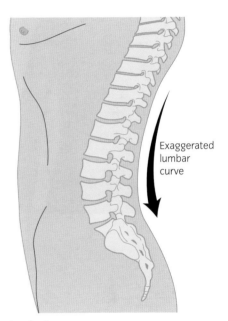

Exaggerated lumbar curve

Lordosis

Scoliosis

Scoliosis is a lateral curvature of the spine in the thoracic region. There are two types: 'C' or 'S' curve.

Scoliosis 'C' curve: there may be one large 'C' shaped curve extending the whole length of spine or two smaller curves: one primary 'C' which occurs near the top of the spine while the other compensatory curve occurs near the base of the spine in the opposite direction to counterbalance the body weight. Most 'C' curves are to the left due to the majority of people being right-handed.

Scoliosis 'S' curve (S for scoliosis and sideways): usually one lumber and one thoracic curve, pelvis tilted down on side of convexity in the lumbar area. Eighty per cent of cases of 'S' scoliosis are due to poor posture.

Causes of scoliosis

These include:

- bad posture – due to faulty sitting habits, common in adolescent girls; results in muscular imbalance between muscles, leading to permanent, long-term changes in body structure
- rapid growth, although rare
- abnormal development of the bones in the spine, which is present at birth
- a variety of conditions affecting the neuromuscular system – nerves and muscles

Symptoms of scoliosis

These are:

- uneven shoulders
- curve in spine
- uneven hips or waistline
- twisted pelvis, with one leg shorter than the other.

Scoliosis

Select equipment and products for electrotherapy treatments

INDUSTRY TIP

Each manufacturer of electrotherapy equipment will provide instructions on how long to use each piece of equipment. As an overview, most body electrical treatments last around 60 to 75 minutes, dependent on the number of pieces of equipment used and the client's treatment objectives.

To achieve the best results, clients will need a course or series of treatments. Throughout the course of treatments you might need to change the equipment you are using to meet the client's needs. You might also need to use more than one piece of equipment to achieve the treatment objectives. It is therefore important that you understand which pieces of equipment work well together and the course of treatments that will suit your clients.

To select the correct piece of equipment you also need to understand:

- how the equipment works
- the electrical current it uses
- what it is used for
- specific contra-indications and contra-actions
- how application to the face and body differs
- how to prepare for the treatment (yourself, your client and your work area)
- how to carry out a consultation to:
    - find out about a client's needs/objectives
    - agree a treatment plan
- carry out a skin analysis and figure diagnosis.

INDUSTRY TIP

In addition to the electrotherapy equipment you will need:

- any accessories that are to be used alongside the machine
- products, tools and equipment for carrying out a body treatment.

Prepare the client for a body electrotherapy treatment

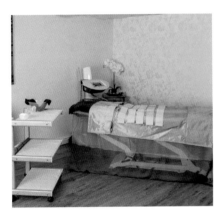

STEP 1 Prepare the treatment room including the equipment.

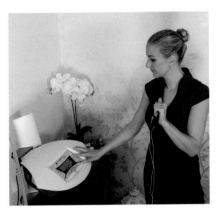

STEP 2 Check that the machine is working properly.

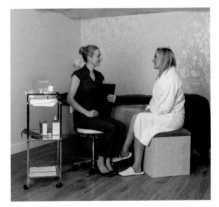

STEP 3 During the consultation, explain the treatment procedure to the client and give them the opportunity to ask questions.

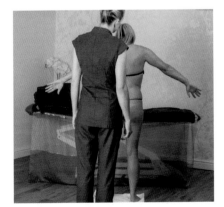

STEP 4 Carry out a body analysis, including body measurements (ie height and weight), a muscle tone test and a cellulite test. The results must be recorded on the client's record card.

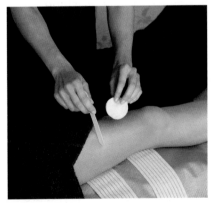

STEP 5 Perform tactile and thermal sensitivity tests on the area to be treated.

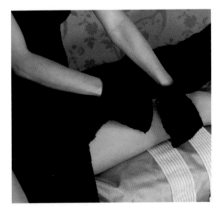

STEP 6 Cleanse the treatment area with a body cleanser and exfoliate as appropriate or wipe over the area with a sanitiser, such as witch hazel.

HANDY HINT

Make sure that the client's body is warm. Ideally the client will have had a sauna or been in a steam room for the best results; however, an infrared lamp can be used instead.

HEALTH & SAFETY

Clean oil off work surfaces and containers quickly, as oil residue is sticky and a great breeding ground for bacteria.

HEALTH & SAFETY

Ask the client to remove all jewellery prior to treatment and insulate any cuts or blemishes with petroleum jelly.

Activity

As a group, discuss with your tutor:

- How do I set up the treatment room?
- What other products/equipment do I need other than machinery?
- How do I check the machines are working?
- How do I carry out a sensitivity test?

Carry out body electrotherapy treatments

In this part of the chapter you will learn about:

- galvanic treatment
- electrical muscle stimulation (EMS or faradic)
- vacuum suction
- G5 mechanical massage
- infrared
- general contra-actions to electrotherapy treatments
- general home-care advice and recommendations for body electrotherapy treatments.

Body electrotherapy uses a range of different currents and frequencies and as a therapist you should ensure that you have good knowledge and understanding of:

- the type of current used and how it behaves
- how the equipment works and can be adapted
- the appropriate products and applicators for each piece of equipment
- the benefits and effects of the treatment to the client
- how to use the equipment effectively to suit the client's needs
- health and safety practices, to include risk assessment.

HANDY HINT

For more on the types of current used in electrotherapy and how they behave, see chapter 304, Provide facial electrotherapy treatments.

Types of electrical current used in electrotherapy treatments

A direct current is used in galvanic treatments, and a modified direct current is used in EMS and microcurrent treatments.

Treatment	Current	Wave form
Galvanic	Direct current – constant direct flow.	**Galvanic wave**
EMS (faradic)	Modified direct current – alters depending upon the machine programme selected for the treatment.	**Faradic wave 1** Brief burst of current, ie pulse (lasting 1 millisecond) Interval when no current flows (lasting 9 milliseconds) **Faradic wave 2** **Faradic wave 3**

Electrical term	Definition
Conductor	A material that transmits electricity, eg metal, saline.
Insulator	A material that does not transmit electricity easily, eg rubber.
Voltage	Force or pressure to push electricity around an electrical circuit.
Amp	Unit of electrical current (the maximum from a power socket is 13 amp).
Ohms	Resistance which slows down the current (= volts ÷ amps).
Watts	Unit that measures the power to run equipment (= volts × amps).
Electrolyte	A substance that conducts electricity when dissolved in a suitable solvent.
Frequency	Number of times per second the current changes direction.

Refer to page 375 for general home-care advice and recommendations for electrotherapy treatments.

Desincrustation

To remove a crust that covers an object.

Iontophoresis

The introduction of water-soluble substances into the skin.

Polarity

Like poles repel each other but opposite poles attract each other

Galvanic treatment

Galvanic treatment improves the skin in two ways:

- **desincrustation** – removal of surface blockages and thorough cleansing of the skin
- **iontophoresis** – this technique is used to push products into the skin.

A galvanic current is a low-voltage, direct current that flows in one direction. It works on the basic laws of polarity (ie like poles repel each other but opposite poles attract each other):

- +ve attracts –ve
- +ve repels +ve
- –ve repels –ve.

Polarity

The galvanic machine has a **polarity** switch for selecting and changing polarity. The machine also has sockets for connecting electrodes. An anode (an electrode with positive polarity) and a cathode (an electrode with negative polarity) are needed for the system to work because opposite poles attract. Products containing positively or negatively charged ions are used during galvanic treatments.

The active electrode (eg rollers) must be the same polarity as the galvanic solution/gel so that products are pushed into the skin.

The active ingredients in galvanic solutions are marked with a plus (+) or a minus (–) to show whether they are positive or negative. Always check that the correct polarity of cosmetic products is used to make sure that an effective treatment is achieved.

The polarity of the products and the machine setting will have an effect on the treatment. It is important to remember that like poles repel so:

- negative (–ve) to negative and positive (+ve) to positive would push away from each other
- positive to negative and negative to positive would be attracted to each other as opposites attract.

Effects of the electrodes in galvanic treatment

Anode (+ve polarity)	Cathode (–ve polarity)
Acid reaction (hydrochloric acid)	Alkaline reaction (sodium hydroxide)
Vasoconstriction	Vasodilation
Pores are tightened	Pores are relaxed
Decreases erythema	Sebum is softened and broken down (saponification)
Soothes nerve endings	Stimulates nerve endings
Decreases lymph	Increases lymph
Skin tightening	Skin softening

Equipment used in galvanic treatment

Equipment	Use
Galvanic body unit	Used for galvanic body treatments.
Carbon electrodes	Used for galvanic body treatments.
Metal plate electrode and sponge envelopes	Used for galvanic body treatments. Body pads are covered with damp sponge envelopes.
Metal-free elastic straps	Used to secure carbon electrodes or plate electrodes to the body during galvanic body treatments.

Different padding sequences

Carbon pads

With body galvanic treatments the electrodes are in the form of carbon pads which are applied to the skin. A positive electrode (pad) is positioned opposite a negative electrode (eg a positive electrode on the biceps and a negative electrode on the triceps). The electrodes have different leads depending on whether they are positive or negative:

- black lead and –ve symbol = negative electrode
- red lead and +ve symbol = positive electrode.

Galvanic products and their uses

Product	Use/benefits
Active solutions (eg gels, creams and serums)	Chosen for specific treatment requirements such as toning, firming, anti-cellulite.
Saline solution	Saline solution used for galvanic body treatments; this acts as a conductor for electrical current on the skin.

Effects and benefits of galvanic body treatments

The following list shows how galvanic body treatments can affect the body and what the benefits are of the treatment:

- has a **diuretic** effect that can be used to increase lymphatic flow and assist during a weight-loss programme
- improves the appearance of cellulite
- improves blood circulation
- stimulates sluggish, sallow skin
- aids the removal of toxins and waste products
- has a stimulating or soothing effect on the nerve endings
- speeds up the metabolism
- disperses fatty deposits.

Precautions

It is important to perform all the following safety checks before carrying out galvanic treatments to avoid the risk of galvanic burns:

- Make sure all jewellery (both client's and therapist's) is removed.
- Cover cuts/blemishes with petroleum jelly.
- Do not exceed 2–3mA on the galvanic unit (as per manufacturer's instructions).

HANDY HINT

Your tutor will have shown you different pad-up techniques. You may need to adapt the sequence depending on the client's needs.

HANDY HINT

You can use 'BIRO' to help you remember the different electrodes:

B – black

I – insertion

R – red

O – origin

INDUSTRY TIP

If the client has oily or congested skin, you can apply direct high frequency for five to eight minutes after extraction and before reversing the polarity. Remember to apply over oxygenating cream and gauze. This will have a healing, drying and germicidal effect.

Diuretic

A drug or substance that tends to increase the amount of urine excreted from the body.

INDUSTRY TIP

The first treatment should never exceed 10 minutes; gradually increase to a maximum of 20 minutes as the sessions progress. Recommend a course of ten treatments with two to three sessions per week. It is recommended that the client follow a healthy eating plan with regular exercise and home-care regime to aid the dispersal of cellulite.

- Make sure that the sponge pockets are not spilt or ripped.
- Make sure that wires are not split or damaged.
- Check that the machine has been PAT tested and that it is still valid.
- Make sure that the client does not have any contra-indications that prevent treatment.

Contra-indications to galvanic treatment

In addition to the general contra-indications listed in the Values and behaviours chapter on pages 30–31, it is important that you are aware of these contra-indications to treatment:

- pregnancy (and post-pregnancy until the postnatal check or GP's advice)
- metal plates and pins
- pacemaker
- epilepsy
- diabetes
- cuts or abrasions in the treatment area
- varicose veins
- kidney disorders due to the diuretic effect of the treatment.

Guide to galvanic treatment application

The purpose of galvanic body treatments is to introduce active substances into the tissues to increase fluid loss and mobilise fatty tissue.

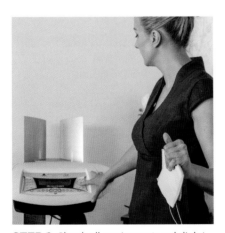

STEP 1 Check all equipment and dials/settings – always follow the manufacturer's instructions.

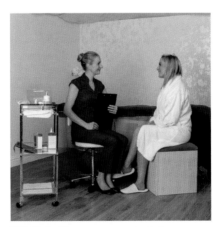

STEP 2 Always carry out a full consultation and check contra-indications.

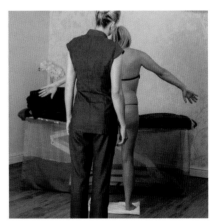

STEP 3 Carry out a body analysis as appropriate. Perform tactile and thermal sensitivity tests in the area to be treated.

 Watch the video of this galvanic body treatment on SmartScreen (unit 305).

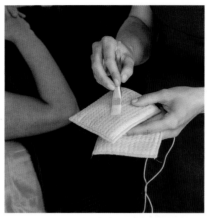

STEP 4 Prepare pads/isolated protectors or pockets – they should be clean and dampened evenly to allow conductivity. (Electrodes must be fully covered by damp sponge protectors or pockets otherwise a galvanic burn may occur.) Apply anti-cellulite gel to the active electrode insulated pad/pocket or affected area only – paste smoothly to ensure even coverage.

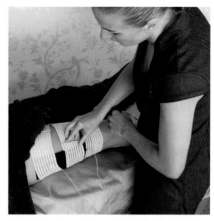

STEP 5 Place the pads in the correct positions for the treatment objective and secure firmly with Velcro straps. (Pads must make full contact with the skin, otherwise it may result in discomfort or a burn.) Slowly increase the current until the client feels a mild tingling/prickling sensation – do not exceed 3mA.

HANDY HINT

At the end of the treatment, turn the dials to zero and make sure there is no current (mA) registering. Switch off the machine at the mains.

HANDY HINT

There is a milliamp meter on the galvanic machine that should not exceed 1.5mA during treatment as the skin's resistance breaks down above this level. It is therefore important to monitor the milliamps throughout the treatment.

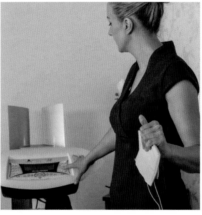

STEP 6 Time the treatment and reverse the polarity for the final 3–5 minutes. Slowly turn down intensity and turn off the current and equipment. Remove pads and any remaining product. Perform any other services as prescribed in the treatment plan (eg lymphatic drainage or manual massage).

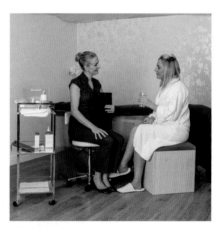

STEP 7 Give your client advice and recommendations to include contra-actions, home care, product and further treatment recommendations. Record and evaluate the treatment.

INDUSTRY TIP

Check product polarity for anti-cellulite gel and select the correct polarity on equipment. (The gel should be the same polarity as the active pad so that they repel.)

INDUSTRY TIP

During a galvanic treatment, tissue fluid is drawn towards the negative electrode (cathode/black). This is known as electro-osmosis and can help to improve the appearance of lumpy tissue/cellulite.

Contra-actions to galvanic treatment

You need to be aware of general contra-actions such as product allergies. However, there are also some contra-actions that are specific to galvanic treatments.

HANDY HINT

Recommend a course of ten treatments with two to three sessions per week.

Contra-action	Description	Action to be taken
Sensitisation due to intensity of the treatment or products	Severe erythema.	Apply a cool compress. If it happens during treatment, reverse the polarity for two to three minutes, then apply a cooling soothing gel.
Galvanic burn	Usually the result of poor practice (eg not applying enough product or over-treating the area). A chemical burn results from a concentration of alkali on the skin. Skin is dark, split and surrounded by an inflamed red ring.	Flush the area with lots of cool water. Apply a dry sterile dressing. Advise client to seek medical advice immediately.
Metallic taste	If the client has fillings or bridge work they may taste metal in their mouth.	Use rubber gum shields to help prevent this.

Home-care advice and recommendations for galvanic treatment

Please see page 397 for general advice and recommendations for home-care for electrotherapy treatments.

HANDY HINT

The normal response to a galvanic body treatment is erythema.

HANDY HINT

Remember to monitor the client throughout the treatment and adjust timings and intensity as necessary. You must increase the current slowly because of the skin's initial resistance.

Electrical muscle stimulation (EMS or faradic)

The first EMS device was patented in 1948 by Dr Sebastian Hawkins (an osteopath and chiropractor).

How EMS treatment works

EMS treatment causes stimulation of the muscles to help tone and strengthen them. An alternating low-frequency, interrupted and surged direct current of electricity is used.

A carbon block (facial) or carbon pads (body) are positioned on the **motor point** of a muscle.

The current stimulates the motor nerves causing a gradual contraction of the muscles, increasing in strength and then gradually decreasing in strength. The surging is controlled by a timing device within the machine.

The client will feel a tingling sensation followed by a gentle muscle contraction as the current is increased. The current then stops, allowing the muscle to relax.

HANDY HINT

Select the correct polarity (if the solution is +ve, the polarity should be +ve and vice versa). Reduce the current slowly. Once the current has reached zero, keep the rollers moving for a moment or two to allow any left-over current to disperse.

Motor point

The part of a muscle that is stimulated and where a visible contraction can be caused with a minimal amount of stimulation.

INDUSTRY TIP

Galvanic should be applied as a course of treatments and can be complemented by additional services such as lymphatic drainage, G5 massage and EMS.

If a contraction is not achieved, it may be due to incorrect positioning or due to layers of adipose tissue hiding the movement.

Muscle contraction due to EMS treatment is different from normal **voluntary muscle contraction** (ie when our brain sends a message via our motor nerves to the muscle). The current from the EMS machine stimulates the motor nerve directly (without going via the brain) causing the muscle to contract. When the current stops the muscle relaxes.

Equipment used in EMS treatment

An EMS unit can be purchased as a single facial or body unit or as a combined facial and body unit.

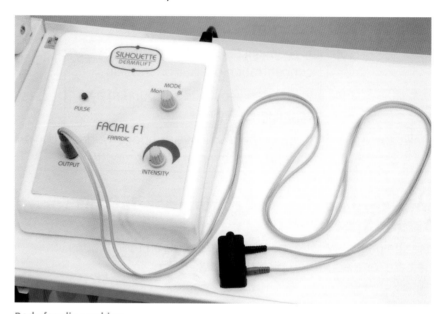

Body faradic machine

An EMS unit produces a low-frequency direct current of between 10 and 120Hz. The EMS unit has a number of controls and settings that the therapist needs to familiarise themselves with.

Control/setting	Description
On/off switch	Usually has a light to show that the unit is switched on.
	If using a body unit there might be a master switch to switch all of the attached pads on or off at once.
Timer	Some units have pre-set times or the programme time can be selected manually and displayed during the treatment.
Frequency control	Controls the number of pulses per second.
	Determines the depth of stimulation.

Voluntary muscle contraction

Muscle contraction that you consciously control.

HANDY HINT

If you are unsure whether a contraction is occurring, place a hand on the muscle to feel it.

INDUSTRY TIP

Make sure that the manufacturer's instruction booklet detailing all the controls and settings is in an easy-to-reach place at all times.

HEALTH & SAFETY

Before use, it is essential to read the manufacturer's instructions explaining what each button on the machine does.

Control/setting	Description
Monophasic pulse sequence	Current flows in one direction.
	Helps to lift muscles.
	The current travels in one direction only from negative to positive. The polarity of the pads remains constant throughout, meaning that there is more strength under the negative pad, which should be placed on the weaker muscle.
	A monophasic pulse sequence is always used during a facial EMS treatment because it flows in one direction only. Only an upward movement of the muscle should be stimulated, as the aim of the treatment is to lift and tone muscles.
Biphasic pulse sequence	The polarity of the pads changes so that the current always travels from negative to positive, but as the pad polarity changes the current runs in one direction and then in the other direction of each pulse.
	Helps with strengthening and toning of the muscle.
	This is best used in longitudinal padding.
Stimulation	The amount of time the pulse of the current will flow for to stimulate the muscle before a rest.
	Usually set between half a second and two-and-a-half seconds.
Relaxation	The length of the rest period when the current does not flow.
	Usually a few seconds to a minute so that the muscle does not become too relaxed before stimulation occurs again.
Mode control	Either constant or variable.
	Controls the sequence of the contractions.
Constant mode	The length of the stimulation period and rest periods remains the same during the treatment.
Variable mode	Varies the length of the stimulation and rest periods during the treatment.
	Ideal for nervous clients as they do not know when to expect the next stimulation so are not able to tense the muscle in anticipation.
	Only used on the body.
Pulse width	Increasing pulse width is similar to increasing the intensity.
	If the pulse width is increased there will be greater stimulation.
Modulated pulse	Gentle stimulation.
	Builds up to its pre-set intensity gradually.
	Causes a more gentle contraction to be produced.
Unmodulated pulse	Intense stimulation throughout the whole stimulation period.
	Ideal for deeper muscles or if there is a large amount of adipose tissue present.
Intensity control	Controls the strength of the current.
	If the dial is turned up, the intensity increases.
Master output control	Can be used to turn up all the current settings at the same time.
	Only used once the client has become used to the contractions.

Electrodes	Description
Block	Used on the face.
	A carbon block with both negative and positive polarity.
	Attached to the EMS unit with a cable.
	Positioned on the facial muscles to stimulate contractions.
Pads	Used on the body.
	Contain carbon.
	Placed on the **origin** and **insertion** of the muscle to achieve a contraction.
	The black pad (or one with a black lead) is placed on the insertion of the muscle.
	The red lead/pad is placed onto the origin of the muscle.
	The black pad has a negative charge which gives a stronger muscle contraction if using the monophasic mode.

Origin

The end of a muscle which is attached to a fixed bone.

Insertion

The end of the muscle that is attached to the bone which moves.

INDUSTRY TIP

If there is no contraction of a muscle or poor contraction, consider whether:

- there is an oily barrier on the skin
- there is too much adipose (fatty) tissue in the area
- the electrode is positioned on the motor point.

Padding

There are three types of padding used for positioning the electrodes on the body for an EMS treatment:

- Longitudinal padding – padding that extends from the top of a muscle to the bottom of a muscle, near its origin and insertion. Pads are placed on the upper and lower motor points of long muscles such as the rectus abdominus, rectus femoris and trapezius.
- Duplicate/dual padding – a pair of pads is placed on the motor points of muscles with similar actions that are adjacent to one another (eg the external obliques and the rectus abdominus).
- Split padding – a pair of pads is split and the electrode is placed on the motor point of the same muscle group on opposite sides of the body (eg right and left pectorals, right and left gluteus maximus).

Other equipment used in EMS treatment

Equipment	Description
Steamer or infrared lamp	The muscles should be pre-heated using a steamer or infrared lamp prior to treatment to get the maximum benefit.
	Relaxes the muscles ready for passive exercise and reduces the risk of injury.
Non-metallic elastic straps	Used to secure the pads to the body during a body faradic treatment.

Products used in EMS treatment

Product	Description
Cleanser	Used to wipe over the area prior to treatment.
	Should be oil free so there is no barrier that would prevent good muscle contraction.
	Witch hazel or an antiseptic wipe can also be used.
Saline solution	An electrolyte which is a good conductor of current.
	Can be used with both facial and body EMS treatments.
	To make a 1% saline solution, dissolve one teaspoon of salt in a pint of hot water.
Exfoliator	Exfoliation prior to treatment may be needed.
	Prepares the skin by removing any barriers to treatment.
Cellulite gel	Applied over areas of cellulite at the end of the treatment.
	Can be recommended to the client for home care.
Antiseptic	For wiping over the electrodes after treatment once they have been washed.

Effects and benefits of EMS treatment for the body

The following benefits and effects are examples of what a client may experience following an EMS treatment:

- increased blood supply resulting in increased oxygen and nutrients to the area
- vasodilation resulting in improved skin colour
- stimulation of muscles improving muscle tone
- spot reduction to specific areas
- increased rate of cellular metabolism
- inch loss due to improved muscle tone
- more efficient removal of waste products as muscular contraction improves lymphatic circulation.

Contra-indications to EMS treatment

Please refer to page 315 for general contra-indications to electrotherapy treatments.

Application of EMS treatment to the body

Carry out steps 1–6 from body electrotherapy preparation (see page 375).

Watch the video of this EMS treatment on SmartScreen (unit 305).

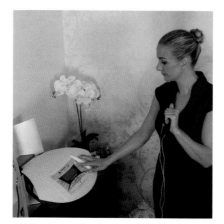

STEP 1 Double-check that the machine dials are all set to zero.

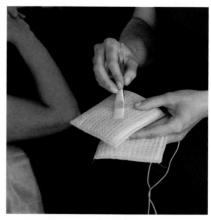

STEP 2 Apply the conductor gel to the area. Alternatively, saline solution can be applied to the electrodes or pad instead.

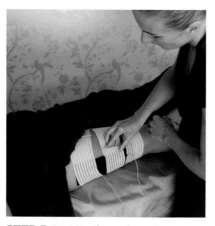

STEP 3 Position the pads on the treatment area identified in the consultation and treatment objectives.

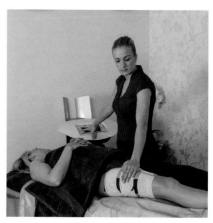

STEP 4 Describe the sensation to the client and explain what they can expect during the treatment when you turn up the machine.

HANDY HINT

Not all units will switch themselves off automatically. If the unit you are using does not have an automatic switch-off function, ensure that it is timed accurately so that you don't under-exercise or over-exercise the muscles.

HANDY HINT

Once the treatment is finished, measure the client again and inform them of their inch-loss results, and then allow the client time to dress in privacy. During the measuring tactfully recommend to them a course of treatments alongside a healthy eating plan to gain the most beneficial results.

With EMS treatment for the body, always remember to:

- Select the programme appropriate to the client's needs.
- Cover the client with a blanket to keep them warm.
- Turn up the intensity until a contraction can be seen. Do this until all the muscles are contracting.
- After ten minutes, turn up the intensity control again to achieve a stronger contraction – depending on the client and how well the muscles contract.

Contra-actions to EMS treatment

Please refer to page 315 for general contra-actions to electrotherapy treatments.

Home-care advice and recommendations for EMS treatment

As with all treatments, advise the client to follow a healthy lifestyle (ie quit smoking, limit alcohol and caffeine intake and take regular exercise). Specific home-care advice related to EMS treatments might include:

- use of an anti-cellulite body product
- **body brushing**
- drinking plenty of water
- following a course of treatments – 10–15 treatments, with two to three treatments in the first week and then an average of two treatments per week
- further monthly treatments once the initial course of treatments has been completed.

Vacuum suction

Vacuum suction is a **mechanical method** of lymphatic drainage treatment.

It is performed using a **ventouse**, which is applied to the skin with a straight and light gliding manner towards the lymph nodes. This encourages drainage of lymph fluid from within the lymph spaces. Although the unit operates by using an electrical current, no current passes through the body or face.

Effects and benefits of vacuum suction

The following list shows the benefits of vacuum suction and the effects of the treatment:

- Aids with the flow of waste products and tissue fluids to the lymph nodes.
- Improves the appearance and tone of the skin.
- Can reduce fine lines.
- Improves fluid drainage and reduces fluid retention.
- Increases circulation.
- Mobilises fatty deposits.
- Helps prevent varicose veins.
- Assists with the removal of comedones and pore blockages.
- Increased blood supply will nourish bones.
- Has a soothing effect on nerve endings.
- Stimulates the lymphatic and circulatory system.

Body brushing

Can loosen and remove any dry skin from the area and increase blood flow. It is a great way to look after your body at home and can be carried out before getting into the shower or bath.

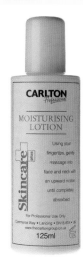

A moisturiser for use after an electrical treatment

Mechanical method

Method using a machine, ie doesn't involve passing an electrical current through the body.

Ventouse

Glass cup used in vacuum suction.

Watch the video of this body vacuum suction treatment on SmartScreen (unit 305).

Application of vacuum suction to the body

Suggested vacuum suction routine:

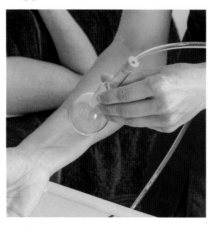

STEP 1 Prepare the treatment room and equipment. Check that the equipment is working properly.

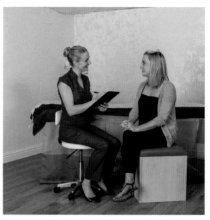

STEP 2 Perform a client consultation, explaining the treatment procedure (demonstrate as appropriate) and allowing the opportunity for your client to ask questions.

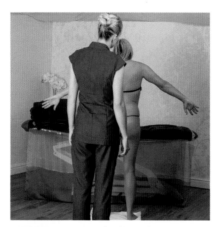

STEP 3 Carry out body analysis and agree treatment objectives/plan.

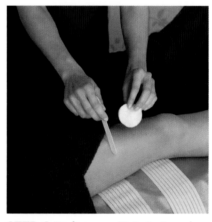

STEP 4 Perform sensitivity tests and check for contra-indications.

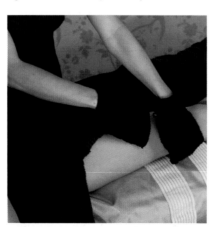

STEP 5 Prepare the area to be treated – cleanse and exfoliate as appropriate. For best results, warm the client's body/area before starting the treatment.

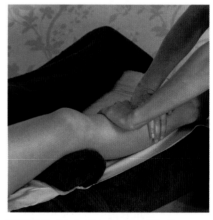

STEP 6 Apply the chosen oil to the area being treated. Ensure the correct amount of oil is used: too little and dragging of skin may occur, causing discomfort; too much and you may have difficulty in controlling the cup.

> **HANDY HINT**
>
> Test on yourself and the client. Do not exceed 20% lift of skin. Loose, soft, fatty areas of tissue require less suction than other areas.

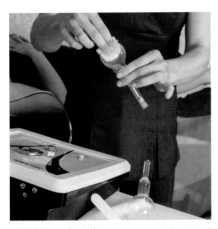

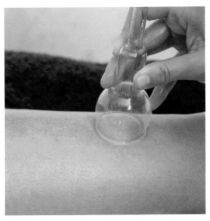

STEP 7 Select the appropriate size cup/ventouse and clean. Cup/ventouse should be selected according to the area being treated; the larger the area, the greater the diameter of the cup.

STEP 8 Carry out the routine on the treatment area identified during the consultation. Always lift and glide towards the nearest lymph node. Do not apply strokes directly over the lymph nodes. Strokes should be well paced, rhythmical and flowing. Overlap each stroke. Keep the skin supported throughout the treatments.

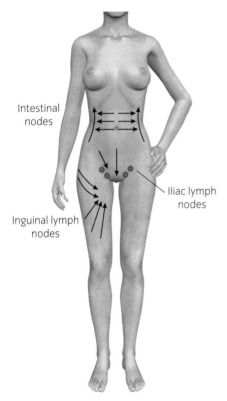

Anterior view of direction of lymph flow using vacuum suction

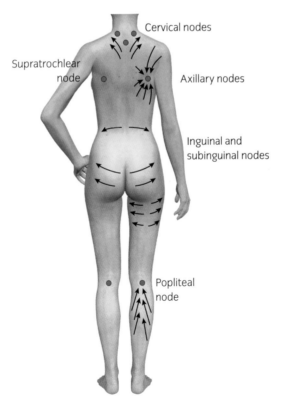

Posterior view of direction of lymph flow using vacuum suction

- Remove any excess oil or massage it into the skin.

- Give advice and recommendations on products and further treatments.

- Explain how to deal with any contra-actions and record the treatment details on the record card.

- Clean and sanitise all equipment and the work area. Wash ventouses in hot soapy water using an antibacterial soap.

Contra-actions to vacuum suction

Please refer to page 315 for general contra-actions to electrotherapy treatments.

Home-care advice and recommendations for vacuum suction

Please refer to page 397 for general home-care advice and recommendations for electrotherapy treatments.

Other electrical treatments

Mechanical massage (G5)

Mechanical massage is the manipulation of the body tissues using gyratory vibration machines.

The most common gyratory massage equipment used in salons, spas and health hydros is the G5 (G = gyratory and 5 refers to the number of detachable heads which are used to achieve different effects and sensations). This kind of massage works deeper into the muscles and is ideal for use on bulky areas of adipose tissue or defined muscle mass. It can be used in conjunction with other treatments to relieve muscle tension and muscle pain, to stimulate the circulation and improve certain skin conditions.

Providing the client is on a reducing diet, the heavier vibrations may help to disperse fatty deposits from specific areas of the body (eg the gluteals, hips and thighs).

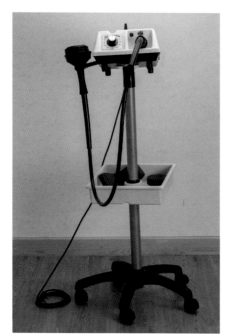

A salon G5 unit

Effects of G5

- Stimulates the circulation providing nourishment to the skin and muscles and improving skin colour.
- Improves lymphatic flow – aids removal of waste and toxins (good for cellulite).
- Desquamates.
- Warms, softens and relaxes tense muscles.
- Eases muscular pain.
- Penetrates deep into subcutaneous layer – so aids dispersal of fatty tissue.
- Motivates clients by helping them achieve desired results in weight reductions and body shaping.

Reasons for using G5

- Less personal than manual massage – ideal for treating male or self-conscious clients.
- Produces a deeper massage, far greater than that of manual massage.
- Spot reduction – gives more depth on problem fatty areas.
- Helps mobilise cellulite.
- Improves poor circulation – both blood and lymph.
- Less tiring than manual massage – reduces fatigue for the therapist.
- Particularly good for weight loss purposes.

HEALTH & SAFETY

To avoid bruising or discomfort do not:
- over-treat an area
- apply too much pressure
- use the wrong applicator heads on certain areas
- use too little medium
- work on contra-indicated areas
- work over bony areas.

How G5 works

The head of the G5 unit has a motor that creates a two-fold movement – it rotates and moves up and down with a vibrating action. Most units have a variable speed selector so that the vibration depth can be adjusted to suit the client's needs.

There is a range of different massage applicator heads that give different effects and sensations.

Application head	Use
Round sponge 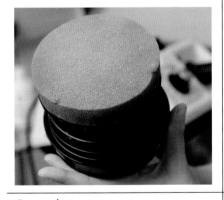	Effleurage applicator designed for use on smaller, sensitive parts of the body. Ideal for gentle massage on delicate areas (eg trunk). Relaxes the client and is used at the beginning and end of the treatment. Use in long one-directional strokes or circular movements towards the head and lymph nodes.
Curved sponge 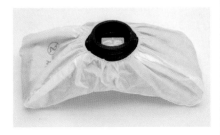	Effleurage applicator designed for use on the neck, shoulders, arms, legs and buttocks. Relaxes the client and is used at the beginning and end of the treatment. Use in long one-directional stoking movements towards the head and lymph nodes.

Application head	Use
Spike applicator 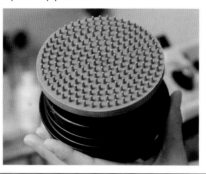	A very stimulating applicator designed to increase the circulation and give a vigorous massage. It has a stimulating effect on nerve endings, creates erythema and desquamates the skin. Can be used on large body areas – not to be used on areas of sensitivity. Use with long sweeping or circular movements. Take care not to over-use as can cause skin irritation.
Cone-shaped applicator (round end point) 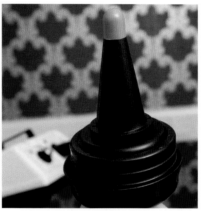	A deep petrissage applicator designed to reduce trigger points and for work on areas of tension. Can be used to stimulate the circulation and to relax muscles. Can be used around the scapula, and for deep work on the trapezius and lumbar muscles. Continually monitor pressure when using this head, as some tension areas can be sensitive.
Multi-prong applicator 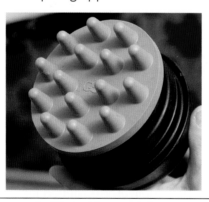	A petrissage applicator designed for vigorous massage and surface stimulation of larger body areas. Can be used on bulk areas to break down adipose tissue and reduce tension (eg thighs, gluteals).
Four ball/egg box applicator 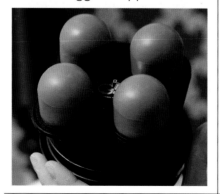	A petrissage applicator designed for deep, heavy-pressure massage on large muscle groups or bulky areas, such as the back, thighs and buttocks. Use circular movements with pressure towards the heart.

Guide to G5 application

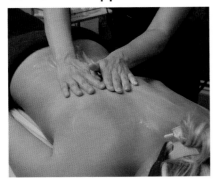

STEP 1 Apply talc-free powder to the treatment area to provide slip and glide for G5 treatment.

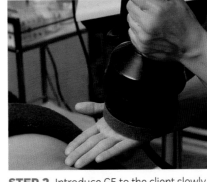

STEP 2 Introduce G5 to the client slowly by using your hand as a guide. The sponge curved applicator can also be used here.

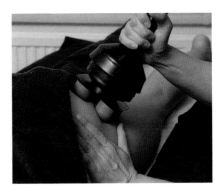

STEP 3 The egg box applicator is a good choice on areas where spot reduction is required such as the thighs.

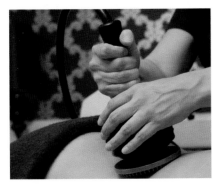

STEP 4 Use a selection of G5 heads to achieve the treatment objectives, building from the sponge head to the hedgehog head.

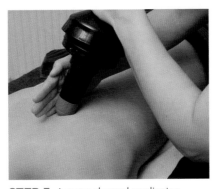

STEP 5 A cone-shaped applicator (pointer) is an excellent choice when working on nodules around the scapula.

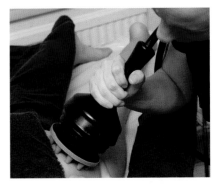

STEP 6 The multi-pronged applicator is a good choice of head for stubborn fatty deposits around the hips or buttocks.

The benefits of using a gyratory massage are the same as for normal massage, but more rapid results can be achieved and a deeper massage applied without putting strain on the therapist. Due to the vibrations and to avoid repetitive strain injury (RSI) in the wrists, it is recommended that you do not use the machine for long periods of time.

G5 can be used as a stand-alone treatment or alongside other electrotherapy treatments. It can be incorporated into a body massage treatment to warm up the muscles first. It is usually concentrated on particular areas of the body, such as the thighs and buttocks, as part of a weight-loss programme. It is also an excellent treatment for the back, to work deep into areas of tension. Another effective treatment is on the backs of the arms, using the sponge and multi-pronged applicator to improve poor circulation. A treatment is always started and completed using a sponge applicator.

 Watch the video of this G5 treatment on SmartScreen (unit 305).

INDUSTRY TIP

Treatment time may be varied according to the area being treated and the effects required (eg spot reduction or full body massage treatment). In some cases only a few massage applicator heads will be selected.

The size of the client will dictate the most suitable applicator heads to be used; do not use or change heads unnecessarily as this breaks the continuity of the treatment.

This is a stimulating treatment and requires greater effort in its application and should be applied at a faster pace than your manual massage therapies.

Infrared treatment

An infrared lamp provides a deep heat from infrared rays from its bulb. These rays are part of the electromagnetic spectrum. Infrared is a heat radiation treatment, and the lamp is also known as a 'non-luminous lamp' as the heat can be felt but the rays cannot be seen.

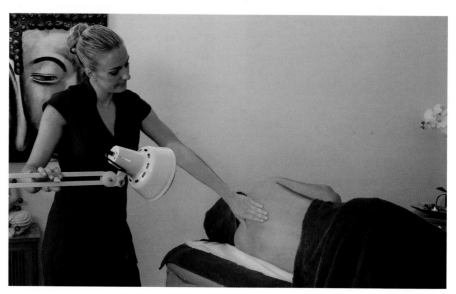

Infrared treatment

Inverse square law

The inverse square law is a principle that expresses the way radiant energy travels through space. The rule states that the power intensity per unit area from a point source, if the rays strike the surface at a right angle, varies inversely accoring to the square of the distance from the source.

The rays emitted from the lamp vary in intensity depending on how close the lamp is to the skin and the duration of the treatment. The **inverse square law** says that the light intensity decreases with the square of the distance from the light source. So the further away the lamp is from the body, the bigger the area it covers and the longer it can be left on. For example, if the lamp is at distance of 40cm, it can be left on for five minutes. If the distance of the lamp is doubled to 80cm, the time it can be left on for is quadrupled to 20 minutes. So if the distance is doubled, the time is multiplied by four. It is much kinder to the skin to have the lamp further away but to leave it on for a longer length of time.

Infrared enhances the treatment by:

- vasodilation, as it increases the body temperature slightly
- softening the muscle tissues and relaxing the muscles
- stimulating the sebaceous glands and lubricating the skin
- its mild heat having a soothing calming effect on sensory nerve endings.

Application of infrared treatment

The most common area treated in this way is the back, so position the client prone, with pillows for support that tilt the body slightly towards the lamp. Ensure the eyes are protected by sunbed goggles, or by draping a towel so that the eyes are shielded.

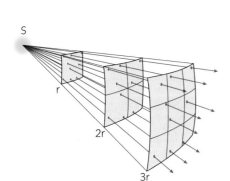

Inverse square law

Following consultation and preparation of the client:

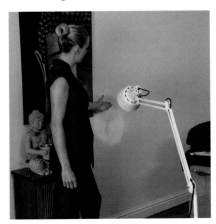

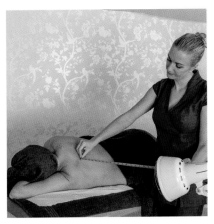

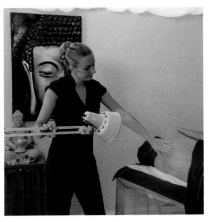

STEP 1 Position the lamp so the light rays hit the area at a 90-degree angle – never put the lamp directly over the client.

STEP 2 Follow the manufacturer's instructions on distance and time. Use a tape measure to ensure that the distance is correct. As a guide, lamps are usually left on for 5–20 minutes at a distance of 45–90cm.

STEP 3 Observe the skin's reaction throughout by looking and touching. You should also ask how the client is feeling. At the end of the treatment, switch off the lamp and place it in a safe area to cool down. Place a towel on the lamp so that you can move it. This also acts as a warning to others that the lamp may be hot.

 Watch the video of this infrared treatment on SmartScreen (unit 305).

General home-care advice and recommendations for body electrotherapy treatments

Following a body electrotherapy treatment, you should give your client suitable advice and recommendations to follow. This advice will help the client maximise the benefits of the treatment.

■ Provide recommendations for the correct skincare routine (eg products that will enhance their treatment).

■ Promote the use of a body brush to the client and explain how to use it.

Encourage the client to:

■ drink plenty of water and reduce caffeine intake

■ quit smoking

■ follow a healthy eating plan

■ take regular exercise.

Encourage the client to book a course of treatments:

■ muscle toning treatments (EMS and microcurrent) – ten treatments with one to two a week and then monthly to maintain the effect

■ vacuum suction, high frequency and galvanic – up to twice a month.

Explain how to deal with a contra-action if one occurs.

HANDY HINT

Body brushing is a great piece of advice to encourage. Suggest to the client that they brush the body in circular motions towards the heart to stimulate the circulation, remove waste and encourage desquamation.

HANDY HINT

It is important to be tidy in your salon. After the client has left, clean and sanitise the machine in line with the manufacturer's instructions and store it away correctly. With the vacuum suction machine, wash the ventouses in hot soapy water, using an antibacterial soap, and leave them to dry before putting them away.

Answers at the back of the book.

1   What range of low-frequency direct current does EMS treatment produce?

   a   0–10Hz

   b   10–120Hz

   c   120–150Hz

   d   25–300Hz

2   What is the maximum time limit for a first body galvanic treatment?

   a   20 minutes

   b   15 minutes

   c   10 minutes

   d   5 minutes

3   What is the recommended maximum percentage that a ventouse should be filled to during vacuum suction?

   a   15%

   b   18%

   c   20%

   d   23%

4   Longitudinal, duplicate and split are all types of pads used in:

   a   EMS (faradic)

   b   Microcurrent

   c   Iontophoresis

   d   Desincrustation

5   During a galvanic treatment, which of the following effects are created at the positive electrode (anode)?

   a   Vasodilation, skin tightening, soothing of nerve endings

   b   Vasodilation, stimulation of the nerve endings, saponification

   c   Vasoconstriction, skin tightening and soothing of nerve endings

   d   Vasoconstriction, stimulation and soothing of the nerve endings

6   What is the purpose of an infrared lamp?

   a   To help with lymphatic drainage

   b   To relax muscles after exercise and treat injury

   c   To relax the muscles ready for passive exercise and to reduce the risk of injury

   d   To cool muscles down before treatment and reduce the risk of injury

7   What is desincrustation?

   a   Stimulation of lymphatic drainage

   b   Removal of surface blockages and cleansing of the skin

   c   Exfoliation and deep cleansing of the skin

   d   Removal of blockages below the surface of the skin

8   What does iontophoresis mean?

   a   To degrease the skin

   b   To push water-soluble products into the skin

   c   To remove the stratum corneum

   d   To perspire

9   In which direction should a client perform body brushing at home?

   a   In circular motions, towards the heart

   b   In circular motions, away from the heart

   c   In long sweeping motions, towards the heart

   d   In short downward motions

10 What is the spike applicator used for in a G5 treatment?

   a   Effleurage of smaller, sensitive areas of the body

   b   Vigorous massage to increase circulation

   c   Deep petrissage to work on areas of tension

   d   Vigorous massage on larger areas of the body

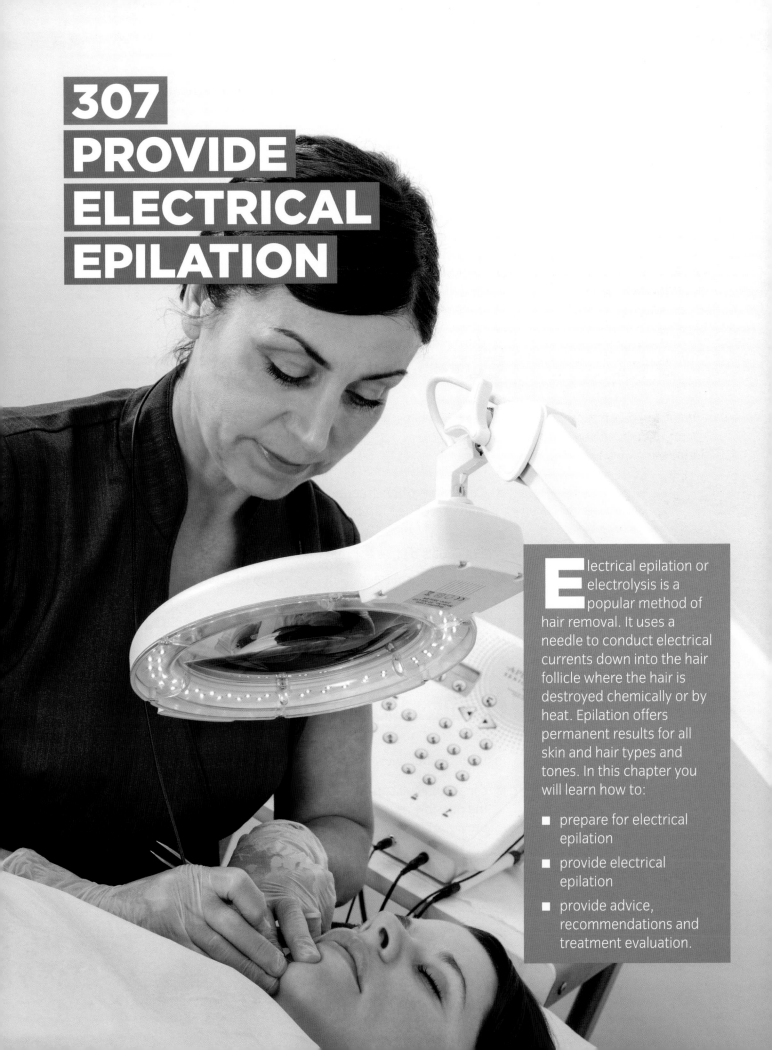

307 PROVIDE ELECTRICAL EPILATION

Electrical epilation or electrolysis is a popular method of hair removal. It uses a needle to conduct electrical currents down into the hair follicle where the hair is destroyed chemically or by heat. Epilation offers permanent results for all skin and hair types and tones. In this chapter you will learn how to:

- prepare for electrical epilation

- provide electrical epilation

- provide advice, recommendations and treatment evaluation.

Electrical epilation

Electrical epilation involves the insertion of a very fine needle or probe (the diameter of the hair) down into a hair follicle to the dermal papilla. The needle can conduct a variety of currents from an epilation machine to the follicle, where it is destroyed by heat or chemicals.

Each hair follicle needs to be treated repeatedly because all hair germ cells in the follicle need to be effectively destroyed to prevent regrowth. By also reducing its source of nourishment (the dermal papilla) the hair becomes weaker, finer and often lighter and eventually the follicle will be unable to produce a hair.

Why clients choose electrical epilation

- Electrolysis has a safe and proven track record.
- Electrolysis has been used safely and effectively since 1870.
- Electrolysis has been proven to be permanent.
- Electrolysis offers freedom from the constant use of temporary methods of hair removal.
- Electrolysis allows freedom from the hair growth which causes individuals distress or that they simply don't like the look of.
- Electrolysis treatment is not restricted to clients with certain hair or skin tones.
- Electrolysis treatment is easier than you think, with a competent operator.

Effective electrical epilation treatment

In order to effectively provide electrical epilation treatment, you must:

- carry out a full consultation to visually assess hair growth, establish the possible reason for hair growth, client's history regarding previous hair removal, medical conditions, area to be treated and the client's availability for regular appointments (see The importance of the consultation, page 402)
- follow strict health and safety procedures in relation to the working area, equipment, products and treatment
- determine the method of electrical epilation to accommodate the type of hair, skin texture and the client's sensitivity
- ensure the accuracy of probing

- adjust and adapt the machine parameters to accommodate effective hair removal
- carry out effective electrical epilation techniques – correct posture, dexterity, good stretch, continuity of hair removal
- remove the hair without resistance
- give effective home-care recommendations and advise the client on management of regrowth.

The history of permanent hair removal

The first safe and effective method of permanent hair removal was devised by an American ophthalmologist, Dr Charles E. Michel of St Louis in 1875. He had been practising electrolysis since 1869 and treated many clients with ingrowing eyelashes by developing a technique of using electrolysis (galvanic current) to remove the hair.

Dr Michel attached a very fine conductor wire to a dry cell battery. The wire was then joined to a surgical needle which was inserted into the lash follicle and the epilated eyelash did not grow back. The current used was 'galvanic', which chemically decomposed the hair follicle making regrowth impossible.

Dr Michel's methods were very effective, but very slow. In 1916, Professor Paul M. Kree improved upon Michel's method by devising a multiple needle galvanic technique which used as many as ten needles at once. This cut average treatment time down from three minutes per follicle to one minute.

The electrolysis treatment began to develop outside the medical profession and this new technique dominated the marketplace in both practice and teaching until the late 1970s.

In 1924 an alternative to galvanic current, called thermolysis, was invented by Dr H. Bordier of Paris and had the advantage over galvanic current by making the treatment time shorter. Thermolysis today can also be referred to as short-wave diathermy, high frequency (HF) or radio frequency (RF). The technique produces heat at the base of the hair follicle to destroy the dermal papillae by coagulation. It became a very popular method of permanently removing hair and is still used today.

In 1945 an electrologist, Henri St Pierre, considered the possibility of combining an alternating current and direct (galvanic) current in one machine for the purpose of removing unwanted hair. He was aware of the advantages and disadvantages for both types of current but consulted with an engineer, Arthur Hinkel, to look at the feasibility of creating a treatment which would combine a high frequency and galvanic current.

The patent was accepted in 1948 along with the blend treatment that is still available today.

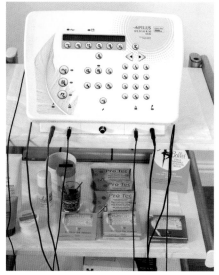

Modern epilation equipment

Electrolysis training became mandatory in the 1970s if studying a two-year beauty therapy programme in further education colleges. It is a vital unit to achieve for any beauty therapist who wishes to be in an enviable position of accommodating the needs of all clientele.

In the 1980s the first computerised epilation equipment was developed and available to the North American market. The treatment had become more accessible and popular with the general public and computerised technology was now able to refine the current application along with improving comfort levels for the client in permanently removing unwanted hair.

The importance of the consultation

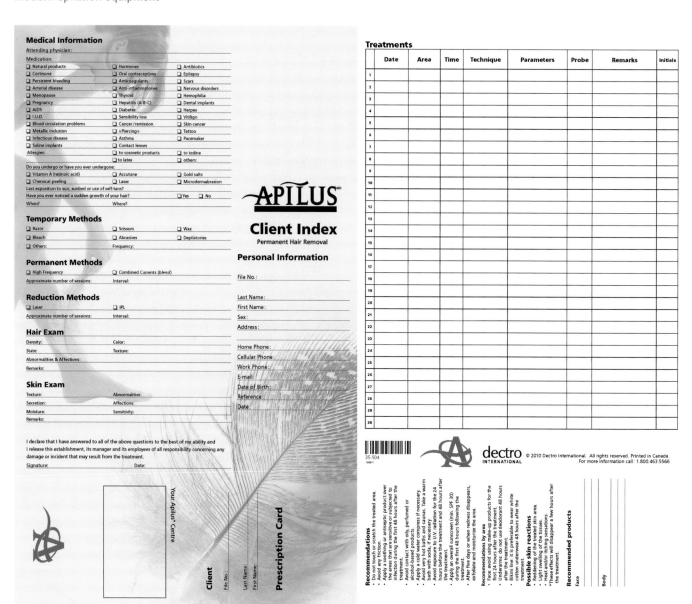

Client record card for epilation treatment

The consultation process is an essential part of the epilation treatment. It will allow you to get to know your client and find out their objectives for the treatment. The very first consultation that you have with a new client will always be more in-depth than subsequent consultations as it is important to establish an accurate assessment of the client's needs. When the client returns for future treatments, a shorter review consultation will take place and the treatment plan amended according to those needs. (Refer to pages 28–30 for more information on the consultation process and communication techniques.)

Proceed with the consultation:

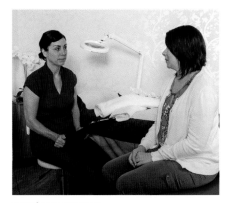
Good eye contact

- Greet the client in a warm, friendly, professional and polite manner.

- Ask the client how they wish to be referred to (ie by first name or by using their title and surname).

- In a private space, position the client so that they are sitting on the same side as you and so that there are no barriers between you (eg the treatment couch) to encourage a better flow of communication and give the client confidence to volunteer necessary information to the questions being asked.

HANDY HINT

Establishing the cause of a client's hair growth is paramount to achieve a successful treatment and manage the client's expectations.

- Explain that all the information you are recording is strictly confidential, and will be stored in line with the Data Protection Act (see pages 83 in the Health and safety legislation chapter).

- With good eye contact, ask to see the area of growth and consider hair type, pattern of hair growth and the length of the hair.

 Watch a video of an epilation consultation on SmartScreen (unit 307).

- Complete the client's record card, addressing the following:

  - name, address, contact numbers and date of birth, doctor's name, address and contact numbers

  - a full medical history to make sure that no contra-indications will prevent you from carrying out the treatment and that the client is in good health (see page 412 for contra-indications).

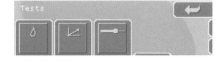

MOISTURE TEST
✓ Verifies the hydration of the skin
• Dry, Normal, Hydrated

Skin moisture gradient plays a key role in electrical epilation

- With open questions (what, why, when, how), establish the history of the client's hair growth (eg how long the unwanted hair has been present and whether it has changed in colour or texture).

- Ask for details of any previous hair removal methods.

Ask your client about their skincare routine and assess the skin type/condition, as this is an important factor which adversely could affect the treatment.

Record any anomalies (eg **telangiectasia**, hyper- or hypopigmentation marks, scarring in the area to be treated), and ask the client about any areas of sensitivity. All details must be recorded on the record card, signed and dated.

Telangiectasia

Permanently dilated capillaries visible through the skin.

Explain the hair growth cycle to the client (see page 158 of the Anatomy and physiology chapter). By explaining the hair growth cycle, you can stress that you will be able to treat all visible hairs above the skin but there may be hairs lying dormant under the skin, which may take weeks to reach the surface. Similarly, if a hair is removed at telogen, then another hair possibly could be visible quite quickly.

Stress the importance of a course of regular treatments to enable you to establish the rate of hair growth to weaken and eventually destroy the unwanted hair follicle. Be honest with the client too as this will help to build a professional relationship, helping the client to develop confidence in the treatment, on you, the electrologist, and more importantly your epilation skills.

Discuss the treatment options available and explain what electrical epilation involves. Describe the sensation that the client can expect to experience.

> **INDUSTRY TIP**
>
> Ask the client's permission to take a photograph of the treatment area so that they can see before and after pictures – attach this to the record card.

HOUSE OF FAMUIR
COSMETIC, HEALTH & BEAUTY

Informed consent for electrolysis treatment.

This agreement is in respect of treatment by electrolysis.

.... and .... Thereafter known as 'the client'

  (Electrologist)   (Client's name)

1. The client understands that electrolysis is a progressively permanent treatment and several treatments will be required.

2. Treatments will need to be on a regular basis as directed by the electrologist.

3. The client understands and undertakes to follow all pre and post treatment recommendations given verbally and in writing by the electrologist.

4. The client has given clear and accurate answers to the questions during consultation to enable the electrologist to establish the cause of growth and create an effective treatment plan.

5. The client understands that there may be immediate post treatment reaction, e.g. reddening and slight swelling in the area treated. Providing the area is not interfered with and aftercare instructions are followed, there should be no long term ill effects.

6. The client agrees to abide by the hair management techniques as discussed and recommended by the electrologist.

7. This agreement will confirm that I have discussed the electrolysis treatment with the undersigned electrologist that I understand that the treatment is progressive and that the hair in the area being treated will require additional treatment.

Signature .... Electrologist .... Date

Signature .... Client .... Date

Informed consent leaflet

Give the client the record card/treatment plan/informed consent leaflet to read and ask them to sign and date it.

At this stage it is highly advisable to ask the client to read and then sign an 'informed consent leaflet for an electrolysis treatment'. A copy should then be given to the client. This confirms that the client has understood the information given regarding the treatment and the advice and recommendations.

At the end of the treatment show the result to the client with a mirror. Emphasise aftercare and the importance of hygiene as the treated area will be more prone to infection. Discuss the recommended aftercare procedures as outlined in the aftercare leaflet which should then be given to the client.

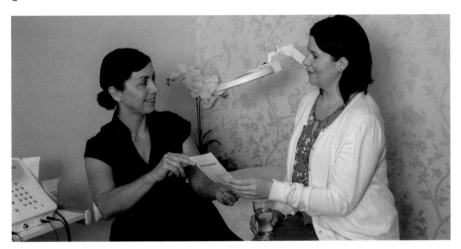

Home-care leaflet

To complete the treatment it is important to accurately record on the reverse of the consultation card the following:

- date of treatment
- method of treatment
- treated area along with any new areas
- needle type and size
- duration, current(s) and intensity
- therapist's comments and signature.

This is a good way to monitor the client's progress and response to the treatment. However, with each treatment the epilation working point must be re-established as the client might be more sensitive to the previous treatment parameters (eg during the client's menstrual cycle).

Moisture gradient

Moisture needs to be present in the dermal tissues before electrolysis can take place. The skin has a natural moisture gradient that encourages the electrolysis action to take place at the base of the hair follicle.

The deeper layers of the dermis have a higher concentration of moisture, gradually decreasing the closer you get to the epidermis.

The moisture content of the skin varies from one person to another and from one area of the body to another. It can be affected by many different factors, for example humidity of the environment, exposure to wind and ultraviolet rays, incorrect skincare, effective exfoliation and general health – diet, illness or certain medications.

Advise the client about the importance of moisturising daily to improve the moisture gradient, which in the long term will assist the effectiveness of the treatment. It is also recommended that the client regularly hydrates by drinking plenty of water.

Oily skin considerations

- Skin texture is often thicker than that of normal or dry skin.
- The surface covering of sebum will act as an excellent insulator.
- The moisture content of the lower follicle is usually good.
- The current should be confined to the lower third of the follicle where it is needed due to the sebum acting as an insulator.
- pH balance possibly affected through the effects of epilation.

Asteatosis (dry) or dehydrated skin considerations

- Small and tight pores.
- Flaky patches evident.
- Dry skins lack sebum and/or moisture.
- Insertion of the needle can be affected by dead cells blocking the follicle opening.
- Dehydrated skin has a low moisture content.
- Client needs to moisturise daily and drink plenty of water to improve the moisture gradient.

Sensitive skin considerations

- Medium to fine pores.
- Thin epidermis with telangiectasia evident.
- Sensitive skins may be dry or oily.
- Responds quickly to the heat generated in the skin during epilation.

Skin and hair types

As part of the consultation, it is important to carry out a detailed analysis of the client's skin type and hair as these will have an impact on the electrical epilation treatment. The table below shows how different skin types and conditions can affect electrical epilation treatments.

Skin type/ condition	Main characteristics	Effect on electrical epilation treatments
Oily	■ Skin texture is often thick and coarse. ■ Pustules and papules present. ■ Imbalance in the pH. ■ Good elasticity so the hair follicles are larger, which makes probing easier. ■ Surface covering of sebum will act as an excellent insulator. ■ Moisture content of the lower follicle is usually good.	■ Current confined to the lower third of the follicle where it is needed due to the sebum acting as an insulator. ■ pH balance possibly affected through the effects of epilation. ■ Care must be taken to prevent cross-infection by avoiding areas where skin disturbances are evident. ■ Using cataphoresis post treatment for two minutes helps to reduce any sensitivity and has a germicidal effect on the skin.
Dry	■ Small and tight pores. ■ Flaky patches evident. ■ Dry skins lack sebum and/or moisture. ■ Very common in post-menopausal women. ■ Advise on effective retail – use an exfoliator regularly with specific night and day moisturisers. ■ Advise to moisturise daily and drink plenty of water to improve the moisture gradient. ■ Promote having regular facials to help improve the skin's texture.	■ Needle insertion can be affected by the dead skin cells blocking the follicle opening. ■ On some machines there is a facility to use anaphoresis at the beginning of a treatment which helps to open up the follicles. ■ Poor elasticity in the skin can also affect needle insertion so it is important to maintain a strong three-way stretch. ■ Due to a lack of sebum there is little insulation against the current. ■ Use insulated or gold needles to reduce sensitivity to the current. ■ Important to monitor the skin's reaction and adjust the working point accordingly. ■ Needle insertions to be spaced apart.
Dehydrated	■ Dehydrated skin has a low moisture content. ■ Can be associated with all skin types and all ages. ■ An internal condition which can be helped by advising the client to drink more water. ■ Advise on effective retail – hydrating moisturisers. ■ Promote regular hydrating facials to help improve this skin condition.	■ Moisture content of the lower follicle is poor. ■ On some machines there is a facility to use anaphoresis at the beginning of a treatment which helps to open up the follicles. ■ Use insulated or gold needles to reduce sensitivity to the current. ■ Important to monitor the skin's reaction and adjust the working point accordingly. ■ Needle insertions to be spaced apart.

Skin type/ condition	Main characteristics	Effect on electrical epilation treatments
Sensitive	■ Medium to fine pores. ■ Thin epidermis with telangiectasia evident. ■ Dry patches can be evident. ■ Sensitive skins can be associated with dry or oily skin types. ■ Skin flushes easily. ■ Recommend retail products to strengthen and soothe epidermis.	■ Responds quickly to the heat generated in the skin during epilation. ■ Use insulated or gold needles. ■ Monitor the skin's reaction and adjust working parameters accordingly – space needle insertions to avoid introducing too much heat to one area. ■ Cataphoresis can be used after treatment to help reduce erythema and cool the skin's tissues.

Ethnic groups

Different ethnic groups possess different skin and hair types and tones. This will impact directly on electrical epilation treatments. Bear in mind that although we have indicated the general types here, many people do not fit easily into one type and so you should treat each client's skin individually on its own merits.

INDUSTRY TIP

Prior to treatment try using pure collagen film sheets for an immediate intensive rehydration.

Black or highly pigmented skin

When treating this type of skin, the following should be taken into consideration:

■ The stratum corneum is thicker in black skin than in white skin and desquamates more easily. Pigmentation is present in the dead and flaking skin cells and so may appear as dark scales on the needle.

■ The sebaceous glands are larger and more numerous than in white skin, with 10% opening directly onto the skin's surface with the remaining 90% opening into the hair follicle. As sebum is an insulator, the current flow can be restricted.

■ The eccrine glands are larger and in a greater number. The sweat gland is not as coiled, with the sweat duct being longer as it reaches the surface of the skin. This type of skin has more sudoriferous glands per square centimetre.

■ It is more difficult to detect erythema when treating black skin; so it is paramount to ensure that the skin is not over-treated, particularly as the skin is often very heat sensitive.

■ The actual number of melanocytes is not larger than in white skin; the melanin granules which it secretes however are significantly larger. There is a greater risk of hyperpigmentation if high frequency is used at high levels.

■ Black skin contains more collagen fibres than white skin, which makes the skin age less quickly; it does however make the skin more prone to keloid scarring.

- The hair follicles in black skin are usually curved, so with this fact in mind and considering that excessive heat can easily cause hyperpigmentation, the blend method is the most suitable electrolysis method to use for black skin.

Afro-Caribbean skin

- Whenever possible, use the blend or galvanic methods so that the heat produced is kept to a minimum and doesn't cause any pigmentation issues.
- Hair growth is usually curly or distorted so short-wave diathermy would not be suitable.
- Use a gold needle for accuracy and sensitivity.
- If short-wave diathermy is the only method available for use, use an insulated needle so that the current is concentrated at the tip of the needle. This reduces the chance of a surface reaction.
- Afro-Caribbean skin is extremely sensitive to heat but it is very difficult to detect erythema. Therefore, you should perform short treatments and needle insertions should be spread out to prevent over-heating the skin tissue.

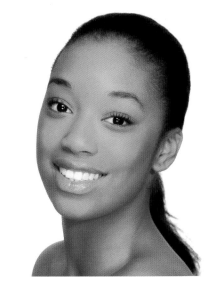
Afro-Caribbean skin

Asian and Mediterranean skin

- Use an insulated needle to reduce surface reaction.
- Asian/olive skin can be sensitive to heat and may have pigmentation variations.
- It can be difficult to detect erythema so short and well-spaced insertions are recommended.
- Avoid over-treatment of the area and allow sufficient time in between appointments for healing.

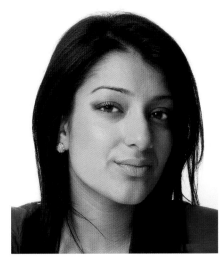
Asian skin

Oriental skin

- Oriental skin is prone to pigmentation marks and can become pitted if over-exposed to heat.
- It is sensitive so a gold needle should be used if possible.
- It can be difficult to detect erythema so short and well-spaced insertions are recommended.
- Leave sufficient time in between appointments.
- The pores are often small and tight so a small-sized short needle (size 2 or 3) is usually required.

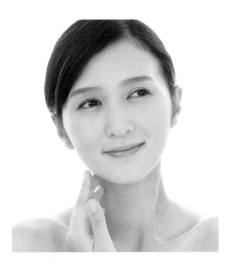
Oriental skin

Anaphoresis and cataphoresis

Anaphoresis can be used as a preparatory treatment and cataphoresis can be given as a recommendation.

Procedure	Description	Effect
Anaphoresis	<ul><li>A roller or electrode acts as a negative electrode on skin. This causes production of sodium hydroxide (or lye), which is alkaline.</li><li>Lye causes vasodilation of the blood vessels – brings blood, fluid and nutrients to the upper layers of the skin.</li></ul>	<ul><li>Opens pores.</li><li>Relaxes the tissues.</li><li>Increases erythema.</li><li>Makes insertions easier.</li></ul>
Cataphoresis	<ul><li>A positive electrode is used on the skin.</li><li>Creates a mild acidic reaction.</li><li>Neutralises the lye created during anaphoresis.</li><li>Causes vasoconstriction.</li></ul>	<ul><li>Closes pores.</li><li>Calms inflammation.</li><li>Soothes nerve endings.</li><li>Restores natural pH.</li><li>Has a germicidal effect on the skin.</li></ul>

Transgender clients

Working as an electrologist is likely to bring you into contact with transgender clients, as one of their objectives will be to permanently remove unwanted hair.

Gender dysphoria is where someone feels strongly from an early age that they were born in the wrong body and should have been born the opposite **sex**. This condition can present many emotional problems, from confusion to frustration. Many transgender people throughout life will have had to 'act out' the gender they were born with while continuously fighting to suppress their true identity.

The distress caused by such feelings can be so severe that the incidence of self-harm and suicide is very high among people with gender dysphoria.

Being transgender is not the same as transvestism, which describes a person who enjoys dressing and acting as the opposite sex.

Male to female transition begins with an extensive analysis by psychiatrists and doctors, who decide whether or not the person is

Gender

Refers to cultural differences between men and women.

Sex

Refers to biological differences between men and women.

suitable for treatment, bearing in mind that the surgery required for gender re-alignment is intensive, difficult and irreversible. Male patients are required to live as a female for up to two years to prove their commitment to the physical change.

Hormones are prescribed (oestrogen and an androgen suppressant) to start the physical transition.

When treating transgender clients please remember:

- Remain professional as the client could be emotional. Be prepared to listen but, as with all clients, it is advisable not to get too emotionally involved.
- A full consultation with treatment planning is exactly the same regardless of the client's gender, the only exception being that male follicles tend to be deeper than those of females.

An important aspect to also discuss with the client is home-care as the hormone medication will change the look and feel of the skin and advice needs to be given with regard to softening and hydrating the skin, either through effective retail and/or professional facial treatments.

Legal, health and safety considerations for carrying out electrical epilation treatments

Any business and therapist(s) carrying out electrical epilation must register with the local authority. It will issue a certificate documenting that the business and therapist(s) have been inspected and approved to carry out this type of treatment. This is a requirement of the Local Government (Miscellaneous Provisions) Act and covers all skin piercing treatments (ie electrical epilation, ear piercing and tattooing).

The premises will be inspected by an inspector who will check to make sure that:

- the equipment is safe and relevant for use
- the equipment has been PAT tested
- needles and other contaminated or hazardous waste are disposed of safely and correctly
- all needles are sterile, used only once and in date
- appropriate sterilisation methods and sanitisation products are being used for equipment and the working environment
- all products are stored correctly and safely according to the manufacturers' recommendations
- there is a washable floor surface
- there are hand washing facilities.

An environmental health officer (EHO) from the local authority will issue a certificate of authorisation if they are satisfied that high standards are being maintained. By displaying this in the reception area, clients will see that the premises have been checked and approved by the local authority. The local authority will carry out further visits to ensure that standards are being maintained at all times. If a salon falls below the required standards it will be issued with an improvement notice. This will state what improvements need to be made and give a timescale in which to make the improvements. If the improvements are not made, then the salon may be prosecuted and may even end up closing down.

In extreme circumstances an inspector may close the premises immediately. This is done only if they feel that there are high levels of danger and that the business needs to close to rectify them.

When carrying out epilation the therapist has a legal obligation to ensure his or her actions (or lack of action) do not put others at risk of injury.

Therefore therapists require a broad range of knowledge regarding legislation to ensure that they are working within the law, that high standards of hygiene and a safe working environment are promoted and that clients receive professional and confidential treatment. For more details on the legal, health and safety, and insurance requirements in the salon, see the Health and safety legislation chapter.

Working with minors

It is a legal requirement that minors under 16 years of age are not treated unless the therapist has gained informed consent from a parent or guardian or a GP. This age may differ nationally and you need to be aware of the situation in your area and also check insurance policy guidelines. Consent should be in writing and the parent or guardian should be present during the treatment process. This is to protect the minor who is deemed unable to make decisions themselves. However, it also protects the therapist when working with minors to have an adult present. It is generally recommended that no one under the age of 16 has an electrical epilation treatment.

Contra-indications

In addition to general contra-indications given on pages 30–31 in the Values and behaviors chapter, the following conditions will prevent an electrical epilation treatment taking place unless medical approval has been given.

The following contra-indications **prevent** treatment.

Activity

Contact your local authority and ask for a copy of the laws relating to skin piercing and any other specific local regulations that might apply.

INDUSTRY TIP

Always check with your insurance company about what you are covered to treat. The list of contra-indications that might prevent or restrict treatment being carried out can vary. Without insurance you are not covered and should not treat.

INDUSTRY TIP

Bacterial infections can result from bacteria entering a follicle due to poor hygiene following electrolysis, by the client not adhering to aftercare advice.

Prevent

Stop treatment going ahead.

INDUSTRY TIP

Skin sensitivity following epilation can occur through exposure to ultraviolet light or taking medication such as antibiotics, etc.

Contra-indication	Reason
AIDS or HIV (human immunodeficiency virus or acquired immunodeficiency syndrome)	▪ Carries a high risk of cross-infection. ▪ The body's ability to heal is restricted. ▪ No insurance cover available.
Anticoagulant drugs (eg warfarin, heparin or asthma)	▪ Might slow the healing process. ▪ Risk of blood spotting due to medication acting as a blood thinner.
Bacterial, viral and fungal infections (eg bacterial (eg impetigo), viral (eg herpes simplex), fungal (eg ringworm – tinea corporis) and infestations (eg pediculosis – head lice)	▪ Risk of cross-infection.
Cancer	▪ Radiotherapy and chemotherapy affect the immune system. ▪ The rate of healing is affected. ▪ More vulnerable to infection. ▪ Most treatment guidelines state that cancer remains a contra-indication for three to five years following the 'all-clear'.
Cardiovascular conditions	▪ Conditions and medications are complex and varied. ▪ GP referral needs to be obtained prior to treatment.
Cochlear implants	▪ Electrical currents may disable and damage hearing devices implanted deep within the ear.
Haemophilia – affects males only	▪ Male haemophiliacs' blood does not clot normally so if the skin is pierced it will continue to bleed. ▪ The gene for this condition can be carried by a female, but the blood of a female carrier clots normally so treatment is not contra-indicated.
Hepatitis A and B	▪ Chances of cross-contamination are high.
Lupus	▪ Skin healing will be compromised.
Minor/young person	▪ Currently, parental consent and GP approval are required if under 16 years of age (in England, Wales and Northern Ireland) and 18 years of age (in Scotland). ▪ Hair growth can be affected but hormonal imbalances can correct themselves during adolescence/puberty.
Moles with hairs	▪ Due to potentially agitating the melanocytes there is an increase risk of melanoma; therefore electrical epilation is not recommended.
Pacemakers	▪ High frequency currents may affect the rhythm of a pacemaker. ▪ In the worst case scenario this might result in a cardiac arrest. ▪ Some models are insulated and may allow treatment but written approval from the GP and manufacturer is required.
Severe skin conditions (eg acne rosacea, acne vulgaris)	▪ Risk of cross-infection from open wounds.

The following contra-indications restrict treatment.

Contra-indication	Reason
Allergies to metals	■ Recommended to use gold needles only.
Anxiety	■ If the client appears agitated during the treatment then damage or injury to the skin could result with the needle – at the consultation stage it is important to reassure the client by explaining the treatment in terms they can understand.
Bruising, swelling, oedema, sunburn	■ Risk of further skin damage.
Chemical peel	■ Depends on the strength and percentage – if low grade, then epilation could be performed 4 to 6 weeks after a chemical peel. ■ Skin is sensitised after a chemical peel.
Dermographia (sensitivity to skin friction)	■ A congenital sensitivity to any form of skin friction which results in swelling of the tissues shortly after treatment. ■ There are no long-term adverse effects and treatment may continue if a client wishes, as the condition usually lasts less than 24 hours. However, treatment time may need to be shortened.
Diabetes	■ Diabetics' skin heals at a slower rate (keep current level low). ■ The client is more prone to infection. ■ GP permission may be required.
Epilepsy	■ Electrical current could trigger an epileptic fit. ■ If controlled by medication and GP approval has been given, treatment may proceed with care.
Keloid scars	■ Electrical epilation could make the problem worse.
Loss of sensation (eg from Bell's palsy, stroke, desensitised nerves)	■ Lack of feeling means the client is unable to give feedback regarding sensation. ■ Skin could potentially be over-treated or damaged.
Metal plates/pins or piercings in the area	■ If present near the treatment area they could cause a galvanic burn due to a build-up of heat in the metal plate or pin, if using the blend method.
Other skin conditions (eg seborrhoea, psoriasis, eczema, cuts, abrasions)	■ Risk of cross-infection from open wounds.
Phlebitis/thrombosis/varicose veins	■ Treatment can be adapted to avoid the affected area. ■ If treatment is required on the affected area the condition should be referred to a medical practitioner prior to treatment.
Recent LASER treatment	■ Assess the skin condition and healing process. ■ If the skin is particularly sensitised then allow two weeks before receiving a treatment.

Contra-indication	Reason
Recent microdermabrasion	■ Skin can be sensitised depending on depth of abrasion. ■ If superficial abrasion has been carried out, allow 7 days before treating with epilation.
Roaccutane (acne medication) Retinal A	■ The medication has a thinning and peeling effect on the skin. ■ Electrical epilation should not be given for six months after the client has finished taking it due to skin sensitivity. ■ Even after six months, the skin could still be sensitive so take more care with current levels.
Recent scar tissue	■ These areas should be avoided due to the risk of cross-infection and sensitivity of tissues. ■ Small surgical scar – avoid for 6 months. ■ Large surgical scar – avoid for 12 months.
Steroid medication (applied to skin or taken by mouth, eg asthma inhalers)	■ Steroid medication might thin the skin. ■ Skin might be very sensitive. ■ Take care when selecting the type of method and current to be used.

Adapt the treatment

There are many conditions (eg non-medicated diabetes and skin that is hypersensitive, or dehydrated skin weakened by chemical peels or medication) that are not necessarily contra-indications.

You need to make a judgement call and a professional decision based on the facts of each individual client. It may be that a GP referral is all that is needed to meet the requirements of the insurance company. You could also consider different ways of modifying the treatment, eg:

■ carrying out treatments over a longer timescale

■ treating over a shorter time

■ leaving greater spacing between individually treated hairs

■ using different methods and techniques.

For example, a cold sore is infectious and therefore a contra-indication to epilation on the upper lip. However, if the client requires electrical epilation in the bikini area or under the arm, this would not be a contra-indication. Even the neck area could be treated, although great care should be taken if working on the chin, as cross-contamination is a real possibility. You should also consider healing after the treatment. If the client has a cold sore then they may be generally unwell which might affect their recovery from the treatment.

Prepare for electrical epilation

Preparation of the therapist

You should ensure the highest levels of hygiene, safety and professionalism when carrying out electrical epilation treatments. High standards of appearance, behaviour and attitude, and excellent communication skills are required. You need to be highly skilled and want to constantly improve your skills, as electrical epilation demands greater levels of skill than many other beauty therapy techniques. It can certainly carry the most risk if not performed correctly.

You should be well presented, with:

- a clean, ironed uniform
- a tidy personal appearance, hair tied back, no false nails, no jewellery, clean fresh breath
- good personal hygiene
- enclosed flat or low-heeled shoes (for safety reasons).

Preparation of the work area

The treatment room needs to be a welcoming and comfortable environment. You need to take into consideration general aspects of comfort (such as temperature, lighting, ventilation) for both you and the client. In addition, there are some special considerations for electrical epilation treatments that you must think about to make sure that treatments are performed effectively and safely.

Lighting

Clear and bright lighting is needed for an electrical epilation treatment as the therapist needs excellent visibility when probing the follicle.

Music

Electrolysis is not a particularly relaxing treatment; therefore relaxing music that you normally play in the salon may be played at a slightly higher level – but not too loudly. (Note: a licence is needed to play music: see page 92).

Equipment

Equipment	Description/use
Couch	■ Adjustable therapy couch. ■ Protected with cover and couch roll. ■ Make sure the client is positioned correctly and is comfortable.
Stool	■ Make sure your posture is correct and comfortable. ■ Adjustable stool for height. ■ Feet must be firmly on the ground. ■ Stool must be accessible and easy to manoeuvre around the couch to reach all areas for epilation.
Trolley	■ Clean trolley. ■ Set up in an organised way for treatment. ■ Trolley should have sufficient space for all your tools and equipment.
Magnifying lamp	■ Essential for clear vision. ■ Magnifies and illuminates the treatment area. ■ Enlarges the appearance of the hair and pores which helps with getting the correct insertion and angle. ■ Acts as a barrier between the client and therapist, protecting the therapist from any splatters of blood or body fluids when working in intimate areas.

Equipment	Description/use
Epilation machine 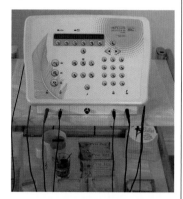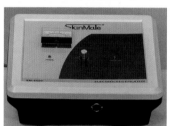	■ Produces an electrical current, either short-wave diathermy, galvanic current or a blend of both. ■ Computerised. ■ A selection of machines to purchase are available.

Tools

Tool	Description/use
Epilation tweezers	■ Have a fine point allowing them to target specific hairs (eg to pick up an individual dark hair which has been epilated from a dense batch of lighter hair). ■ Have a few pairs of high-quality tweezers available to allow you to continue treatments while those you have already used are sterilised.
Gloves	■ Non-latex and powder-free gloves. ■ Protects the therapist and client from any contamination which may occur due to blood-spot/needle-stick injuries.

Tool	Description/use
Consumables	■ Needed throughout the treatment, eg cotton wool, tissues, face mask.
Towels	■ To cover the client to keep them warm. ■ To protect the client's modesty.
Mirror	■ For use in consultation before treatment and to show client results after the treatment. ■ Ideally should have magnification function.

Hygiene

Equipment	Description/use
Sharps box	■ A yellow-coloured secure container for disposal of used needles and contaminated waste. ■ Needles and contaminated waste are collected by a special company that is licensed to dispose of and incinerate the waste.

Equipment	Description/use
Sanitiser	■ Fluid used for keeping spare instruments, chuck caps and tweezers during treatment. ■ All metal tools must be placed in an autoclave after treatment to ensure sterilisation is complete.
Autoclave	■ For sterilising metal tools/equipment. ■ Uses steam to sterilise equipment. ■ After a treatment, wash equipment (eg tweezers and chuck caps) with hot soapy water (a soft toothbrush is ideal) to remove any microscopic particles of tissue fluids, inner root sheaths or skin cells that may have become attached to the instruments. ■ Then rinse and place into the autoclave for sterilising.
Glass bead steriliser	■ Reach temperatures between 190°C and 300°C. ■ Temperature has to be maintained for 30–60 minutes. ■ Holds only very small items and these have to be made of high-grade stainless steel.

Preparation of the client

Unwanted hair growth can be a cause of embarrassment to the client and can affect their whole mental and physical well-being. To protect their privacy, it is vital to carry out a detailed consultation in a quiet, private location. The client will then feel able to discuss fully and openly their requirements, concerns about the treatment and their hopes and expectations. They will also feel more comfortable about showing you the area of unwanted hair growth. The more relaxed and comfortable the client is made to feel the more at ease they will be.

Prepare the electrical epilation needle holders

Needle holder

The needle holder is the means by which current travels down the needle.

There are two main types of needle holder:

■ switched

■ unswitched.

Switched needle holder

Switched needle holders are controlled by a button that is operated with the index finger. When the button is pressed, the current is able to flow.

Unswitched needle holders

Unswitched needle holders are controlled by use of a foot pedal. When the foot pedal is pressed, the current is able to flow. The needle holder is a smooth pen (with no button).

The benefits of this type of holder are:

■ the hand remains totally steady as no movement is required (ie the index finger is not required to press the button)

■ less risk of repetitive strain injury, carpal tunnel syndrome or other similar hand and arm conditions as there is no hand movement

■ the needle holder can be held in a more flexible way for use in areas that are hard to reach.

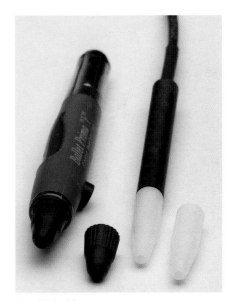

Needle holder

Chuck caps

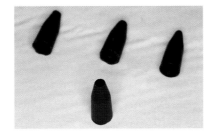

Chuck caps

Used with some needle holder designs, chuck caps are screwed gently onto the tip of the needle holder. They:

■ protect the shank of the needle

■ hold the needle in place during treatment

■ are made from ground glass and plastic.

Sanitise chuck caps in the manufacturer's recommended product and keep in an ultraviolet cabinet.

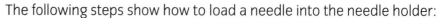

The following steps show how to load a needle into the needle holder:

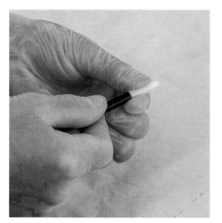

STEP 1 Loosen the chuck cap.

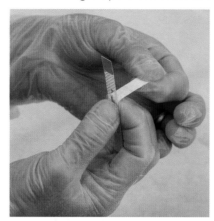

STEP 2 Tear open needle packet and expose shank of needle only.

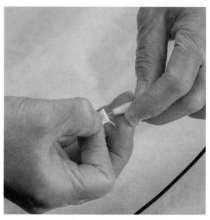

STEP 3 Insert the needle, together with its protective sleeve, fully into the chuck and needle holder.

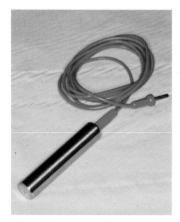

STEP 4 Gently remove the secure packaging, exposing the needle, and tighten the chuck cap.

Prepare the epilation needles

It is advisable to wear appropriate PPE (ie gloves) before aseptically loading the needle into the needle holder. Tighten the chuck cap and proceed with the treatment. After the treatment has finished, always dispose of the needle by removing it with a pair of tweezers and place the needle into a sharps box.

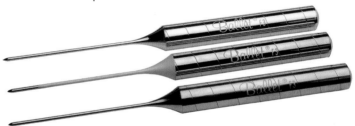

Epilation needles

Types of needle

One-piece needles

These are manufactured from one piece of metal. This allows for more rigidity and a smoother surface to the needle. This rigidity allows more precision and feedback sensation for the electrologist while carrying out an insertion. Sizes range from 001 to 006.

Two-piece needles

These are made from two pieces of metal. The needle wire is crimped to the shank. This needle is more flexible than a one-piece needle and is used for finer hairs and where accessibility to the follicle is restricted. Sizes range from 002 to 006. Two-piece needles are available in different shaft lengths – short is 0.48cm and regular is 0.63cm. The length is shown on the packaging with an S for short or R for regular. They are also available in different shank sizes – F and K. F is the standard size in the UK and has a larger diameter than K.

An electrode is a metal bar (a positive/indifferent electrode) attached to the epilation unit. This is needed to complete an electrical circuit if using the galvanic or blend method

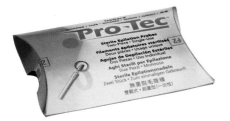
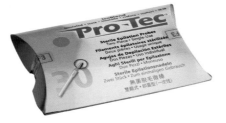
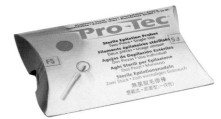

One-piece and two-piece epilation needles in various sizes

Gold needles

A gold needle is a stainless steel needle that is coated with 24-carat gold. The benefits of gold needles are:

- Smoother insertion – gold is a very smooth metal, which allows the needle to glide into the follicle. This results in less erythema and more comfort for the client.

- Gold is a good conductor of electricity, which sometimes allows the current to be reduced, resulting in less erythema.

- Gold is hypoallergenic and therefore suitable for those with allergies to other metals and those with sensitive skin.

- Reduced trauma to the skin so healing is quicker.

- Results can be achieved more quickly – as the treatment is more comfortable for the client, each treatment session can last for a longer amount of time. As a result, fewer sessions are required.

- Flexibility for the client – as there is less erythema, the client can book a treatment at a time that suits them without fear of obvious erythema afterwards.

Gold needles

Insulated needles

Insulated needles are stainless steel needles that are coated with a medical-grade insulation material. Only the tip of the needle is left exposed.

Insulated needles are recommended for use with short-wave diathermy or computerised flash methods as they intensify and target the current at the tip of the needle facilitating the use of lower current levels than with standard needles. They have the following benefits:

- They protect the epidermis as the current is targeted at the tip of the needle.

- They concentrate the heat generated at the tip of the needle.

- They give a more comfortable treatment as the heat does not rise to the surface of the skin.

- They produce less erythema on the surface of the skin as the heat is contained at the base of the hair follicle.

- There is a faster healing time as the trauma to the skin is limited to the area being treated.

Standard insulated needles are not recommended for the blend method as galvanic current needs to flow from the entire length of the needle; however, some manufacturers produce a specific needle for the blend method which has less insulation than a standard insulated needle.

Needle diameters

It is important to ensure that you use the correct diameter of needle to make sure that the treatment is effective. The diameter of the needle must be equal to the diameter of the hair that is being treated. The diameter of the needle affects the heating pattern produced at the tip.

A larger diameter needle has a bigger surface area, which generates a wider spread of current flow. A smaller needle diameter concentrates the current flow at the tip of the needle. Selecting a needle which is too small will require far more current to have the same effect as a needle that fits the follicle.

Through experience you will learn which needle to use on each type of hair. To begin with it is easy to just look at the hair and place the needle next to it. If you select a needle that is too large it will not fit comfortably into a smaller hair follicle.

Needles are available in six main sizes (diameters).

INDUSTRY TIP

The diameter of the needle must match the diameter of the hair.

Needle size	Use
1	Very fine vellus
2	Fine, vellus, facial hair
3	Fine, shallow, terminal facial hair
4	Average terminal hairs on the face and body
5	Coarse terminal hair, most commonly used on the body
6	Thick, coarse hair (eg pubic hair)
10	Not used for hair removal, used for advanced electrolysis techniques
12	Not used for hair removal, used for advanced electrolysis techniques
TEL F3	Not used for hair removal, used for advanced electrolysis techniques

Types of hair

The type of hair and hair growth rate will affect the method of electrical epilation you use and the intensity and timing of the treatment. There are three types of hair:

- lanugo
- vellus
- terminal.

Within vellus and terminal hair types, the hair can be curly, straight or have compound hairs (see page 426).

Lanugo hair

This is soft fine hair that covers a baby in the womb. It disappears a few months after birth and is replaced by vellus hair. Lanugo hair does not have a medulla.

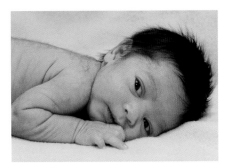
Lanugo hair

Vellus hair

This is the fine, soft downy hair that is found all over the body with the exception of the palms of the hands and soles of the feet. These hairs do not usually grow more than 2cm in length. Generally they do not contain a medulla or dermal papilla unless they develop into terminal hairs (eg as a result of a medical condition).

Vellus hair

Terminal hair

At birth this type of hair is found on the scalp, eyelashes and eyebrows. During times of hormonal change (eg puberty) terminal hair can replace vellus hair in certain areas. This type of hair is coarse and long. It has a well-developed root and bulb with a strong blood supply. The hair follicle extends deep into the dermis during anagen growth. Terminal hair is visible:

- on the scalp
- under the arms
- on the legs
- in the pubic area
- on the face.

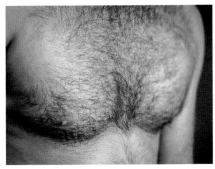
Terminal hair

Terminal hair has three layers:

- the cuticle
- the cortex
- the medulla.

Terminal hair can be subdivided into three types:

1 Asexual: terminal hair that is present at birth

2 Ambisexual: terminal hair growth at puberty

3 Sexual: eg hair growth due to the male hormone androgen.

Shapes of hair follicles

Terminal hair can vary in length, texture, shape and diameter. Below are some examples of unusual hair growth that you may encounter during your career as an electrologist.

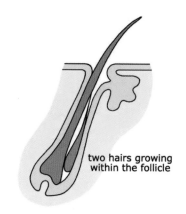

two hairs growing within the follicle

Pili multi-gemini or compound hairs

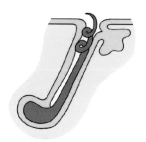

Curly or corkscrew hairs

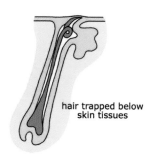

hair trapped below skin tissues

Embedded hairs

Club hairs

A club hair has a club end due to the disintegration of the hair bulb during the telogen stage of hair growth.

Pili multi-gemini or compound hairs

A compound hair is where the hair follicle has two or more dermal papillae. As a result at least two hairs grow from the same follicle. When using a direct current (either galvanic or blend method), treat the larger hair with the current as this may affect both hairs. If only the larger hair is removed, and you are using the blend method, after completion of the treatment try to remove the hair gently using tweezers. If you are unable to remove the hair using tweezers, assess the condition of the skin and treat it again if appropriate.

Curly or corkscrew hairs

The hair follicle has been distorted by waxing or plucking or is naturally curly or curved. The only electrical epilation methods that will offer successful results are the galvanic or blend methods. Lye (or sodium hydroxide) is formed by a chemical process that takes place during epilation and can reach the full depth of the follicle.

Embedded hairs

The hair doesn't come through the skin and remains embedded in the skin. Embedded hairs can be seen as small bumps on the skin. Embedded hairs are caused by friction on dry skin (eg tight-fitting clothes rubbing an area). If the hair is not infected, ease the hair out so that it is showing on the skin's surface. Epilate if appropriate. Allow the natural hair growth and healing processes to take place. Good homecare advice should be offered, eg regular exfoliation.

Ingrowing hairs

Here, hair shafts grow under the surface of the skin. They can be caused by hair breakage, friction or dead skin cells blocking the pore. If the hair is not infected treat it in the same way as an embedded hair.

Lanugo comedones (bundle hairs)

This is a bundle of lanugo hair protruding from a follicle or follicles, resembling a comedone. They are held together by sebum, as they often stem from the sebaceous gland. They are usually found in oily, seborrhoeic skin and can be removed from the pore by tweezers without traction.

Tombstone hair

When a new anagen hair is in the same follicle as an old telogen hair, which has been treated with epilation, the telogen hair is removed and the anagen hair as it progresses to the surface becomes thicker and darker than normal. Resulting tombstone hairs can naturally either fall out as a result of the prior treatment or thorough skin cleansing; otherwise tweezing will remove them.

Hair growth rates

The rate of hair growth/regrowth will have an effect on the frequency of treatments. The rate of hair growth/regrowth varies depending on, for example, the type of hair, area of growth and hormonal factors. The average rates of growth/regrowth can vary considerably from individual to individual.

Region	Hair line	Eye brows	Upper lip	Chin	Under arms	Arms	Bikini	Legs
Anagen	2–6 years	4–8 weeks	16 weeks	1 year	4 months	13 weeks	2–4 months	16 weeks
Anagen %	85%	10%	65%	70%	30%	20%	30%	20%
Depth	3–5 mm	2–2.5 mm	1–2.5 mm	2–4 mm	3.5–4.5 mm	2.5–4 mm	3–5 mm	2.4–4 mm
Telogen	3–4 months	3 months	6 weeks	10 weeks	3 months	18 weeks	12 weeks	5–6 months

Changes in hair growth

Hair growth and changes in hair growth can be caused by a number of different factors such as:

- congenital factors – present from birth
- topical stimulation
- systemic changes.

Congenital factors

Genetics will determine hair growth, hair colour and the type and the amount of hair we have. When hair becomes excessive it is called hypertrichosis.

Hypertrichosis causes superfluous hair growth. It is the growth of coarse, terminal hair that is considered excessive for a particular age, gender and/or ethnicity. It can affect both men and women and describes a general overgrowth of terminal hair affecting the entire body surface. Not considered hormone dependent, it results primarily from ethnic or genetic predisposition for heavy hair growth.

Topical stimulation

Topical stimulation (eg plucking, threading and waxing of hormonally influenced areas) can cause excess hair growth over time, as can friction, eg from plaster casts.

Systemic changes

Normal systemic hair growth can be stimulated by hormonal changes, for example puberty, pregnancy or menopause.

Abnormal systemic hair growth is primarily caused by either hormonal imbalance or endocrine disorders.

Excessive hair growth in a male-type pattern on the face and body in females is referred to as hirsutism. It may also be accompanied by other male characteristics due to the excess of male sex hormones, androgens, in the blood. This causes dormant (inactive) hair follicles to grow hair and existing vellus and terminal hairs to become well established, due to the increased sensitivity of the hair follicles to androgen stimulation.

Causes of hirsutism can include:

- natural normal hormonal changes, eg puberty, pregnancy or menopause
- medications – reaction to certain drugs, eg steroids, the contraceptive pill, hormone replacement therapy (**HRT**)
- stress and anxiety
- anorexia nervosa or bulimia
- surgical intervention, eg hysterectomy
- disease or disorders of the endocrine system – caused by dysfunction or tumours or cysts within specific endocrine glands.

HRT

Medications (synthetic or bio-identical hormones) prescribed by a doctor to alleviate the symptoms of the menopause.

Endocrine system

You were introduced to the endocrine system in the Anatomy and physiology chapter on page 235. The endocrine system is especially relevant to electrical epilation, as many diseases and disorders of the endocrine system can result in excessive hair growth.

Diseases and disorders of the endocrine system

The following are examples of diseases/disorders that a client could present with during a full consultation. To maintain good working practice and not affect the outcome of an epilation treatment, medical permission regarding any of the following must be obtained by the client from a consultant or GP before receiving any epilation.

Endocrine gland	Hormone	Hypersecretion	Hyposecretion	Description
	Growth hormone (GH)	Giantism		Excessive growth of bones and internal organs.
	Growth hormone (GH)	Acromegaly		Can occur later in life. Bones and soft tissue thicken, with coarse facial features and large hands.
Pituitary gland (anterior)	Growth hormone (GH)		Lorain-Levi syndrome (dwarfism)	Deficiency of GH in childhood: caused by either genetic abnormality, tumour or cause is unknown.
	GH, follicle stimulating hormone (FSH) and lutenising hormone (LH)		Fröhlich's syndrome	Deficiency of GH, FSH and LH: in adults obesity and sterility are main symptoms. Caused by a tumour or in most cases unknown.
Pituitary gland (posterior)	Anti-diuretic		Diabetes insipidus	Kidneys unable to regulate water reabsorption. Caused by damage to hypothalamus, eg trauma, tumour.
	Thyroxine (T4)	Hyperthyroidism or thyrotoxicosis		Increased metabolic rate. Symptoms include increased mental and physical activity, overactive sweat glands, weight loss and raised pulse.
	Thyroxine (T4) and triiodothyronine (T3)	Graves' disease		Autoimmune reaction to thyroid tissue. Symptoms above would be evident with protrusion of the eyeballs (exophthalmos).
Thyroid gland	Thyroxine (T4) and triiodothyronine (T3)		Hypothyroidism: cretinism – children	Found in children. Dwarfism with mental deficiency and slow heartbeat. To correct the disorder, treatment must begin very early in life.
			Hypothyroidism: myxoedema – adults	Causes swelling of the thyroid gland (goitre). Symptoms include low metabolic rate, reduced mental and physical activity, tiredness and coarse, dry skin and hair. Caused by prolonged iodine deficiency or genetic abnormality.

Hypersecretion

Overactivity of an endocrine gland.

Hyposecretion

Underactivity of an endocrine gland.

Amenorrhoea

Absence of menstruation.

INDUSTRY TIP

If a client has diabetes, remember that as a therapist you need to be aware of some of the complications that can occur. The treatment might need to be adapted or restricted.

Endocrine gland	Hormone	Hypersecretion	Hyposecretion	Description
Parathyroid	Parathormone (PTH) or parathryn	Hyperparathyroidism – kidney stones		Raises calcium levels in the blood due to reabsorption of calcium from bones.
				Symptoms are formation of kidney stones, renal failure or calcification of soft tissue.
			Hypoparathyroidism – tetany	Caused by benign tumours of the gland.
				Painful spasms of skeletal muscles caused by diet low in calcium.
Adrenal glands – adrenal cortex	Glucocorticoids	Produces too much cortisol – Cushing's syndrome		Affects both men and women but more common in women over the age of 30.
				Symptoms for females: **amenorrhoea**, develop male characteristics – hirsutism. Weight gain on the chest, stomach and face – 'moon-like' face with high colour and acne, hypertension, diabetes may develop.
			Addison's disease	Adrenal glands cease to work due to autoimmune processes, ie the body's defences react against the glands' tissue.
				Symptoms are hyperpigmentation, menstrual irregularities, loss of body hair, electrolyte imbalance, feeling exhausted, weight loss, lack of energy, low blood pressure, dehydration.

Endocrine gland	Hormone	Hypersecretion	Hyposecretion	Description
Pancreas – Islets of Langerhans	Insulin		Diabetes mellitus – type 1	Occurs in children and young adults. Inherited or genetic abnormality. Unable to control the metabolism of carbohydrates (sugars) and fat. Treatable (but not curable) with careful monitoring and insulin injections.
			Diabetes mellitus – type 2	Most common form of diabetes. Insulin secretion might be below or above normal levels. Treatment might include changes to diet and medication or insulin injections to control the symptoms. Possible long-term side effects with both types. Symptoms are extreme thirst, frequent urination, weight loss, tiredness/irritability, irregular periods. Possible changes to blood capillaries – weakened. Nerve endings affected – pins and needles/numbness to hands and feet. Prone to skin infections. Vision disturbances. Thinning of the skin – healing ability compromised.
Ovaries	Androgens	Polycystic ovary syndrome or Stein-Leventhal syndrome		Enlarged ovaries with follicular cysts. Cysts form either by the failure of the ovary to release an egg during ovulation or higher than average levels of male hormones. Symptoms are hirsutism – apparent from puberty onwards, irregular and/or light menstruation, infertility, thinning of hair, acne, increase in weight. Cause unknown, possibly a hereditary link.

'Normal' endocrine conditions affecting hair growth

Hormone balance is an important function of the endocrine system and the body is constantly trying to maintain a state of equilibrium, ie homeostasis. There are certain stages in life when the adrenal cortex and the reproductive organs secrete large quantities of steroid hormones into the circulatory system.

Stage	Description
Puberty	Puberty begins on average between the ages of 12 and 14.
	Start of the reproductive years.
	Breasts develop.
	Uterus, fallopian tubes and ovaries mature.
	Ovulation begins.
	Menstrual cycle begins to occur at regular intervals.
	Pubic and axillary hair begins to grow due to the increased level of androgens.
	Pelvis changes shape and there are increased deposits of fat around the buttocks and hips.
Pregnancy	Increase in hormonal activity.
	Fine hair growth on the lip, chin and sides of the face can be evident due to excess androgens being produced.
	Hair growth is usually temporary and will disappear at the end of the pregnancy.
Menopause	This marks the end of the fertile years.
	Menopausal symptoms start between around the ages of 45 and 55 where levels of oestrogen and progesterone start to decline.
	This is due to ovarian tissue becoming less responsive to FSH and LH.
	Facial hair often develops during the menopause due to the increased sensitivity to the dominant male androgen hormones.
	For symptoms see page 251 in the Anatomy and physiology chapter.
Stress	Chronic stress of any kind produces increased production of cortisol (a glucocorticoid) from the adrenal cortex which helps maintain resistance to stress. However, continuing high levels of glucocorticoids may cause:
	■ in women, menstrual problems which could lead to amenorrhoea and increased growth of superfluous hair.
	■ Ulcer formation.
	■ High blood pressure.
	■ A reduction of the body's ability to resist infection.

Provide electrical epilation treatment

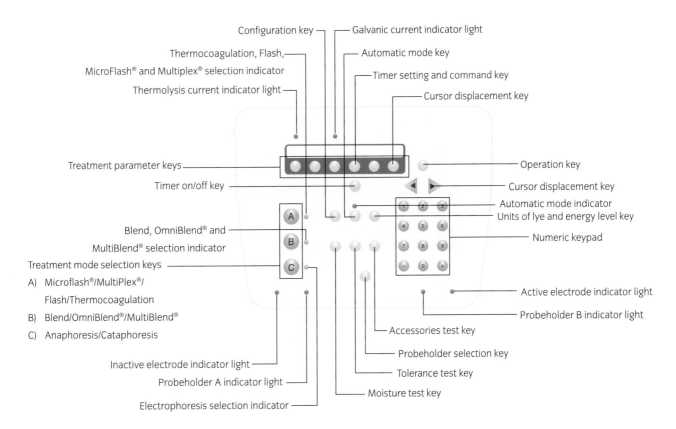

Configuration key
Thermocoagulation, Flash, MicroFlash® and Multiplex® selection indicator
Thermolysis current indicator light
Galvanic current indicator light
Automatic mode key
Timer setting and command key
Cursor displacement key

Treatment parameter keys
Timer on/off key
Operation key
Cursor displacement key
Automatic mode indicator
Units of lye and energy level key
Numeric keypad

Blend, OmniBlend® and MultiBlend® selection indicator
Treatment mode selection keys
A) Microflash®/MultiPlex®/Flash/Thermocoagulation
B) Blend/OmniBlend®/MultiBlend®
C) Anaphoresis/Cataphoresis

Inactive electrode indicator light
Probeholder A indicator light
Electrophoresis selection indicator

Active electrode indicator light
Probeholder B indicator light
Accessories test key
Probeholder selection key
Tolerance test key
Moisture test key

Diagram of control panel of Apilus computerised epilator

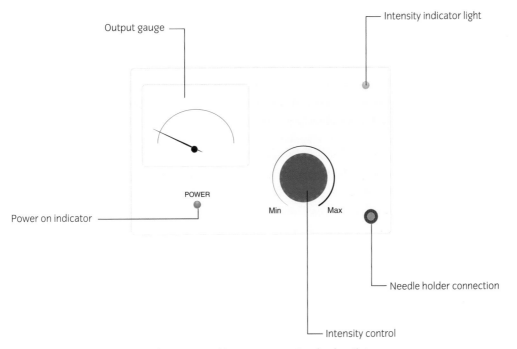

Output gauge
Intensity indicator light

POWER
Power on indicator
Min
Max
Needle holder connection
Intensity control

Diagram of control panel and operational buttons on a standard epilator

Methods of electrical epilation

In this part of the chapter you will learn about:

- methods of electrical epilation
- how to carry out an electrical epilation treatment
- probing techniques
- home-care advice and recommendations for electrical epilation treatments
- contra-actions to electrical epilation treatments.

There are three methods of electrical epilation:

- the galvanic method
- thermolysis
- the blend method.

The method chosen will depend on many factors: hair type, skin type/condition and previous methods of hair removal. Electrical epilation is only effective when the hair is in the anagen stage of hair growth (ie the active growth stage where the dermal papilla is still attached to the blood supply).

The method may change over a course of treatments. During a course a variety of methods can be used for their different benefits – either at the same time on the same area or on different areas of the face or body.

The galvanic method

Galvanic epilation uses a direct current (see page 319 in chapter 304) that flows from a positive electrode to a negative electrode. During galvanic epilation the client needs to hold an indifferent electrode to complete the electrical circuit. The needle holder is the negative electrode (cathode) and the indifferent electrode is the positive electrode (anode).

When a direct current is passed through the saline solution (water (H_2O) and salt (NaCl)) found in the hair follicle, the salt and water break down into their chemical elements and form different substances. These substances are:

- sodium hydroxide (NaOH)
- chlorine gas (Cl_2)
- hydrogen gas (H_2).

Sodium hydroxide (also known as lye) is a caustic agent that causes tissue destruction. It is the lye that destroys the hair bulb and cuts off the blood supply to the hair. The amount of lye needed varies according to the hair type. Fine hairs are likely to require about, for example, 15 units of lye and very coarse hairs may require 80 units of lye, but this is dependent on the type of machine being used.

This method of electrical epilation was the first method used and is very effective but slow. Each hair takes a minimum of ten seconds to treat.

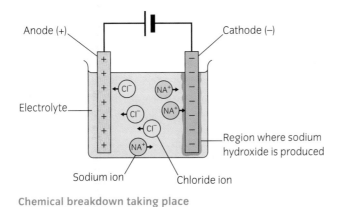

Chemical breakdown taking place

INDUSTRY TIP

If a client has a poor pain threshold, the galvanic method can be used at a low level of current over a longer time (eg 30–60 seconds per hair) for a more comfortable treatment.

The short-wave diathermy method

Short-wave diathermy uses an oscillating alternating current with very high frequency (2–30MHz or 2–30 million cycles per second) and low voltage. The high-frequency current creates vibrations which agitate (or disturb) water molecules present in the hair follicle. This agitation within the tissues causes friction which produces heat. It is the build-up of this heat at the base of the hair follicle that causes the destruction (coagulation) of the tissue.

Short-wave diathermy is precise and is focused on the dermal papilla so it doesn't damage any surrounding tissue.

INDUSTRY TIP

Short-wave diathermy is a good method to use on a new client before the re-growth pattern is established and because the hairs being treated are unlikely to be in the anagen growth stage.

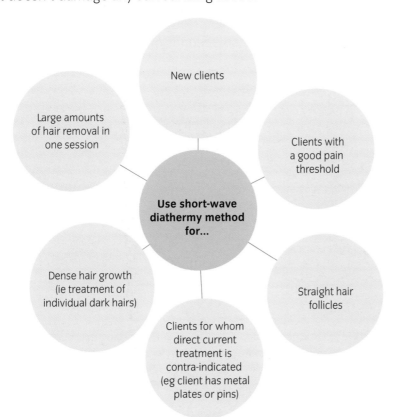

The reaction of an alternating current on the skin (as used in the short-wave diathermy or thermolysis method of electrolysis) follows a pattern starting with the current and ending with either coagulation or cauterisation (advanced epilation) of the tissues as the flow chart below illustrates. To achieve a safe treatment, with no detrimental effect on the skin, the desired result in hair removal is coagulation of the dermal papilla, which, when repeatedly treated in this way, results in the eventual destruction of the hair. Cauterisation is used in advanced electrolysis techniques to achieve highly specific and desired results.

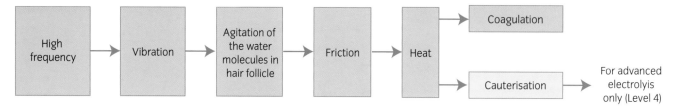

The blend method

This is a mixture of both short-wave diathermy (alternating current) and the galvanic method (direct current). Lye is produced as a result of the direct current used in galvanic and the alternating current used in short-wave diathermy produces heat. The heat speeds up the reaction of the lye. As lye is heated it becomes more effective and is capable of reaching every part of a distorted lower hair follicle. The blend method:

- uses a higher level of current for a shorter period of time (ie relatively high levels of current for five seconds)

- uses a lower level of current for a longer period of time (ie slightly lower levels of current for six seconds or more)

- is **'treat and leave'**.

'Treat and leave'

Describes a technique recommended for blend or galvanic when treating hair growth that is distorted. Groups of hairs are individually treated with the epilation needle using blend or galvanic. After several hairs have been treated, the operator then removes all hairs at the same time with tweezers – this allows extra time for the 'lye' (sodium hydroxide) to take effect on distorted hair follicles.

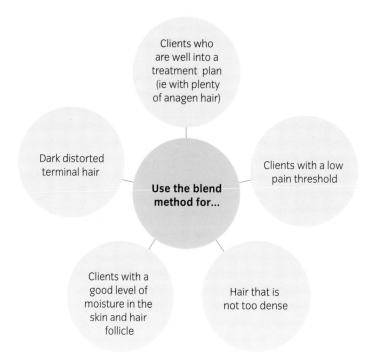

Carry out a professional electrical epilation treatment

Carry out the following before the treatment:

- Fully prepare the room and work area. Make sure that all tools and equipment are sterilised and sanitised and that the work area is clean and tidy.

- Carry out a thorough consultation, explaining the treatment and allowing the client the opportunity to ask questions. Prepare the client and ask them to remove jewellery from the area to be treated and their hand if they are going to be holding an indifferent electrode.

- Wash and dry your hands thoroughly and apply a pair of gloves. Sanitise the gloves using antibacterial hand sanitiser.

- Position the magnifying lamp over the treatment area.

- Sanitise the treatment area using a skin sanitiser or an antiseptic wipe.

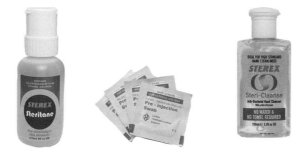

Ensure that the treatment area is sanitised and free of dead skin cells and harmful microbes

- Assess the hair growth pattern and direction.

- Load the needle holder in front of the client so the client can see that you are using a fresh sterile needle.

- Place the tweezers in one hand and the needle holder in the other and switch on the magnifying lamp.

- Remember to position yourself so that you are comfortable and so that you can reach the equipment easily, without having to over-stretch. If you are right-handed, sit on the right-hand side of the client. If you are left-handed, sit on the left-hand side of the client. You can move around to access difficult treatment areas.

The following images show epilation being carried out on different parts of the body.

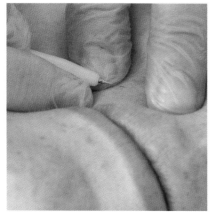

Lip

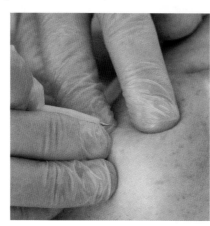

Chin

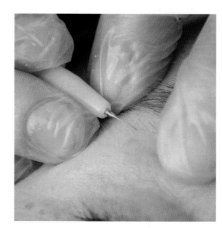

Eyebrow

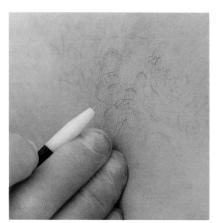

Underarm

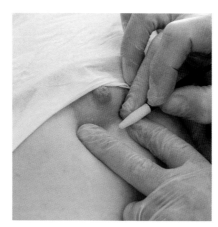

Breast

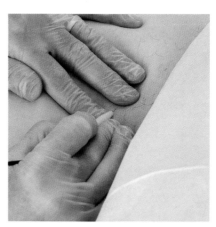

Bikini line

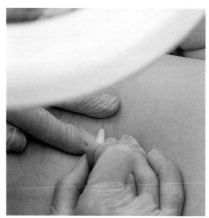

Abdomen

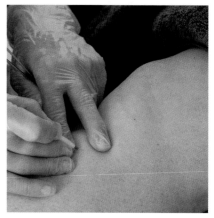

Leg

Perform electrical epilation

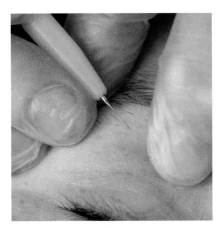

STEP 1 Wipe the treatment area over with sanitiser and blot with tissue to remove any excess moisture. Using either the two-way or three-way stretch insert the needle (probe) and allow the current to flow for the required number of seconds. Remove your finger from the button or foot from the foot pedal and remove the needle. Gently slide the hair out using a pair of tweezers.

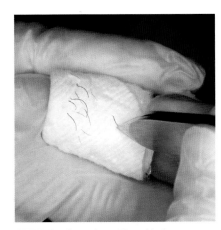

STEP 2 Place the epilated hair on a cotton pad. If the hair does not slide out easily, check the accuracy of your probing and the depth of insertion. If the probing is accurate then consider using an alternative method, for example blend.

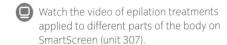

Watch the video of epilation treatments applied to different parts of the body on SmartScreen (unit 307).

INDUSTRY TIP

An effective 'working point' can be achieved by considering the following:

- lengthening the application time
- changing the type of current for example to blend
- changing the 'modality' if using a computerised machine.

Always remember to take into consideration the client's skin tolerance, hair type, area being treated, length of time between appointments, etc. The intensity must only be increased in line with the manufacturer's instructions. It is recommended to increase the time and not the intensity. If using the blend or galvanic methods the 'treat and leave' method could also be applied.

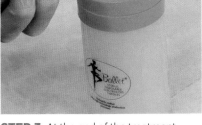

STEP 3 At the end of the treatment, dispose of the needle by loosening the chuck cap on the needle holder and tapping the used needle into the sharps box.

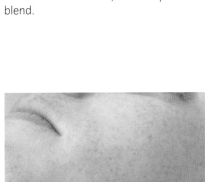

STEP 4 Apply aftercare lotion/gel/cream to a piece of cotton wool and then gently wipe over the treatment area. Show the client the results in a mirror and show them the removed hairs on the cotton pad. Advise on home-care and management of hair growth.

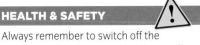
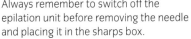

HEALTH & SAFETY

Always remember to switch off the epilation unit before removing the needle and placing it in the sharps box.

Probing

Stretch the skin

'Stretch' is one of the most important things to get right. If the skin is correctly stretched, the follicle opening is enlarged and allows for easy access and provides for accurate insertions – a well-supported stretch helps the client feel secure. Applying pressure top and bottom of the follicle opening will only elongate it, ie make it thin like a slit.

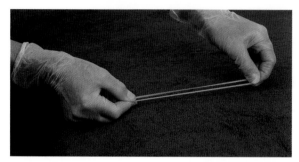

Applying pressure top and bottom will make the follicle thin

This makes it difficult to insert the needle into the follicle. When this happens, some therapists stretch even harder, making the 'slit' even thinner, which makes insertion impossible. The recommended stretch is in three directions to aid accurate insertions.

Three-finger stretch

Stretch the skin using the index (first) and middle (second) finger of the hand that is not holding the needle holder, and with the assistance of the middle or fourth finger of the hand holding the needle holder, stretch the skin with a gentle pulling pressure downwards. This technique opens up the follicle to allow easy entry.

Two-finger stretch

An alternative method is the two-finger stretch. During insertion, stretch the skin using the index (first) and middle (second) finger of the hand not holding the needle-holder.

Whenever possible, aim for a steady, supportive three-way stretch position to make sure that your probing is accurate and that the treatment is as comfortable for the client as possible.

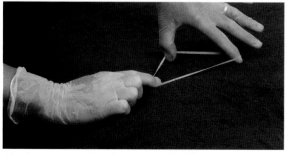

Aim for a supportive three-way stretch

Insert the needle or probe

- Insert the needle parallel to the hair growth. As a guide, look at a small group of hairs in the area to see the direction of growth for that area. However, take care to observe closely as each hair is individual.

- Study carefully the angle of the hair at pore level as it leaves the follicle. This is the angle of insertion. Once you have established the direction of hair growth and the angle of the hair, you can insert the needle.

Position the needle parallel to the hair and slide it into the follicle. Using either the two- or three-finger stretching technique, depending on the area, insert the needle gently, being sure not to apply any force. Make sure that you don't cause any depression or puckering of the skin. When you feel a slight resistance to the needle, you have reached the correct depth and the current can be applied. Remember to keep observing the skin for any reaction or loss of colour in the area – these are signs of incorrect probing.

> **INDUSTRY TIP**
>
> Follicle feedback – if the needle is not inserted correctly, the surface of the skin will indicate dimpling or puckering, loss of colour in the area being probed or even the reflection of light from the needle changes.

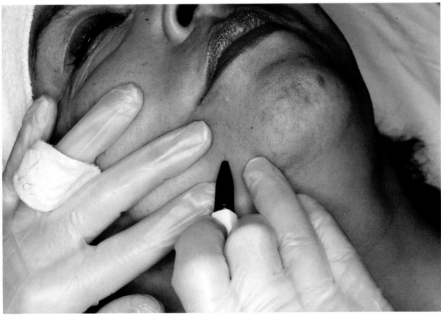

Probing

Inaccurate probing could result in:

- damage to the surrounding tissues
- blood spotting
- discomfort for the client
- an ineffective treatment.

It is therefore very important to make sure your probing is accurate. If any skin damage is caused, adequate healing time must be allowed before any further treatment is given.

Incorrect probing	Effect of incorrect probing
Probing is too deep 	▪ Will hurt the client and may rupture a capillary, resulting in a blood spot. ▪ Destruction of the follicle will not take place and skin damage may occur. ▪ Bruising can occur and if eyebrow hair is probed deeply could result in a black eye. ▪ Scabs can also be caused by probing too deeply.
Probing is too shallow 	▪ Could cause skin damage (eg surface burns). ▪ Hypo- or hyperpigmentation. ▪ Client will experience discomfort. ▪ The treatment will be ineffective.
Incorrect probing angle into follicle wall 	▪ Will cause surface burns and capillary damage. ▪ The treatment will be ineffective. ▪ Discomfort to the client. ▪ Blanching and bruising could occur. ▪ Could result in the formation of scabs. ▪ Blood spotting.
Applying the current while inserting or removing the probe – current released into the incorrect area 	▪ Healing time extended. ▪ An ineffective treatment with only partial destruction of the follicle (as the current has been released into the surrounding tissue). ▪ Pigmentation, scabbing.

Advice and recommendations

It is important to give the client precise, accurate and complete advice and recommendations, which should include both verbal and written aftercare instructions. The client should adhere closely to these to ensure that the tissues are allowed to heal promptly, preventing any adverse reaction occurring and to support the treatment with appropriate management of hair growth between treatments.

Watch a video of epilation advice and recommendation on SmartScreen (unit 307).

The following advice should be explained clearly:

- Avoid touching the area, to reduce possibility of bacteria entering open follicles.
- Apply recommended aftercare preparation for the next 24 hours using a fresh cotton wool pad, or longer if the skin is slow to recover.
- Avoid using any form of perfumed products, eg soaps, shower gels, talcum powders and creams in the treatment area for 24 hours to prevent infection or irritation.
- Do not wear make-up on the treated area for 24 hours following treatment, due to the risk of clogging pores which may result in bacterial infection.
- Sunbathing or the use of sunbeds is not recommended due to the risk of hyperpigmentation in treatment area.
- If treating the underarm area, no deodorant is recommended for 24hours, to prevent the risk of infection and irritation.
- Generally no heat treatments of any type are recommended for 24 hours following electrolysis treatment due to the risk of irritation and inflammation.
- Avoid excessively hot baths or showers for 24–48 hours after treatment.
- Avoid products containing AHAs or chemical peels for two weeks before and after any treatment.
- Avoid stimulation to the treated area (eg facial electrical).
- Avoid using bleach or any depilatory creams on the treatment area as this could infect and sensitise the area.
- Swimming in chlorinated water or salt may also irritate skin tissues.
- Exercise after treatment may lead to perspiration salts entering open follicles and causing infection.
- Tight clothing should be avoided in the area of treatment due to the risk of irritation.
- Report any scabs or pustule infection to the salon. Do not pick or rub the skin as this may lead to scarring.
- Hair growth management advice should be given between treatments. Advise to trim hair growth with nail scissors or shave occasionally between services.

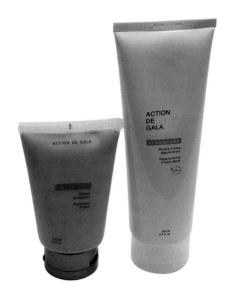

■ Clients should be advised to use retail products that will help to hydrate and maintain the moisture gradient of the skin as well as drinking 2 litres of water daily.

Suitable aftercare products are any antiseptic cream, gel or lotion. The aim of aftercare products are to:

■ encourage the client to look after the treatment area following electrical epilation treatment

■ provide an antiseptic barrier to prevent infection occurring in the follicles, reduce inflammation and cool the skin tissues

■ promote healing of skin tissues

■ cool skin tissues.

Methods of evaluating treatment

The therapist can evaluate the effectiveness of the treatment given through using a range of methods, which include:

■ visual – assessing the appearance of the skin and hair growth during and following treatment

■ verbal – gaining feedback from the client on how they felt during treatment process and about the effects and results of treatment

■ written – client questionnaire or written testimonial

■ repeat business – client returns for regular treatment and adds additional treatments, recommends friends to therapist.

Contra-actions

A contra-action is an adverse reaction which may occur during or following treatment.

The therapist should be aware of what is considered a normal reaction or abnormal reaction during or following treatment.

Normal skin reaction following electrical epilation

The client should be told what to expect:

■ localised redness (erythema)

■ localised swelling within the tissues, around individual follicles

■ localised warmth within the area

■ any reaction subsides very quickly lasting from 20 minutes to a few hours, rarely lasting longer depending on skin sensitivity and healing ability.

Activity

Design an advice leaflet giving clear instructions to the client on post-treatment care of the area being treated.

Generally the skin will heal quickly, although occasionally minute pinkish-brown scabs may form. If this occurs, scabs should drop off within a few days.

Abnormal skin reactions following electrical epilation

Contra-action	Cause	Action required
Blanching of the skin	Insertion is too shallow so the electrical current is released too close to the skin surface and burns the skin. The intensity of the current is too high. The length of time that the current is applied for is too great. The needle used is too small in diameter, allowing heat to rise to the surface of the skin.	Keep the area dry and use an antiseptic lotion. Recommend continued use of a product containing aloe vera to aid cellular renewal and regeneration. If hypo-/hyperpigmentation results it may fade over time (although it can be permanent). Once healed, exfoliate the area regularly, massage the area to encourage the blood supply and use good quality skin products to promote healing.
Blood spotting or bleeding	Incorrect insertions – angle or depth. Forcing the needle through the skin and not following the line of the follicle into the skin. The needle used is too large which can damage the sides of the follicle and cause bleeding.	Apply a dry cotton wool compress with slight pressure. Dispose of the contaminated needle into the sharps box. Dispose of the contaminated cotton wool into the sharps box. Change gloves. Apply antiseptic solution to the area once bleeding has ceased. Ensure accurate insertions using the correct diameter of needle. Perform a depth test to judge the depth of the hair.
Bruising	The needle has penetrated through the base or side of the follicle resulting in damage to a superficial capillary – poor probing technique or using too large a needle during treatment.	Apply pressure immediately with a cold compress to prevent blood spreading under the skin. Carry out a depth test if in doubt (eg eyebrows require very superficial insertions). Ensure the correct diameter needle is being used. Check accuracy of insertions. Be gentle with an elderly client or client with sensitive or thin skin.

Contra-action	Cause	Action required
Bending or damaging the needle	Incorrect angle of needle insertion. Damage to needle as a result of knocking it against equipment (eg magnifying lamp).	Replace the needle immediately. Never try to straighten it. Find out the cause and put it right (eg if the needle was damaged on the magnifying lamp, alter the position of the lamp).
Excessive erythema	Intensity of the current is too high. Current applied for too long. Over-working an area (ie insertions too close together). Insertions are too deep or too short.	Apply cataphoresis to the affected area for at least two minutes post treatment. Apply a cool compress to cool the tissues and reduce erythema. Use a soothing aftercare product. The use of gold needles or insulated needles is recommended. During treatment, reduce current intensity, application time or treatment time.
Excessive oedema	An allergic reaction to the metal content of the epilation needle or products used. Insertion too deep – particularly on the eyebrows. Over-treatment – insertions too close in an area of dense hair growth. Intensity too high. Length of treatment too long.	Stop the treatment and apply a cold compress to cool the tissues and reduce oedema. Apply cataphoresis to the affected area for at least two minutes post treatment. Use a soothing aftercare product. Increase space of insertions on areas of dense hair or sensitive skin. Keep within the time limits for the treatment and treat sensitive areas for less time. Use gold needles as they are hypoallergenic.
Hyperhidrosis – excessive sweating	Client may be nervous. Illness. Recent exercise. Hot weather conditions. Hot flushes – menopause.	Allow client time to compose themselves and offer them a glass of water. Reduce the temperature of the treatment room but make sure it is still comfortable. Gently wipe the skin (if appropriate). Ensure current levels are as low as possible. If using short-wave diathermy, use an insulated needle to help prevent the heat rising.
Hyper- and/or hypopigmentation	Inaccurate probing. Level of current is too high. Changes in the skin tissue due to exposure to ultraviolet light following treatment.	Reflect on your technique. Consider using the blend technique if the follicles are distorted. Emphasise the importance of aftercare to the client.

Contra-action	Cause	Action required
Palpitations	Can be caused by a variety of medical conditions. Can be triggered by stress or panic.	Stop treatment and try to calm the client. Raise the couch into a more upright position and adjust your working angle. Provide the client with a cold glass of water.
Pitting and scarring	Over-treatment over a period of time. Repeatedly inaccurate insertions. Insertions too deep. Current applied when inserting or removing the needle. Needle used is too large a diameter. Level of current used is too high. Current applied for too long. Continued use of short-wave diathermy on unsuitable hair (eg distorted follicles).	Change your technique and ensure you do regular CPD. Keep the area dry and use an antiseptic product. Once healed, exfoliate the area regularly, massage the area to encourage the blood supply and use good quality skin products to promote healing.
Weeping follicles	Too much galvanic current has been used, causing excessive chemical decomposition of the skin tissues.	Apply a cold compress and an antiseptic aftercare product. If a blister forms, ensure it stays dry and clean. Advise the client not to irritate it (ie pop or pick it). Use a lower intensity current or use for a shorter length of time.

Electrical epilation moving forward

Computerised technology has enabled current application to become so refined that clients have benefited from improving comfort levels along with an extensive selection of epilation methods to treat and remove unwanted hair permanently.

Manufacturers today offer newly qualified or existing electrologists a range of equipment from basic diathermy units to advanced computerised machines offering in some cases three modalities in one. This offers the discerning practitioner more options to treat a range of hair types with effective results.

Flash®, MicroFlash®, AdvanceFlash®, PicoFlash®, Multiplex®, Synchro®, Pulsing blend® and Multi-blend® are all examples of different methods available on computerised machines today. The computer controls the output and timing precisely, allowing a powerful high intensity, high frequency current to be passed for very short periods of time – for example the Apilus Platinum®. This operates at speeds of one thousandth of a second. This method is suitable for straight follicles as the heat pattern is intense and precise at the tip of the needle. The sensation from this current is less than with other methods; this is because the current passes for such a short period of time that the heat nerve receptors do not have time to register the sensation.

Extensive research by dermatologists in Canada have proven that by using the MicroFlash® technique, which treats the papilla and bulge during insertion, re-growth is finer and softer than with original conventional methods. This offers the client confidence in achieving their objective and establishes enthusiasm to continue with treatments as they are able to see effective results quicker and promote the benefits of epilation to their friends. This proven technique works on the principle that the computer will be set to send two pulses after the needle is inserted into the follicle, with the release of the first pulse at the papilla and in a controlled and timed manner the second pulse is released further up the follicle where the stem cells are located in the bulge. The computer controls the current output; it also allows the time to be adjusted between the two pulses according to the electrologist's speed and experience. Some computerised epilators automatically and proportionally reduce the power of the second pulse to ensure that it is safely contained within the follicle.

Hairs that are strong and deep with very distorted follicles will require warm lye to be created in the follicle but today's computerised technology offers the addition of a flash of high frequency to distribute the lye to the distorted areas and will minimise discomfort levels, thereby providing an opportunity for the therapist to cover larger areas to minimise the unwanted hair.

Many clients are not aware of the importance of maintaining the moisture gradient in the skin during a course of epilation treatments. However, new technology developed by Dectro International has accommodated this ongoing problem by allowing the electrologist to confidently treat distorted follicles in a dry/dehydrated skin safely and effectively, by offering another type of epilation method besides the blend method aimed at follicles with only slight distortion. This method is called the Multiplex® technique and provides a low-intensity high-frequency current to be passed for around one second; this pre-warms the follicle. An automatic high-intensity micro-flash of high frequency is then passed for another fraction of a second. This allows the heat pattern to spread slightly further away from the needle than with standard computerised flash and has the effect of producing a 'longer' heat pattern which will be directed around the slightly distorted follicles. Computerised technology allows all hair types to be treated quickly and efficiently with minimal disturbance to the client's skin and lifestyle.

INDUSTRY TIP

Advanced technology now even offers a moisture sensor, to assess the moisture at different depths of the follicles in various regions of the body too.

INDUSTRY TIP

Computerised epilation offers more choice of current settings and timings to suit the needs of your clients, while successfully treating all types of follicles.

Industry study

The client is transgender (male to female). She has male pattern facial hair growth (a beard), which is strong, coarse, dense terminal hair. Initially, she was having a two-hour treatment once a week. She began taking prescribed female hormones, which helped a little in weakening the hair on the body but made only an insignificant improvement to the coarse, dense facial hair.

To start with, the therapist used short-wave diathermy because it produced quick results within the time allowed and enabled them to treat a large amount of hair. This was the method the client requested. Many transgender people are very knowledgeable about hair removal and electrolysis. The currents were initially about a quarter of the output of the machine and a size 5 needle was used.

The therapist concentrated on removing the dark hairs only, leaving the white hairs because they were less noticeable. The client decided that this was the best course of treatment. This had the benefit of naturally spacing out treatment within an area of dense hair growth and prevented overtreatment. The client's upper lip was her main concern so the therapist concentrated on this area and spent any additional time removing areas at the side of the face.

The client shaved in between treatments. Although I advised her against this, it was necessary for her emotional well-being.

The client has now been having treatment for a year and the hair growth has been visibly reduced. She now comes for one hour every other week. Over time the hair growth has not only decreased but also the regrowth has become finer and lighter. The therapist has been able to go down 2 needle sizes. Eventually the client should be able to attend for short 'tidying-up' appointments using a size 2 or 3 needle every month.

The client's confidence has grown considerably as a result of having electrical epilation. The female hormones have also continued to make a huge difference to her appearance and she has become more confident and comfortable in her own skin. She has decided to proceed to the next stage in her journey and explore the option of sexual reassignment surgery. The therapist feels privileged to help her on her journey to becoming a happier person who can hold her head up high and rejoice in her new-found confidence.

Answers at the back of the book.

1 What type of current is used in short-wave diathermy?

   a High frequency

   b Interrupted alternating current

   c Direct

   d Interrupted direct

2 Vellus hair is usually:

   a Fine and long

   b Dark and thick

   c Dark and long

   d Fine and downy

3 A prohibition notice can be issued if:

   a A salon presents a danger

   b A salon follows health and safety

   c A salon follows some health and safety

   d A salon does not offer epilation

4 What is another name for 'lye'?

   a Hydrochloric acid

   b Sodium carbonate

   c Sodium chloride

   d Sodium hydroxide

5 What are the chemical constituents of saline?

   a $NaCl + CO_2$

   b $Na + Cl$

   c $H_2O + NaCl$

   d $CO_2 + H_2O$

6 When carrying out an epilation treatment on an area of very dense hair growth, which one of the following is it most important to treat?

   a All the hair

   b The dark hair

   c The finer hairs for comfort

   d The white hair

7 Follicle walls can also be known as:

   a Stratum corneum

   b Inner root sheath

   c Outer root sheath

   d Stratum lucidum

8 The most suitable needle to use on a client with a nickel allergy is:

   a An insulated needle

   b A stainless steel two-piece needle

   c A stainless steel one-piece needle

   d A 24-carat gold plated needle

9 Hirsutism is an increased sensitivity to:

   a Adrenaline

   b Growth hormone

   c Androgens

   d Thyroxine

10 Which one of the following is a technique used when using the blend method?

   a Higher for longer

   b Shorter for lower

   c Lower for longer

   d Higher for wider

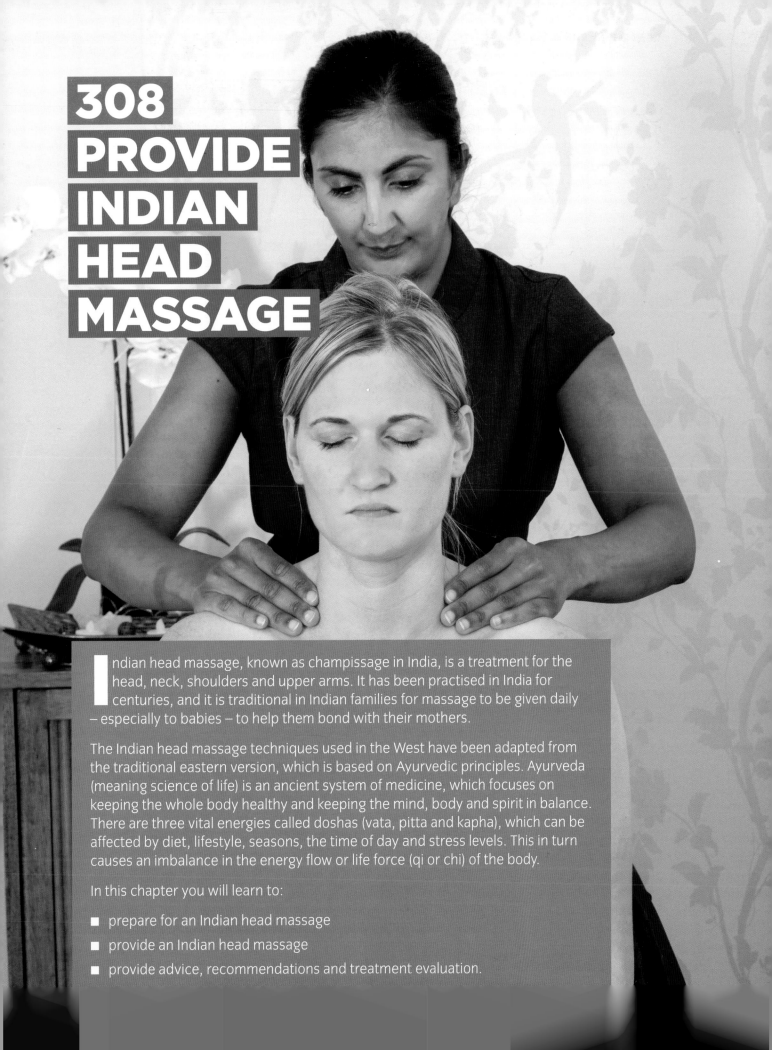

308 PROVIDE INDIAN HEAD MASSAGE

Indian head massage, known as champissage in India, is a treatment for the head, neck, shoulders and upper arms. It has been practised in India for centuries, and it is traditional in Indian families for massage to be given daily – especially to babies – to help them bond with their mothers.

The Indian head massage techniques used in the West have been adapted from the traditional eastern version, which is based on Ayurvedic principles. Ayurveda (meaning science of life) is an ancient system of medicine, which focuses on keeping the whole body healthy and keeping the mind, body and spirit in balance. There are three vital energies called doshas (vata, pitta and kapha), which can be affected by diet, lifestyle, seasons, the time of day and stress levels. This in turn causes an imbalance in the energy flow or life force (qi or chi) of the body.

In this chapter you will learn to:

- prepare for an Indian head massage
- provide an Indian head massage
- provide advice, recommendations and treatment evaluation.

Prepare for Indian head massage

You should make sure you are familiar with the:

- structure of the skin and hair
- structure, function, position and action of the muscles of the body
- location, function and structure of the bones of the body
- location, function and structure of the circulatory and lymphatic systems and the location of the lymph nodes in the head and neck.

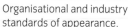
HANDY HINT

Remember to incorporate your understanding of anatomy and physiology into your massage practice.

Preparation of the therapist

As a therapist you will be working in close proximity to the client throughout this treatment. It is very important that you are dressed and presented in a professional manner. See the Values and bahaviours chapter for more information.

Before you start any treatment you should make sure you are fully prepared physically by doing the hand exercises in chapter 303, Provide body massage, page 257, and that you are mentally focused. The client is paying for your time and 100% attention so you should avoid any distractions.

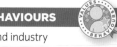
VALUES & BEHAVIOURS

Organisational and industry standards of appearance.

Preparation of the treatment area

The treatment area should be fully prepared before the client arrives. You should make sure that all work surfaces have been cleaned and are tidy and organised. Make sure that any equipment or products that you need are ready and easily accessible within reach before you start, so that you do not have to interrupt the flow of your treatment to go and get anything.

VALUES & BEHAVIOURS

Effective, hygienic and safe working methods.

The treatment environment

The client needs to be comfortable during their treatment. Additional information on preparing the treatment environment can be found in chapter 303.

Equipment and products

Treatment couch

A treatment couch may be useful for the client to rest up against during treatment. Pillows can be placed at the end of the couch for the client to lean forward onto. Only encourage this if it comfortable for both of you to do so.

Treatment chair

A height-adjustable chair will is ideal. This should have a low back so that the client's upper back is accessible and no arms to allow the therapist full access to the client during treatment. The chair should also have no wheels so that the client remains in a static, secure position throughout the treatment. You may choose to use a special Indian head massage chair; however, only do so if it does not put strain your back and you can fully access around the chair.

Trolley

The trolley should be positioned within easy reach. Position all the products you know you will need on the top shelf so you can access them easily. The trolley should be cleaned with a suitable cleaning product. Protect the surface with a piece of couch roll to mop up any oily residue.

Lined bin

This should preferably be a pedal bin, so you do not have to touch it with your hands. Use it to dispose of waste as soon as possible and prevent any cross-infection.

Towels

A freshly laundered towel will be required for the client to rest on. A rolled towel or prop is also needed to place behind the client's neck for support while you are treating the head and face.

Skincare products

As the client will be having their face treated as part of the Indian head massage, you will need a suitable cleansing product to remove their make-up before you start the treatment.

Consumables

You will also require some consumables:

- cotton wool to remove cleanser
- tissues
- couch roll to protect towels and maintain hygiene
- spatulas, to decant products hygienically.

Accessories

The following accessories will be useful:

- Comb or brush – to comb or brush through the client's hair at the start and finish of the treatment. This will help to make sure you can get your hands through the hair during the treatment and will also remove any loose hair before you start. These items should be sterilised before and after use to avoid cross-infection.

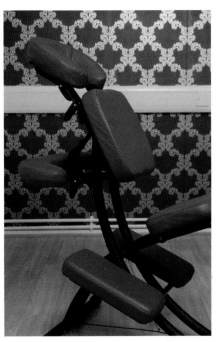

An Indian head massage treatment chair

INDUSTRY TIP

If you have a large bust, you may find using a pillow rolled over at the end more comfortable than having the client rest their head back into your chest during the treatment of the face and scalp.

INDUSTRY TIP

Try to avoid using make-up remover wipes, as these often contain mineral oils that can cause skin congestion. Many clients and therapists use them because they are quick and easy and seem more economical, but in the long term they are not always cost-effective or beneficial to the skin. Many are also not environmental friendly.

■ Hair clips – if the client has long hair, it is a good idea to clip it out of the way while you work on the back, neck, shoulders and arms.

Indian head massage mediums

A selection of massage mediums is available, including various carrier oils, waxes, creams and pre-blended products. See chapter 303, Provide body massage, for more information about the different massage mediums.

Traditional treatment oils

There are a variety of oils that may be used during Indian head massage treatment – these are not only used to help with contact during treatment but also for their particular properties. Make your choice according to the client's treatment objectives, hair and skin type, allergies and preferences. It is important to carry out a patch test (see chapter 303) if you have any concerns about product allergies. For skin types and conditions and how to recognise them, see chapter 302, Anatomy and physiology.

HANDY HINT

Fractionated coconut oil is often clear and liquid, unlike traditional coconut oil which is semi-solid.

Treatment product	Uses	Hair/skin type
Sesame oil (vata oil)	Traditional oil widely used in India, due to its anti-inflammatory and nourishing properties. May help reduce swelling and muscular aches and pains.	Dry hair and skin. It is thought that sesame oil can help to delay the onset of grey hair.
Olive oil (vata oil)	A rich, nourishing oil. Anti-inflammatory.	Dry or dehydrated skin.
Mustard oil (kapha oil)	Traditional Indian head massage oil which is strong-smelling. Has a warming effect on tissues; good for use in winter. May cause sensitisation in some clients due to the vasodilating effect.	Good for muscular aches and pains, joint stiffness and sporty clients. More suitable for male clients.
Coconut oil (pitta oil)	Semi-solid at room temperature, this oil needs warming before use – this can be done by working into the hands. Has a pleasant aroma.	Dry, brittle, over-processed or coarse hair. Skin/hair in need of moisturising and softening.
Grapeseed oil	A light-textured oil with very little aroma. Mixes well with thicker oils to give a better working consistency.	Suitable for all skin types, but particularly sensitive or oily skins.

Treatment product	Uses	Hair/skin type
Almond oil (vata oil)	A light, nourishing oil. Reduces pain and stiffness. Has a high vitamin E content.	Suitable for all skin types, but particularly dry and mature skins.
Cream	Can be used on clients who do not like the feel of oil on their skin. Can be used on the face and chosen according to skin type.	Different types according to product.
Powder (talc free/cornflour)	Ideal if a client does not want oil in their hair. Apply to the hands only, to help them slide easily through the client's hair.	Oily hair.
Wax	Beeswax or jojoba. Almost solid, this product liquefies when warmed. Waxes can be a base product or have additional ingredients added.	Different types according to the product.

Preparation of the client

The consultation

A detailed consultation to establish the client's priorities and needs must take place before every treatment. For more information on the consultation process, see the Values and behaviours chapter.

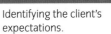

VALUES & BEHAVIOURS

Identifying the client's expectations.

Communicating with clients.

Contra-indications to Indian head massage

A description of each of the following conditions can be found within the relevant system in chapter 302, Anatomy and physiology. You should be familiar with all of the contra-indications to this treatment, ie diseases and disorders that will impact on your treatment to the back, neck, shoulders and head.

 Watch a video of an Indian head massage consultation on SmartScreen (unit 308).

You should prevent treatment in the case of the following:

- contagious skin diseases (fungal, bacterial, viral, infestations)
- severe eczema
- severe psoriasis
- severe skin conditions
- thrombosis
- during chemotherapy

Labyrinthitis

Infection of the inner ear.

- during radiotherapy
- **labyrinthitis**.

You should restrict treatment in the case of the following:

- broken bones
- recent fractures and sprains
- cuts and abrasions
- recent scar tissue
- skin disorders
- skin allergies
- product allergies
- epilepsy
- uncontrolled diabetes
- high/low blood pressure
- metals pins or plates
- piercings
- pregnancy
- medications
- lumps and swellings (eg sebaceous cysts)
- migraine.

The client should then be prepared in the following ways:

- The client should remove all jewellery, including earrings, necklaces and facial jewellery. Ask them to place these in their bag. If the client needs to remove glasses, ask them to place them in a safe place such as their bag or on the trolley if they prefer. If the client is wearing a hairpiece, it will need to be removed before the treatment.
- Indian head massage is usually applied over light clothing. The ideal item of clothing for the client to wear is a T-shirt (advise the client about this when they book). Bulky clothing and collars are best avoided as they will get in the way.
- If the client is removing their outer clothing, make sure they understand what needs to be removed. Female clients can leave their bra on but just hook their arms out of the straps. They can then be given a towel or wrap to protect their modesty.
- Provide the client with a sterile comb so that they can comb through their hair – or you may prefer to do this as part of the treatment ritual. It is important to do this before you start to remove any loose hair and to make sure the hair is tangle free.
- Position the client on a chair or stool. You should encourage the client to sit up, with their back straight, for the first part of the treatment until you need to work on the face and scalp – if they lean

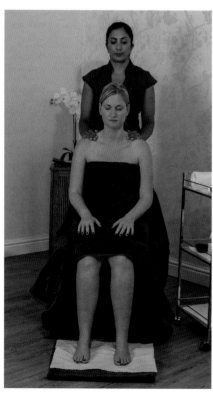

Make sure you are positioned correctly before starting the treatment

forward this will make it difficult for you to access them without over-reaching and straining your back.

■ It is important that both the client's feet remain in contact with the floor during the treatment. You need to consider both the height of the client and your ease of access so that you are both comfortable before you start.

■ The client should rest their hands unfolded in their lap.

HEALTH & SAFETY

Clean oil off work surfaces and containers quickly, as oil residue is sticky and a great breeding ground for bacteria.

History and philosophy of Indian head massage

Indian head massage (IHM) does not solely originate from Asian Indian treatments but also has roots in Native American traditions. However, it is the Asian form that worked on the parts of the body incorporated in the treatment used today.

Indian head massage is part of traditional Indian grooming and has been used in the family as an expression of love for others for generations. The treatment is based on a traditional medicine system called Ayurveda. Ayurveda means science of life or knowledge of life. The aim is to achieve balance of mind, body and spirit. These must be in harmony within oneself to achieve well-being. Narendra Mehta was key in bringing this wonderful treatment to England and in the development of Indian head as a popular treatment.

What is Ayurveda?

Ayurveda is the traditional healing system of India and Sri Lanka dating back more than 200 years. It is a holistic system with a variety of different components aimed at improving emotional, physical and mental health. Ayurveda health involves harmonious interactions between emotions, intellect, body actions, behaviour and environment.

Doshas

It is believed that we are all composed of three vital energies called doshas. The doshas are central to the Ayurvedic philosophy. Our individual constitution is governed by all three doshas in varying degrees, but most of us are governed by one or in many cases two dominant doshas. The three doshas are:

1 vata (translated means to move, to enthuse)

2 pitta (to heat or to burn)

3 kapha (to embrace, keep together).

To achieve health the three doshas must work together in harmony.

Provide Indian head massage

As Indian head massage can be performed with the client fully clothed, it is considered a non-invasive treatment. It is a great introductory treatment for clients who have never had a massage and may feel embarrassed about undressing. It is also a very portable treatment – all you need is a chair or stool, so it can be performed in virtually any environment, for example at a desk in an office. Indian head massage can also be incorporated into a facial treatment.

The physical, physiological and psychological effects of treatment

A detailed list of physical, physiological and psychological effects of massage can be found in chapter 303, Provide body massage. However, there are some specific benefits related to Indian head massage, shown in the following table.

Benefit	Explanation
Improved skin and hair texture	Techniques used will desquamate the skin.
	Oils and creams will nourish and condition the skin and hair, especially if left on for some time after the treatment.
	Improved circulation will improve the skin and hair growth.
Improved skin and scalp condition	An increase in circulation will help bring nutrients to the cells.
	Techniques used will desquamate the skin.
Improved muscle tone	Stimulating techniques will cause the muscle fibres to contract, causing a very temporary change in muscle tone.
Improved memory and concentration	Stimulating techniques will help improve circulation to the head and brain; being relaxed will also improve memory.
Reduce tension headaches	Techniques used will help to aid relaxation, which will in turn reduce tension headaches.
Reduce tinnitus	Tinnitus is a ringing or 'shushing' sound in the ear – it is believed that relaxation helps to reduce it.
Improved sleep patterns	General relaxation of the body and mind will help sleep patterns.
Reduce sinus problems	Congested sinuses will benefit from the increased circulation over the face and scalp and pressure point massage will stimulate the flow of energy in the area.

Indian head massage techniques

The massage movements used during an Indian head massage treatment are:

- effleurage
- petrissage

- tapotement
- frictions
- vibrations.

See chapter 303, Provide body massage, for more detailed information on these. There are also some techniques that are used specifically in Indian head massage, shown in the following table.

Technique	Application	Effects
Champissage – tapotement	This is a traditional movement. Hold the hands together as if praying, with the thumbs overlapped for support. Strike the skin with the fingertips in a tapping action.	This is a stimulating movement; the effects are similar to hacking.
Petrissage – chopping	Hold the hands flat to the skin side by side. Slide the hands together, chopping and pushing the skin tissue up in between them.	Similar to tapotement.
Marma pressure points	Specific pressure points applied to the scalp and face. Apply pressure using either the thumbs or fingertips (one or more) systematically over the skin's surface. Apply pressure and hold it in time with the breath. Breathe in, apply pressure, hold, breathe out and then release the pressure.	Stimulating to both the circulatory and the lymphatic systems.

Marma points

Marma points are specific points located throughout the head and body where energy flows. Pressure is applied to these during treatment to help balance the flow of energy.

Marma points are all over the body and are points through which vital energy (prana) flows. They are positioned on the body where veins, arteries, tendons and bone meet. They are also junctions where vata, pitta and kapha meet and correspond to the major chakras.

Marma points are grouped according to regions of the body and there are 107 in total. These points are similar to acupressure points and have similar origins. Marma points are larger and easier to find than acupressure points. Like acupressure points, they are sensitive to pressure and massaging them is highly beneficial to health. There are 37 marma points in the IHM treatment area. Pressure is applied on the marma point to ease poor posture, injury, emotional blocks and trauma.

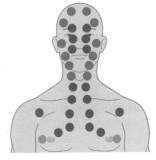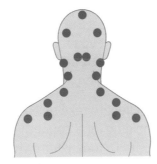

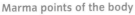
Marma points of the body

Chakras

Chakra is a Sanskrit word, meaning wheel. There are said to be 88,000 chakras. Most therapy practices involve only the seven major chakras.

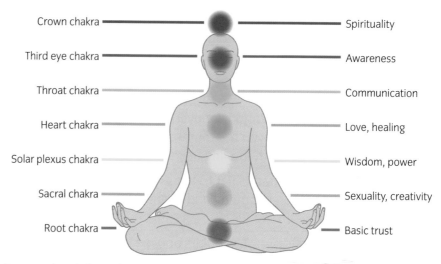

Crown chakra	Spirituality
Third eye chakra	Awareness
Throat chakra	Communication
Heart chakra	Love, healing
Solar plexus chakra	Wisdom, power
Sacral chakra	Sexuality, creativity
Root chakra	Basic trust

Seven major chakra points

Watch a video of chakra balancing on SmartScreen (unit 308).

Chakras are thought of as emotional centres linked to the physical body through the endocrine glands and organs situated in the location of the chakra. The energy that travels through the chakra can become disrupted due to emotional disturbances or stress. The resulting imbalance is believed to cause physical illness. Chakras are said to spin (some clockwise, some anticlockwise) and the speed at which each spins can either increase or decrease depending on the state of health. Harmony can be achieved by balancing the chakras. Chakras react to light energy, causing them to vibrate at a certain frequency. This frequency relates to a specific sound and colour.

Chakras are said to resemble a flower blossom, each chakra having a different number of petals. The petals represent energy channels. The stem of the flower connects and bonds with the spine and the energy channel which moves up the spine (within the spinal fluid) to the top of the head.

Chakra balancing

An IHM treatment begins and ends with a short period of time focusing on and balancing the chakras. This time helps to create a sense of peace, calm and well-being. As you become more experienced you may be able feel the sensation of the chakra energy spinning. It is important that you remain focused and clear your mind as you perform this part of the treatment. Both you and the client should be balanced with feet firmly on the floor.

Ask the client to take three deep breaths, breathing in through their nose, holding for a count of two and then breathe out through their mouth. Try to tune your own breathing with the client's.

Chakra name	Location	Colour
1 Root or base (Muladhara) 4 petals	Base of spine, lower pelvic areas	Red
2 Sacral (Svadisthana) 6 petals	Pelvic area	Orange
3 Solar plexus (Manipura) 10 petals	Upper abdomen below sternum	Yellow
4 Heart (Anahata) 12 petals	Centre of chest by the heart	Green
5 Throat (Vishudda) 16 petals	Middle of throat	Blue/ turquoise
6 Third eye, Ajna or brow (Ajna) 96 petals (divided into 2)	Middle of forehead	Indigo
7 Crown (Sahasrara) (1000)	Top of head	Purple/ violet

Meet treatment objectives

The techniques that you use will need to be altered and applied according to the objectives of the treatment. Details of the treatment objectives for all massage treatments can be found chapter 303, Provide body massage. Below are some that relate specifically to Indian head massage.

- Relaxation – increase effleurage and keep techniques slow and flowing, in particular any petrissage techniques. Reduce tapotement and frictions, keeping them near the start of the treatment.

- Sedation – movements should be slow and rhythmical. Repetitive stroking and effleurage will also help to sedate both physically and mentally. Avoid tapotement techniques unless carried out very early in the treatment.

- Stimulation – increase the use of tapotement and frictions to stimulate the client both physically and mentally. Keep movements brisk and firm.

- Invigoration – make techniques firm, brisk and bracing to enliven and revitalise the client both physically and mentally.

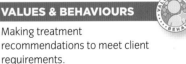

VALUES & BEHAVIOURS

Making treatment recommendations to meet client requirements.

Position the client

Make sure the client is sitting comfortably. Their feet should be flat on the floor with their shoes removed for comfort. If the client is very short you may need to place a box under their feet so that they are comfortable. You need to be able to comfortably move around the back and sides and not over-stretch. Massage chairs are great for client comfort but are difficult to adjust for taller therapists so a normal chair may be more suitable. You should maintain your posture throughout treatment. Make sure that when you work on the face you place a support behind the client's neck so this needs to be easily accessible. The client's head should remain in normal aligned posture (ie chin tucked in) it and should not be pulled back so that you can reach the face, as this is uncomfortable and will strain the client's neck. Your body weight can be used to help increase the pressure of your techniques by gently leaning in; this will also prevent excessive strain on your joints.

The normal sequence of treatment starts with chakra balancing, massage to the upper back, shoulder, arms (hands), neck, scalp, face and finishing with final chakra balancing.

Treatment timing

A commercial Indian head massage treatment is usually between 30 and 45 minutes long, depending on the routine. On-site massage, for example in an office, may be shorter.

Treatment routine

The following is a suggested treatment routine. Once you are ready to start, excuse yourself to wash your hands. Return and proceed to cleanse the client's face. Leave a few minutes before you start to balance and ground both yourself and the client. This is shown in the following four steps.

Grounding and breathing techniques

To start the treatment you and the client need to be focused and relaxed. The following grounding and breathing relaxing techniques will help to achieve this.

> **HANDY HINT**
>
> Make sure you comb through hair carefully before you start with a wide-toothed comb, especially if the hair is curly. This will prevent discomfort caused by the hair catching in the fingers.

> **INDUSTRY TIP**
>
> If offering Indian head massage in a workplace such as an office, the treatment may be as short as 15 minutes.

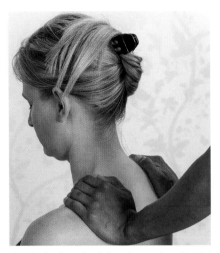

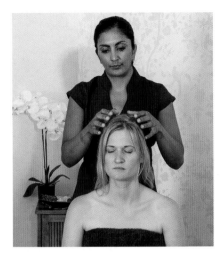

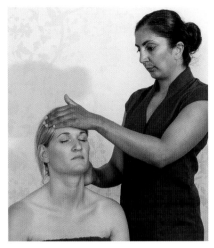

STEP 1 Place both hands on the client's shoulders; ask the client to take a deep breath and exhale slowly – do this three times.

STEP 2 Holding – place both hands over the top of the head with a gap between the hands. This will be over the crown chakra. Take deep breaths for one minute.

STEP 3 Stand to the side of the client and place one hand on the occipital bone and one hand over the third eye chakra (centre of forehead). Hold for one minute. Stand behind the client and place a hand over the throat chakra and hold for one minute.

Apply oil

Gently rake your fingers or a comb through the client's hair. Place the fingers together with the thumb to form a circle and place on the crown of the head. Pour warm oil into the finger circle using a container with a funnel or a squeezy applicator. This will enable you to control the application and will prevent the oil running down the face. Work the oil through the hair and over the treatment area.

If the hair is long, clip it up on the top of the head out of the way.

Indian head massage techniques

It is expected that you will be given a routine by your tutor to follow. The following images show you how to apply some of the techniques used within an Indian head massage. Remember to maintain good posture throughout your treatment.

HANDY HINT

When balancing the crown chakra, the hands should be apart to allow the energy to flow in.

HANDY HINT

Make sure you tell the client about the benefits that the oil will have on their hair. It is a really excellent conditioner and will help strengthen the hair shaft. Make sure you give the client clear instructions on how to remove the oil from their hair following treatment.

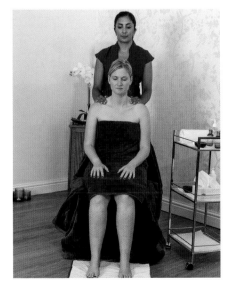

Watch a video of this Indian head massage treatment on SmartScreen (unit 308).

Good posture

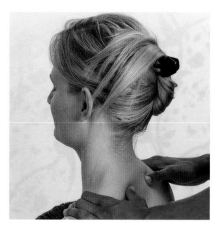

STEP 1 Thumb sweeps, keeping the fingers static on the shoulders. Sweep the thumbs up over the top of the trapezius to meet the fingers.

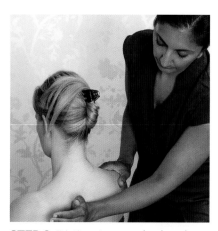

STEP 2 Frictions to upper back and shoulders over the trapezius and rhomboids using the heel of the hand.

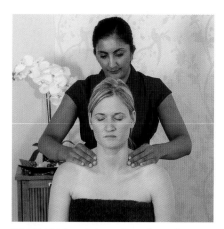

STEP 3 Thumb kneading along the trapezius.

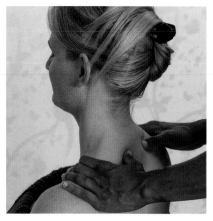

STEP 4 Thumb pressure either side of the spine along the erector spinae.

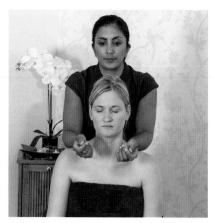

STEP 5 Using forearms, apply pressure across the top of the shoulders. Roll hands left to right to roll forearms to massage across the trapezius. Apply slight pressure with body weight into the forearms to push the client's shoulders down.

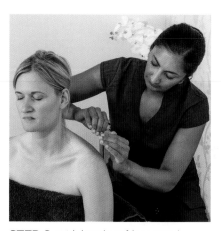

STEP 6 With hands softly cupped, apply alternating cupping to the trapezius, rhomboids, levator scapula and deltoids.

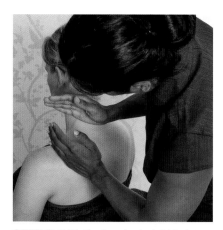

STEP 7 With the hands straight but relaxed, apply hacking to the trapezius, rhomboids, levator scapula and deltoid.

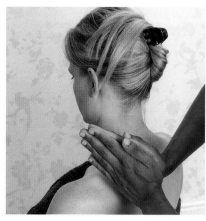

STEP 8 Champissage to the upper back and shoulders.

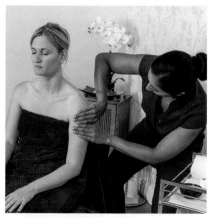

STEP 9 Work down the arm over the lower deltoid, triceps and biceps, using the fingers and thumb to apply compression/to gently squeeze the muscles.

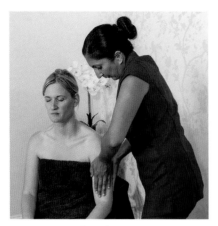

STEP 10 Work each arm separately and apply compression pressure the arm over the lower deltoid, triceps and biceps using the palms on opposite sides of the arm to squash the muscles.

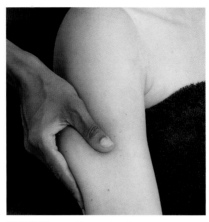

STEP 11 Working on both arms using the heels of the hand, roll the hands forwards from the triceps to the biceps (posterior to anterior).

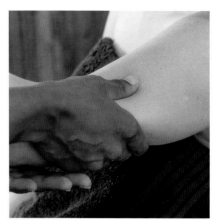

STEP 12 Palmar knead the biceps and triceps.

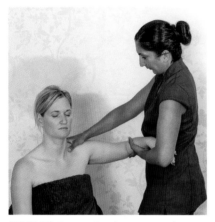

STEP 13 Supporting the arm, gently mobilise the shoulder joint. Gently mobilise the arm.

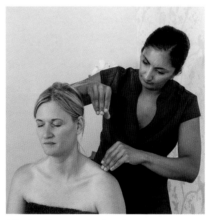

STEP 14 Using the fingertips and thumbs in an alternating plucking action, apply pincemont to the top of the trapezius. Can also be used along the biceps and triceps.

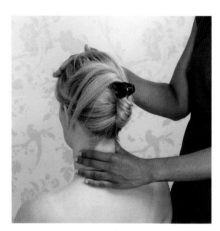

STEP 15 Supporting the head, gently and slowly rock it backwards and forwards. Pick up the muscles of the neck between the fingers and thumbs; squeeze and lift.

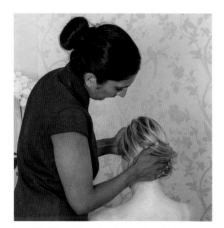

STEP 16 Using the fingertips, finger frictions to the back of the neck along the top of the trapezius, levator scapula and occipital area.

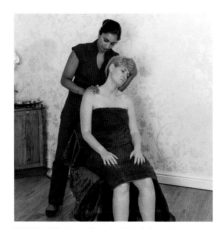

STEP 17 Standing behind the client, support the head with one hand. Gently stretch the head to one side while applying pressure down the arm on the top of the opposite shoulder to stretch the sternocleidomastoid, scalenes and trapezius and levator scapula.

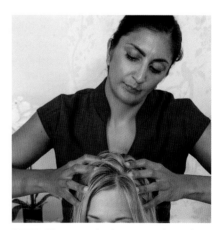

STEP 18 Using the fingertips through the hair as if shampooing to knead all over the scalp.

HANDY HINT

The scalene muscles are three muscles located on each side of the neck.

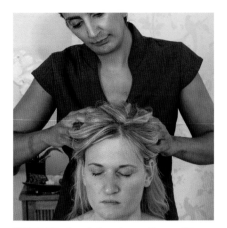

STEP 19 Carefully grip sections of the hair and lift to pluck the hair until the whole scalp is covered.

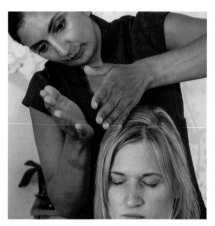

STEP 20 Hacking gently to tap over the scalp.

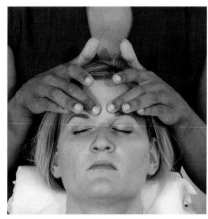

STEP 21 Apply firm pressure using the middle fingertips to the corrugator and frontalis muscles of the forehead. Apply pressure as you breathe out; hold for a breath in and release.

HANDY HINT

Do not overload the hair with oil; it only needs a superficial coating. Saturating the hair will be a waste. Do however make sure that the ends of the air are covered well as this is often the area that suffers the most from dryness.

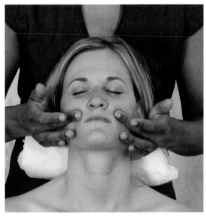

STEP 22 Pressure points to the zygomaticus along the cheekbone. Apply pressure as you breathe out, hold for a breath in and release.

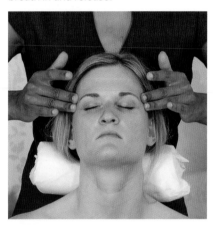

STEP 23 Slow firm circular kneading to the temples using either the fingertips or the heel of the hand.

HANDY HINT

It is really important that you do not have rings on your hands as you will find that the client's hair will get caught, making it an uncomfortable experience for the client.

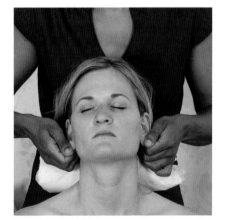

STEP 24 Thumb and finger knead with pressure along the earlobes and pinnas.

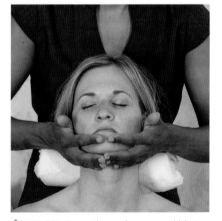

STEP 25 Smoothing along mandible to relax facial muscles.

HANDY HINT

Some clients find it hard to relax. Encourage the client to keep their eyes. This will help the client to relax and avoid distractions that might be in the treatment room.

When you have finished, step back from the client so that you move out of their personal space. Check they are feeling okay and offer them a drink of water. Allow the client to relax for a few minutes and to gather their thoughts before getting up.

Provide advice, recommendations and treatment evaluation

Contra-actions

A contra-action is an adverse reaction that happens either during or as a result of a treatment. Therefore you need to be aware of what to look out for and how to deal with a reaction if one occurs. In chapter 303 you will find a list of contra-actions and actions to take, which are also applicable to Indian head massage.

The contra-actions for pre-blended oils also apply to those used in Indian head massage.

Recommendations and advice

There is a comprehensive list of recommendations and advice in chapter 303. In addition to this, there is some advice that is specific to an Indian head massage treatment.

Advise the client to leave the oil in the hair for as long as possible to condition and nourish it. They should sleep with a towel over their pillow to prevent staining if they wish to leave it in overnight.

To remove the oil from the hair, advise the client to wet their hair and then place some shampoo in the palm of their hand, add water and mix it with the fingers. They should then apply the diluted shampoo to the hair and scalp and work the shampoo into the hair well. Then rinse the hair well.

Make sure your always consider any personal needs that your client might have and advise them accordingly. This might be related to products or further treatment.

For information on client records, feedback and evaluation, see the Values and behaviours chapter.

VALUES & BEHAVIOURS

Being courteous and helpful.

Maintaining customer care.

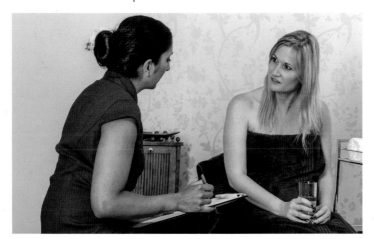

 Watch a video of Indian head massage advice and recommendations on SmartScreen (unit 308).

Informing the client how to wash the oil out of their hair is an important part of Indian head massage advice and recommendations

Answers at the back of the book.

1 Which one of the following describes a marma point?
   a Nerve ending
   b Energy wheel
   c Chakra site
   d Pressure point

2 Mustard oil is used to do which one of the following?
   a Calm and soothe the skin
   b Decongest the skin
   c Warm the tissues
   d Reduce sensitivity

3 Which one of the following is an absolute contra-indication to treatment?
   a Scar tissue
   b Baldness
   c Impetigo
   d Ear piercing

4 Which one of the following is not a traditional Indian head massage medium?
   a Grapeseed oil
   b Almond oil
   c Olive oil
   d Sunflower oil

5 Which one of the following is the main benefit of leaving the oil on the hair after treatment?
   a To nourish the hair shaft
   b To maintain the hair colour
   c To hydrate the hair follicle
   d To stimulate growth

6 What is the colour of the root chakra?
   a Red
   b Orange
   c Yellow
   d Green

7 Indian head massage is part of which tradition?
   a Buddhist
   b Chinese
   c Ayurvedic
   d Western

8 Which three chakras are balanced at the beginning of an Indian head massage?
   a Crown, third eye and throat
   b Third eye, heart and solar plexus
   c Solar plexus, crown and third eye
   d Heart, throat and crown

9 Coconut oil is in what state in its natural form, when cool?
   a Gel
   b Wax
   c Semi-solid
   d Solid

10 Which one of the following is a traditional Indian head massage technique?
   a Pressure point
   b Hacking
   c Frictions
   d Champissage

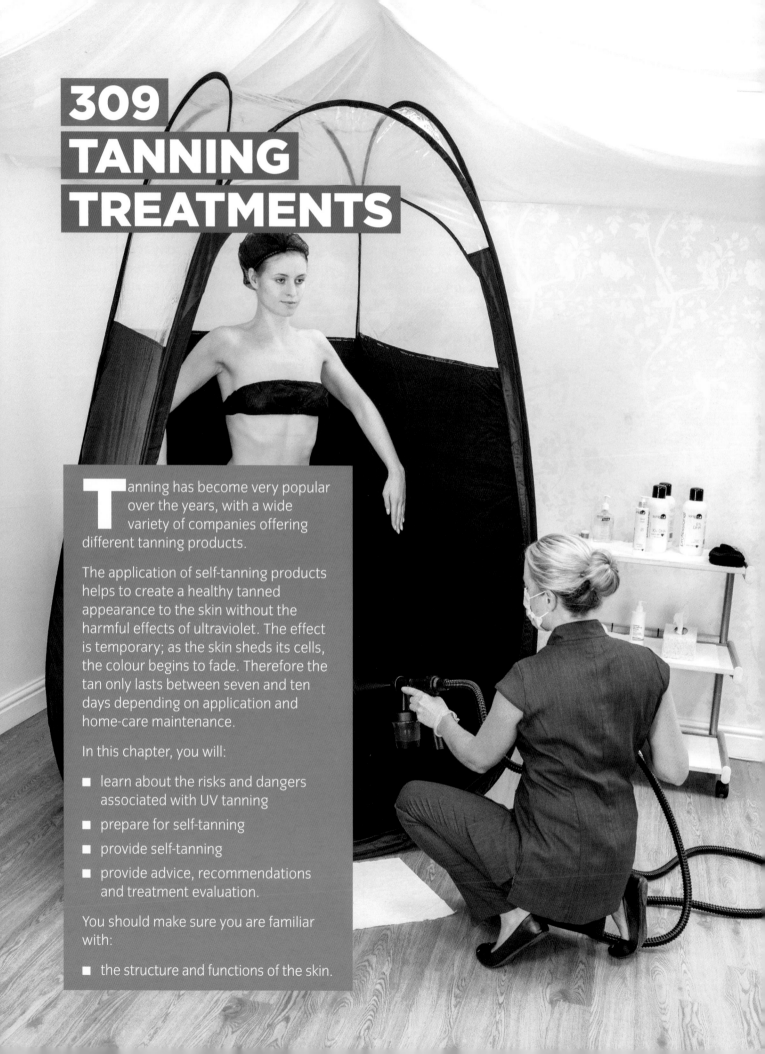

309 TANNING TREATMENTS

Tanning has become very popular over the years, with a wide variety of companies offering different tanning products.

The application of self-tanning products helps to create a healthy tanned appearance to the skin without the harmful effects of ultraviolet. The effect is temporary; as the skin sheds its cells, the colour begins to fade. Therefore the tan only lasts between seven and ten days depending on application and home-care maintenance.

In this chapter, you will:

- learn about the risks and dangers associated with UV tanning
- prepare for self-tanning
- provide self-tanning
- provide advice, recommendations and treatment evaluation.

You should make sure you are familiar with:

- the structure and functions of the skin.

Self-tanning treatments

Self-tanning is achieved by the application of a solution to the skin, in the form of a lotion, mousse, cream or gel. This can be applied either by hand or using a spray gun and compressor while standing in a spray booth.

The active ingredient used in most self-tans on the market is a colourless sugar derived from fructose called **dihydroxyacetone** (DHA) which reacts with the bacteria and amino acids of the stratum corneum skin cells, creating the tanned look. Different results occur from individual to individual and even on different areas of the body of the same person.

Dihydroxyacetone (DHA)

The main ingredient in self-tanning solutions, made from sugar beets and sugar cane.

Prepare for self-tanning treatments

Preparation of the therapist

You should present yourself in a professional manner and in line with salon policy. For more about this, see the Values and behaviours chapter.

You will also be working in close proximity to the client throughout this treatment, and personal protective equipment (PPE) appropriate to the treatment must be worn.

PPE	Description
Gloves	Disposable gloves that are talc and latex free protect the hands from discoloration.
Apron	Plastic apron – wear this to prevent the tanning solution from staining your uniform.

PPE	Description
Mask	Disposable face mask – this is optional. However, if you are using a lot of self-tan it will help prevent inhalation and protect the respiratory system.

Preparation of the client

In order to check the client's skin tolerance to the self-tan product, it is important to carry out a patch test 24–48 hours before the treatment is carried out.

1 Apply a small amount of product behind the ear with a cotton bud.

2 Leave for 24 hours.

3 Record the date and area on the client's record card.

4 If the client reacts to the patch test, the therapist will not be able to carry out the treatment.

When a client books the treatment, either in the salon or over the phone, you should advise the client to do the following:

■ Remove all make-up prior to the treatment.

■ Remove all perfumed products, including body lotions and antiperspirant/deodorant.

■ Exfoliate the skin 24 hours prior to tanning using an oil-free exfoliator.

This will ensure that there is no barrier left on the skin prior to the self-tan application.

■ Ask your client to carry out any hair removal such as waxing or shaving 24–48 hours before self-tanning.

■ Get your client to wear loose black clothing (no silk as this could permanently stain) and bring flip-flops with them to wear after the treatment.

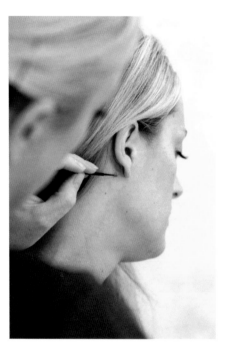

Patch test behind the ear

Activity

It is necessary to have had a patch test to ensure you are not allergic to the tanning solution before carrying out the following activity. Using the three different shades of tan, take a cotton bud and apply a small amount of each to an area on your body such as the arm. Let it fully develop and then record the results by taking a photograph. This will give you a full understanding of how the different tan strengths look when fully developed.

Preparation of the treatment area

All tools and equipment need to be disinfected before and after treatment to reduce the risk of cross-infection.

- The treatment area needs to be wiped down using a disinfectant, and trolleys and therapy couches will need protecting with disposable couch roll or a plastic couch cover to avoid any over-spray from the tan.

- Flooring needs to be of a type that can be wiped clean using hot water and disinfectant; carpet is not suitable in the treatment area, as it cannot be cleaned properly. It is also advisable to have a dark-coloured floor rather than cream or white, due to the staining which will occur from prolonged use of tanning ingredients in the area.

- Where possible, use disposable sticky feet for the client to stand on. As these are sticky, they will not blow around like tissue paper would. Adhesive foot-shaped disposable cardboard cut-outs, available in left and right shapes, stick to the client's feet throughout treatment and are ideal. These prevent discoloration of the soles of the feet, which can often happen during tanning treatments, as well as providing hygienic foot protection to reduce the risk of cross-infection.

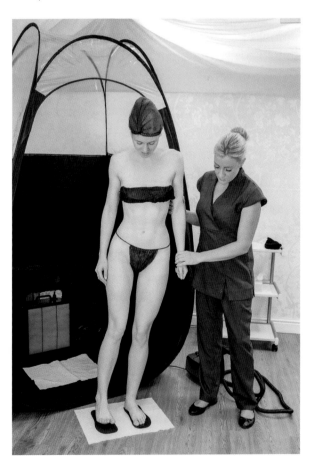

Therapist assisting the client on to the sticky feet

- There needs to be adequate ventilation to allow for exchange of oxygen and to prevent a build-up of tanning solution in the air. This will also prevent the odour of the tanning solution from lingering.

- Lighting should be bright and even so that it does not cast any shadows – this will help you achieve an even application of the tanning products. Some tanning tents now have plastic windows in them to allow more light in.

- The room needs to be warm enough for the client to feel comfortable throughout their treatment. If it is too hot, this may cause the client to perspire and could affect the consistency of the end result.

- The room in which the treatment is taking place needs to be private, as the client will be in a state of undress.

- If music is playing it needs to be at a noise level acceptable to all, and appropriate for all clients from young to mature.

- A lidded, lined waste bin should be in the room for disposal of any waste products, eg tissue or cotton wool. This waste bin should be emptied between clients into a bin liner, which will be sealed and placed in the outside bin every evening.

- Clean the self-tanning tent out in between each client by filling up the spray gun with water. This will also clean the self-tanning gun through to prevent any blockages in the nozzle of the gun. This also prevents different coloured tanning solutions mixing together to produce an undesirable result. As the tanning solution contains DHA, which is a sugar, the mechanism can become blocked if the self-tan unit is not cleaned thoroughly. This will prevent it working correctly and may lead to a spotting effect during application. The self-tan compressor also needs to be portable appliance tested (PAT) annually, and have a label displaying this.

Consultation

A consultation must take place before the self-tanning treatment is carried out on the client. This is to ensure that the treatment is suitable for the client and also to identify the client's needs and requirements. It is important that adequate time is allowed for the consultation when the client makes the appointment.

Always remember the following:

 Watch a video of a tanning consultation on SmartScreen (unit 309).

1 Greet the client with a smile and warm sincere welcome. Introduce yourself by name to the client and use the client's name.

2 Explain to the client that you need to ask some questions which will help you to decide on the best treatment plan for them, as well as assessing whether the treatment is suitable for them and that there are no contra-indications. Take them to an area where you have some privacy.

3 Client questioning during consultation is vital to enable the therapist to carry out the treatment professionally. Personal details such as name, address, contact number, medication, reason for treatment and as much detail as necessary should be recorded.

4 Encourage the client to ask any questions at any time so that they feel confident in the treatment process.

5 Explain what the treatment involves, how long it will take and what home-care and aftercare are required.

6 Keep records of the treatments for future reference and the colour/percentage you have used.

Treating minors

While treating clients in beauty, anyone under the age of 16 is classed as a minor, so you will need to obtain parental consent to allow them to be treated.

Parents should be also present during the treatment. This is a legal requirement for insurance.

Contra-indications to self-tan

It is important to check for any contra-indications that may prevent or restrict treatment. These are described in the following tables.

Prevent	Reason
Skin diseases, eg impetigo (bacterial), ringworm (fungal), shingles (viral), scabies (infestation)	Risk of cross-infection.
Severe skin disorders, eg severe eczema or psoriasis	The condition could be worsened.
Eye infections, eg conjunctivitis	Risk of cross-infection, and the condition could be worsened.
During chemotherapy or radiotherapy	Medication will alter the effects of the treatment, and these clients should also avoid unnecessary exposure to chemicals.

Restrict	Reason
Skin disorders, eg rash	May irritate.
Undiagnosed lumps and swellings	May aggravate the condition, and the underlying issue is unknown.
Recent fractures and sprains	Work around any dressing/ bandages.
Product/skin allergies	Allergic reaction may occur.
Respiratory disorders	The condition may be aggravated; ensure the client has any necessary medication with them.
Broken bones	Will stain the cast.
Recent scar tissue	May irritate.
Cuts and abrasions	May irritate.
Contact lenses	During a self-tan the mist may settle on the lenses.
Pregnancy (especially during the first three months)	Hormonal changes may affect the colour of the tanning treatment.

Tools, equipment and products

Certain essential products, tools and equipment are used in all self-tanning treatments.

Product, tools and equipment	Description	Use
Therapy couch	Cushioned treatment couch	May be used for the client to lie on during hand application of tan or during exfoliation treatment.

Product, tools and equipment	Description	Use
Cleanser	Oil-free solution.	Used to remove any barriers from the skin prior to treatment.
Exfoliator	Mitt form or cream/liquid.	Removes dead skin cells, especially around drier areas such as knees and elbows, and helps to achieve a more even colour.
Pre-tan moisturiser	Oil-free solution.	Applied to areas where the tan may 'grab' such as knees, elbows and heels; helps give a more even coverage.
Barrier cream	Thick protective cream.	Applied to the palms of the hands and soles of the feet and finger- and toenails to prevent staining.

Product, tools and equipment	Description	Use
Tanning solution	Solution which contains DHA in varying percentages to achieve differing depth of colour.	Liquid for self-tan and cream for hand application; applied all over the treatment area to achieve a healthy-looking tan.
Self-tan tent and self-tan booth	Two types: ■ pop-up tent which can be folded away after use ■ mechanical booth in which the client stands.	The client stands in the tent while the therapist self-tans them. The client stands in the booth and a pre-measured dose of tanning solution is automatically sprayed on to them.
Self-tan **compressor**	A pump which produces a stream of compressed air; sometimes called a pig due to its shape.	Releases the self-tan, which is being pushed along a hose by the compressor.

Compressor

A machine used to supply air or other gas at increased pressure.

Product, tools and equipment	Description	Use
Self-tan gun	Gun-shaped, with a trigger.	Forces the tanning solution out of the gun to give a fine mist application to the face/body.
Air hose	Plastic tubing.	Attaches the self-tan gun to the compressor.
Protective hair covering	Disposable cap or hair net.	Protects the client's hair from the tanning solution.
Disposable underwear	Disposable fabric briefs which are available as a brief, g-string or boxer short; also available as a backless bra.	Prevents the client's own clothing from being damaged by the tanning solution/ products.

Product, tools and equipment	Description	Use
Sole protectors (sticky feet)	Woven fabric or card foot shapes which stick to the client's feet.	Reduce the risk of staining to the feet during self-tan application.
Consumables	Cotton wool, cotton buds and tissues.	Used to remove cleansers and excess tan from areas such as eyebrows and the palms of the hands.
Disposable gloves	Latex- and talc-free gloves.	Prevent staining of the therapist's hands.
Sanitising products	Solutions such as witch hazel, pre-tan wipes.	These are used to clean the area prior to treatment if there is no shower available; usually in a wipe form.

It is essential to make sure that all tanning equipment is working before you carry out the procedure. You need to keep it well maintained and cleaned in order to prevent the spray gun getting clogged. Always clean your equipment according to the manufacturer's instructions and report any broken equipment to a manager.

Provide self-tanning treatments

Machine application of self-tan

Ask the client to:

Watch the video of this tanning treatment on SmartScreen (unit 309).

- take out their contact lenses or remove their glasses, if wearing them
- remove all jewellery and other accessories
- cleanse the face of any make-up
- put on a hair net to protect the hair.

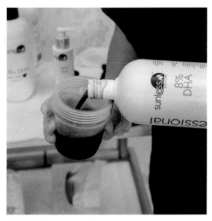

STEP 1 Decant the product into the spray container.

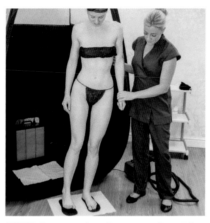

STEP 2 Assist the client onto the sticky feet.

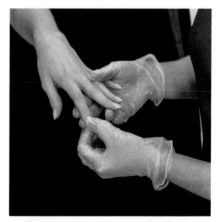

STEP 3 Apply moisturiser/barrier cream to the fingernails, elbows, knees, toenails and any dry areas.

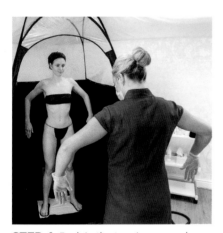

STEP 4 Explain the tanning procedure to the client and advise them on how to stand during the treatment.

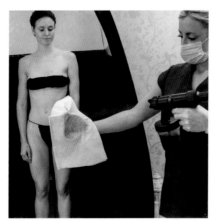

STEP 5 Test the spray before application (using a tissue to see the density of the colour).

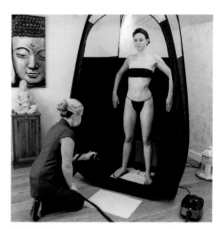

STEP 6 Crouch down and start by spraying the client's legs.

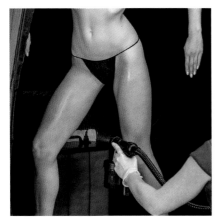

STEP 7 Ask your client to turn to the side and spray the legs.

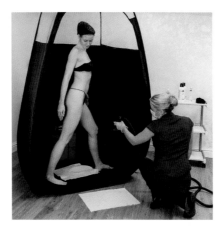

STEP 8 Ask your client to turn to the other side and repeat.

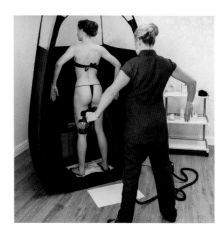

STEP 9 Ask your client to turn to the back and spray the backs of the legs.

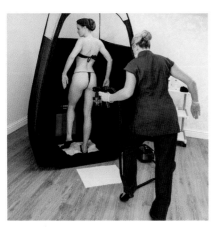

STEP 10 Ask your client to raise their heel so you can spray under the buttocks. Carry out the procedure again with the other heel raised

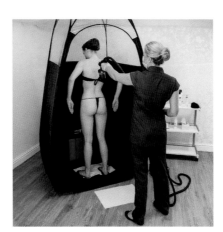

STEP 11 Spray the upper body, remembering to overlap each stroke for an even coverage.

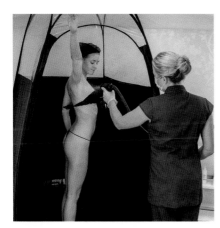

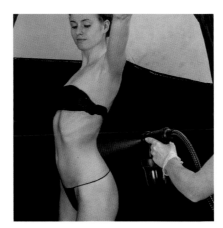

STEP 12 Ask your client to turn to the side and raise the arm.

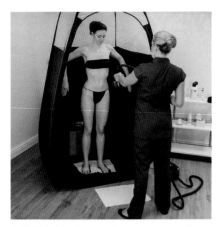

STEP 13 Ask your client to turn to the front and spray the abdomen and legs.

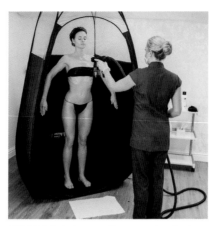

STEP 14 Ask your client to raise their chin and spray the décolleté and under the chin.

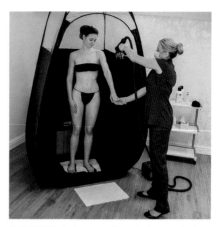

STEP 15 Ask your client to lower their arm and spray over the top.

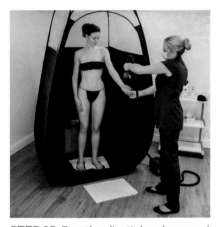

STEP 16 Turn the client's hand over and spray the inside of the arm.

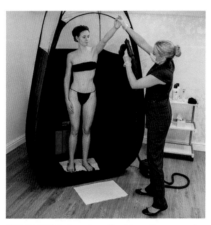

STEP 17 Raise the client's arm up again and spray underneath. Repeat steps 15–17 for the other arm.

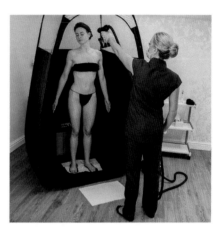

STEP 18 Ask your client to close their eyes and take a deep breath while you spray over the face.

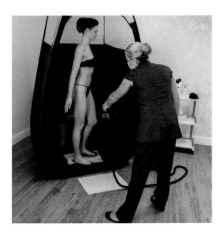

STEP 19 Finally spray over any areas of the body that look lighter. Ask your client to turn around as you do so.

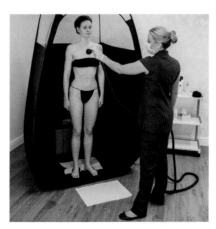

STEP 20 Remove the gun and dry the body with the air from the nozzle.

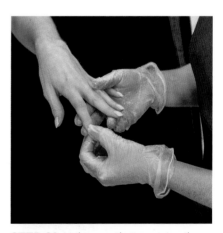

STEP 21 Make sure that you wipe the client's fingernails at the end of the treatment, to avoid build-up of colour or staining.

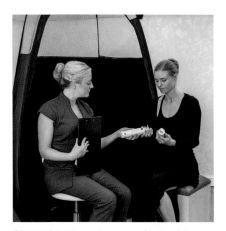

STEP 22 Now give your client advice and recommendations, and advise on any retail products available.

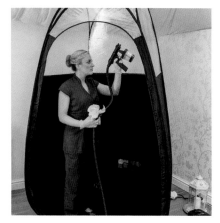

STEP 23 Clean the tent thoroughly as explained earlier in the chapter.

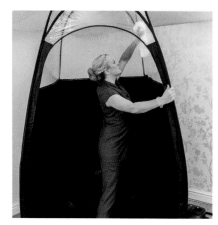

STEP 24 Dry with couch roll.

To ensure an even application, make sure that you:

- always hold the spray gun straight and at right angles to the body
- always follow the same routine
- always spray lightly on hands, elbows, knees and feet
- never spray too close to the body – the manufacturer's instructions should suggest the best distance to spray from.

Hand application of self-tan

Always follow the manufacturer's instructions to ensure that you achieve the optimum effect – these will vary between products. Wear gloves to prevent your skin getting stained where there is contact with the product.

The product may be applied with the client lying down or standing, depending on the available facilities and their preference. The procedure for manual treatment application should be carried out as follows:

Hand-applied routine

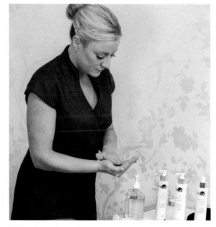

STEP 1 Start by sanitising your hands.

Watch a video of this manual tanning treatment on SmartScreen (unit 309).

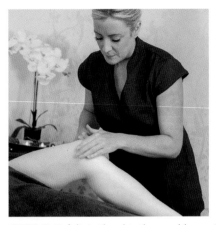

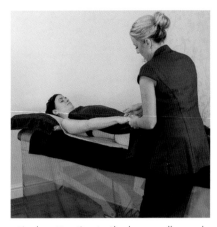

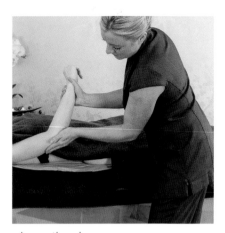

STEP 2 Exfoliate the skin thoroughly, paying particular attention to the knees, elbows, hands and any other dry areas.

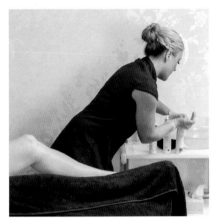

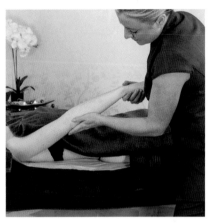

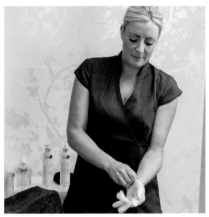

STEP 3 Remove the exfoliator by either cleansing with sponges or asking the client to take a shower.

STEP 4 Apply moisturiser to the feet, ankles, knees, elbows and wrists and barrier cream to the palms of the hands and the soles of the feet.

STEP 5 Put on your gloves to protect your hands from staining.

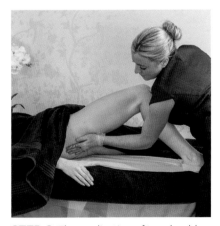

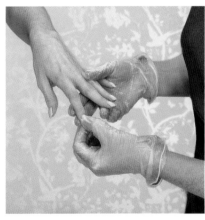

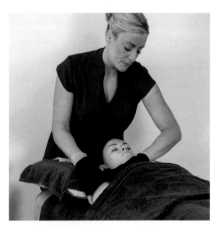

STEP 6 The application of tan should be methodical. Ensure that all the body parts are covered and that you have achieved an even application.

STEP 7 Any tanning products must be removed from the client's eyebrows and nails, the palms of their hands and the soles of their feet.

STEP 8 Use a buffing mitt if recommended by the manufacturer to gently rub away any streaky patches. Follow the same aftercare routine and advise on any retail products.

Troubleshooting

If the client has not prepared the skin properly, or too much tanning product is applied, the tanning application may become streaky or patchy. There are tanning remover wipes that you can use to remove excess, and these should be used as soon as you notice any problem areas. However, if your client complains of streakiness, suggest to them that exfoliation will help to improve the appearance of the finished tan.

Common self-tanning problems include:

- patchiness/streaking – use exfoliator and blend tanning solution with moisturiser to create a 50/50 solution, then reapply
- spotting – if you do over-spray and the tan forms 'spots', lightly dab with a tanning mitt or feather over with tissue
- green patches – If you experience any green areas, you should wash the area off (this is where the tan has reacted with deodorant and will not develop)
- discoloration of bleached/highlighted hair – wash hair thoroughly as soon as possible.

INDUSTRY TIP

Allow time for the product to dry thoroughly.

Activity

Look in beauty magazines or on the internet, and see how many brands of self-tanning products you can find. Check which ones have associated retail products to go with the self-tan.

Advice and recommendations

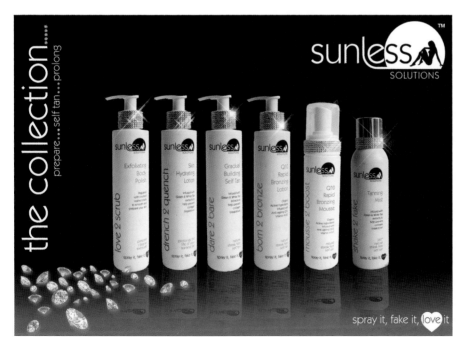

Sunless products

It is important to advise the client what to do after their treatment, as the development time of a self-tan can be up to 24 hours. If they do not follow the advice and recommendations, the treatment result may be affected.

Colour guide

A colour that shows up on the skin so you can see where you have applied the tan. The colour guide wears off as the tan develops.

 Watch a video of tanning advice and recommendation on SmartScreen (unit 309).

Ask the client to do the following:

- Avoid showers and baths for at least 8 hours to allow the product adequate time to react with the skin.
- Avoid any activity that makes you sweat immediately following treatment as this will dilute the product and affect the finished result.
- Avoid wearing tight clothing immediately following the application to prevent product removal and marking of clothes.
- Do not apply deodorant, perfume, body products or make-up while the **colour guide** is still on the skin.
- Moisturise daily to prevent the skin from becoming dry. This will help maintain the tan longer.
- Exfoliate after three days to make sure the tan wears evenly.
- Avoid chlorinated pools, heat treatments and excessive bathing as this will cause the tan to fade quickly.
- If a contra-action occurs, contact the salon for advice as soon as possible.
- Be aware that the tan may stain delicate fabrics.
- Re-book for the next tanning appointment in approximately seven to ten days.

Contra-actions

Contra-actions are rare, but they do happen. It is the therapist's job to ensure that the client is aware of contra-actions and how to deal with them.

Contra-action	Comments
Irritation/allergic reaction	An allergic reaction may occur if the client has an allergy to a product used during the treatment. Remove the product straight away and apply a cool compress. If the problem persists for longer than 24 hours, ask your client to seek medical advice. If a skin allergy occurs at home, advise your client to remove the product straight away and consult their GP, and to let the salon know the outcome.
Skin/hair discoloration	Hair discoloration is most common on bleached or very blonde hair. If this happens, advise the client to shampoo their hair straight away to prevent staining. If the skin discolours and the tan becomes patchy, advise your client to exfoliate to remove the patchiness. As long as your client wears a hair net during application this problem should be avoided.

Client feedback

It is important to gain feedback from the client. Some manufacturers recommend that their cream tan is applied quite thickly, which will not reflect the end result once the guide colour is washed off. Make sure the client is aware if this is the case, as part of their consultation, so it does not come as a shock. Show the client an area where the tan has not been applied, such as the demarcation line of their underwear, so they can compare the depth of colour. Ask open questions to ensure that you get a clear idea of the client's opinions about the result. You want their feedback to be constructive to help you improve. If the client is happy with their tan, hopefully they will come back to the salon and ask for you. Always thank the client for their feedback, whether negative or positive.

Methods of gaining feedback

Feedback can be gained by:

- asking questions verbally
- observation – is the end result as smooth and even as can be expected (depending on the products being used), with no streaks or patches?
- handing out written questionnaires.

An excellent and very simple method of reviewing client satisfaction is to see how many of your clients re-book.

Complete records

You must keep records of the treatments you carry out. The make, type and percentage of tan used should be noted, along with any adaptations and anything that the client specifically requested. Contra-actions should also be noted if they occur. These client records must be stored safely and confidentially in line with the Data Protection Act (see the Health and safety chapter), and will useful for reference on future visits.

UV tanning

This section will explain what happens when you tan under UV light and the risks associated with this.

Sunbeds give out ultraviolet (UV) rays that increase your risk of developing skin cancer (both malignant melanoma and non-melanoma). Many sunbeds give out greater doses of UV rays than the midday tropical sun.

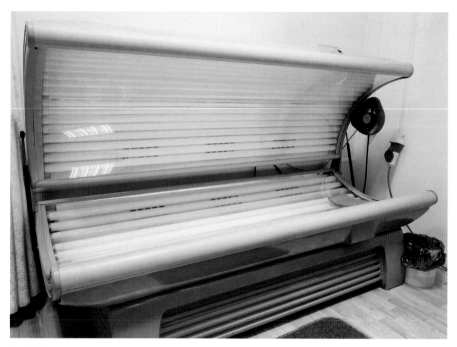

Sunbed

Activity

Find out more about the Sunbeds (Regulation) Act 2010 and present your findings in an interesting way.

The risks are greater for young people. Evidence shows that:

- people who are frequently exposed to UV rays before the age of 25 are at greater risk of developing skin cancer later in life
- sunburn in childhood can greatly increase the risk of developing skin cancer later in life.

It is illegal for people who are under the age of 18 to use sunbeds. The Sunbeds (Regulation) Act 2010 makes it an offence for someone operating a sunbed business to permit those under 18 to:

- use a sunbed at the business premises, including beauty salons, leisure centres, gyms and hotels
- be offered the use of a sunbed at the business premises
- be allowed in an area reserved for sunbed users (unless they're working as an employee of the business).

The GOV.UK website has further details about the Sunbeds (Regulation) Act 2010.

UV rays from sunbeds

Sunbeds, sunlamps and tanning booths give out the same type of harmful radiation as sunlight. UVA rays make up about 95% of sunlight. They can cause your skin to age prematurely, making it look coarse, leathery and wrinkled. UVB rays make up about 5% of sunlight and burn your skin.

A tan is your body's attempt to protect itself from the damaging effect of UV rays. Using a sunbed to get a tan isn't safer than tanning in the sun. It may even be more harmful, depending on factors such as:

- the strength of UV rays from the sunbed
- how often you use a sunbed
- the length of your sunbed sessions
- your skin type – for example, whether you have fair or dark skin
- your age.

In 2006, the Scientific Committee on Consumer Products concluded the maximum ultraviolet radiation (UVR) from sunbeds should not exceed $0.3W/m^2$, or 11 standard **erythema** doses, per hour. These 11 standard doses are the same as exposure to the tropical sun, which the World Health Organization (WHO) describes as extreme.

Erythema

Reddening of the skin (here caused by sunburn).

Damage from UV rays

Prolonged exposure to UV rays increases your risk of developing malignant melanoma, the most serious form of skin cancer.

You can't always see the damage UV rays cause. The symptoms of skin damage can take up to 20 years to appear.

UV rays can also damage your eyes, causing problems such as irritation, conjunctivitis or cataracts, particularly if you don't wear goggles.

Advice about using sunbeds

The Health and Safety Executive (HSE) issued advice on the health risks associated with UV tanning equipment, such as sunbeds, sunlamps and tanning booths. They recommend clients should not use UV tanning equipment if they:

- have fair, sensitive skin that burns easily or tans slowly or poorly
- have a history of sunburn, particularly in childhood
- have lots of freckles and red hair
- have lots of moles
- are taking medicines or using creams that make their skin sensitive to sunlight
- have a medical condition made worse by sunlight, such as **vitiligo**
- have had skin cancer or someone in their family has had it
- already have badly sun-damaged skin.

The HSE advice also includes important points to consider before deciding to use a sunbed. For example, if your client decides to use a sunbed, you should advise your client about their skin type and how long they should limit their session to.

Vitiligo

A long-term skin condition caused by a lack of a pigment in the skin called melanin.

Activity

Write a booklet for clients at your spa/salon comparing UV tanning sessions with spray self-tanning services, to help them make a decision. Remember to include HSE advice and legal requirements for sunbed use, where necessary.

Answers at the back of the book.

1   What is the sugar that makes the tanning solution work?
    a   AHD
    b   ADH
    c   DHA
    d   HAD

2   What are the three parts of a self-tanning unit?
    a   Hose, solution, booth
    b   Compressor, booth, gun
    c   Solution, hose, compressor
    d   Gun, hose, compressor

3   Which of the following cells create pigment in the skin?
    a   Erythrocytes
    b   Melanocytes
    c   Leucocytes
    d   Phagocytes

4   What is tanning solution absorbed into?
    a   Sebaceous glands
    b   The epidermis
    c   Sweat glands
    d   The dermis

5   How long does the application of a self-tan, including drying time, usually take?
    a   10 minutes
    b   15 minutes
    c   20 minutes
    d   60 minutes

6   Which of the following would restrict a self-tan treatment?
    a   Impetigo
    b   Ringworm of the body
    c   Shingles
    d   Cuts and abrasions

7   What is the layer of the epidermis that is shed during exfoliation called?
    a   Stratum lucidum/clear layer
    b   Stratum germinativum/basal layer
    c   Stratum corneum/horny layer
    d   Stratum spinosum/prickle cell layer

8   Which of the following is not a method of tanning?
    a   Using a sunbed
    b   Applying exfoliator
    c   Using a self-tanning lotion
    d   Sunbathing in the sun

9   A professional self-tan usually fades within how many days?
    a   1–2
    b   3–5
    c   7–10
    d   12–13

10 Which one of the following is a contra-action to a self-tan?
    a   Streaking
    b   Itching
    c   Uneven patches
    d   Stained soles

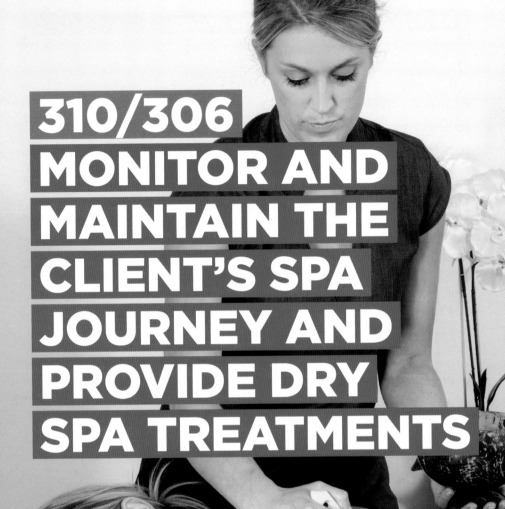

310/306
MONITOR AND MAINTAIN THE CLIENT'S SPA JOURNEY AND PROVIDE DRY SPA TREATMENTS

The word spa is thought to come from the Latin phrase *solus per aqua* which means health from water. The history of spa therapy can be traced back thousands of years to China, India, Greece and Italy. Today's spa industry focuses on therapeutic treatments combined with the use of water in some form (sometimes from the sea or a natural spring), to bring health benefits to the client.

Spa facilities need to be maintained to a high standard and meet clients' expectations of a high-quality, luxury service. The spa area needs to be prepared, monitored and maintained in a way that ensures staff and clients are not put at risk as a result of poor health and safety practice and treatments need to be carried out to the highest standard. As a therapist it is your responsibility to help ensure that the spa is maintained to a high level and that clients' experiences are positive.

In this chapter you will learn how to:

- prepare for and provide spa treatments
- monitor and facilitate a client's spa journey
- provide advice, recommendations and treatment evaluation.

Monitor and maintain spa areas

In this part of the chapter you will learn about:

- environmental and sustainable working practices
- health and safety working practices
- preparation of equipment.

Environmental conditions

Aroma

Smell.

For most clients a spa treatment is a memorable experience that should start as soon as they enter the spa environment. The decor, lighting, music and **aroma** should set the scene and prepare clients for their experience. This memorable experience should continue into the treatment areas (including the changing rooms, which should have secure lockers so that clients feel happy leaving their belongings there). You should also:

- provide disposable footwear and robes
- make sure that the area is at the right temperature (ie it is warm enough so that the client feels comfortable when they have undressed).

The spa's relaxation area needs to be an area of calm with:

- comfortable furnishings
- relaxing music
- relaxing lighting
- a good supply of drinking water and refreshments.

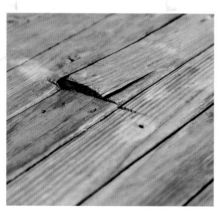

Broken boards

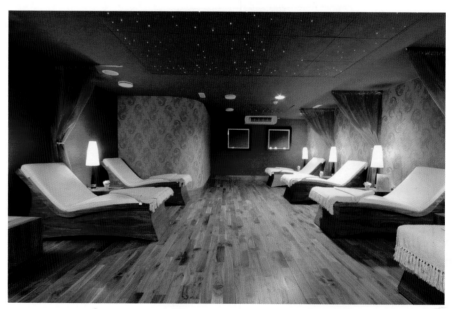

A spa relaxation area

Sustainability practice within a spa

Sustainability is a major influence in today's global economy. It is increasingly important to embrace the local resources available and embed these into the spa treatments and services offered. Spas need to change their working methods to consider the environment by:

- minimising pollution
- reducing and managing their waste
- reducing energy usage.

This can be done through reducing water consumption in treatments, recycling and reusing using paper disposables not plastic, buying local products and organic ingredients, using solar panels for energy and being aware of the health of our planet.

Activity

List 10 steps to help the environment that should be considered when working in a spa.

HANDY HINT

The Environmental Protection Act 1990 is an Act of Parliament of the United Kingdom that as of 2008 defines, within the UK, the structure and authority for waste management and the control of emissions into the environment.

Health and safety working practices

The spa environment needs to be kept clean at all times. Areas for showering need to:

- follow all health and safety guidelines for cleanliness
- have a regular supply of clean laundered towels and robes
- have a regular supply of complimentary toiletries for the client to try (that reflect the products and brand used in the spa).

The wet area in a spa is an ideal breeding ground for harmful **micro-organisms** due to the use of warm temperatures and water within treatments. It is therefore essential that the area is sterilised, disinfected and that standards of health and safety are maintained on a daily basis:

- **Disinfect** the duck boards and check for damage.
- Wipe down floors and surfaces with an appropriate disinfectant cleaner.

Micro-organisms

Very small living things (bacteria or viruses) that can only be seen through a microscope.

Disinfect

To inhibit the growth of micro-organisms.

INDUSTRY TIP

You can maximise retail opportunities by providing complimentary toiletries.

Preparation of equipment

To reduce the risk of **cross-infection**, you need to follow the manufacturers' instructions for cleaning equipment. When preparing the equipment and work area you also need to carry out the following tasks in the sauna/steam room:

- Air personal sauna/steam cabinets in between clients.
- Disinfect sauna pods after each client – make sure they are disinfected at least once every day.
- Remove any water and leave the door open overnight to allow the cabinet to dry out.
- Disinfect larger communal saunas every day and leave the door open to air dry overnight.
- Check and change water filters on spa pools regularly according to the manufacturer's instructions.
- Disinfect the edge of the spa bath daily.
- Clean hydrotherapy bath jets and shower heads daily.

Other best practice tips

- For each piece of equipment, make sure notices are displayed that explain:
  - how to use each piece of equipment
  - what the effects of the treatment are
  - when the equipment should not be used.
- Only use towels and gowns once. They should be washed after each use.
- Provide shower caps for clients, especially if they have recently coloured their hair to prevent the colour from contaminating the spa water.
- Use disposable tissue where possible.
- Provide the client with flip-flops which can be washed after use, or disposable spa footwear.

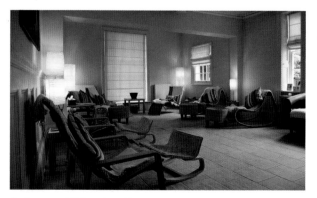

A clean and tidy relaxation area

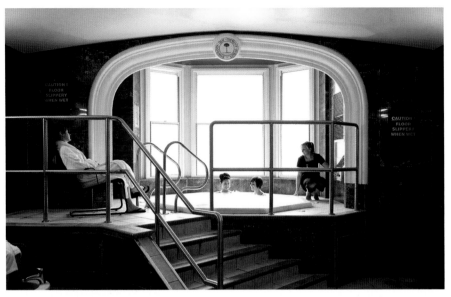

A clean spa area being used by clients

Activity

Carry out a risk assessment of the spa area in your college or workplace. Refer to SmartScreen for a risk assessment sheet.

Activity

Make a list of all the personal protective equipment (PPE) that a spa therapist might need.

Preparation for spa treatments

In this part of the chapter you will learn about:

- preparation for spa treatments
- consultation to identify the client's objectives
- contra-indications and well-being in the spa area.

In addition to the advice in the Health and safety chapter on how to reduce the risk of cross-infection and cross-contamination, the following measures should also be taken:

- Clients need to shower before and after each treatment to remove any products and degrease their skin to reduce the risk of any oils contaminating the water.
- Clients with long hair should tie it up so that it is not in the water. Long hair may become trapped in filters.
- Clients need to remove plasters before they use the spa so that they do not become loose and end up in the water.

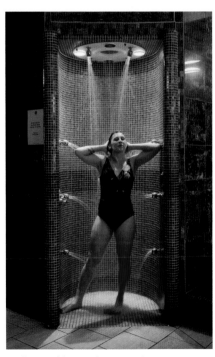

A client taking a shower prior to a spa treatment

Watch a video of spa treatment consultations on SmartScreen (unit 310).

Consultation

A spa therapist needs to ensure that the 'client journey' exceeds all their expectations. Key questions would be around:

■ What spa treatments have you had before?

■ What are your expectations of the spa treatment?

■ Are there any areas of your body you would like to improve?

From a thorough consultation, a treatment plan can be devised for the initial visit with any recommendations for further treatments.

Client spa journey

Having some guidelines on how to use the spa facilities and the type of treatments available will make the client's spa experience more enjoyable.

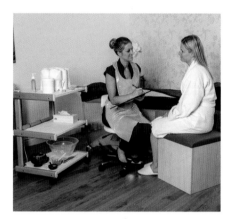

Carrying out a consultation prior to a treatment

From the reception area the client should be taken through to the changing areas where a locker is provided containing slippers and gown for the client to change into and store their personal belongings away safely. They should then be shown where the spa pool/thermal area is and how to use it. If the client is going to have a treatment afterwards, then they should be told where to wait for the therapist to come and greet them.

The International Spa Association (ISPA) defines the 10 elements of the spa experience as:

1 Water – internal and external use of water.

2 Nourishment – feed ourselves.

3 Movement – exercise, stretching, fitness.

4 Touch – connectivity and communication though touch and massage.

5 Integration – relationship between mind, body, spirit and environment.

6 Aesthetics – appreciation and search for beauty.

7 Environment – location, water, healthy.

8 Cultural expression – sense of place in the community.

9 Social contribution – cycle of giving and receiving.

10 Time, space, rhythms – perception of time and space and its relationship to natural cycles.

Relaxation room

This area can be used by clients before or after treatments and should be an area of quiet, softly lit, deeply cushioned beds or chairs where the client can relax and refresh themselves with juice or fruit and simply sit back and appreciate peace and quiet.

Contra-indications

In addition to the general contra-indications listed in the Values and behaviours chapter (pages 30–31), there are a number of contra-indications that are specific to spa treatments:

In addition to the general contra-indications listed in the Values and behaviours chapter (pages 30–31)

Contra-indication	Treatment	Restricts/ prevents treatment	Reason
Recent Botox	Massage	Restricts	Avoid massage treatments for 24 hours to prevent movement of the injected product.
Body piercing	Massage	Restricts	Avoid the pierced area until it is fully healed.
Claustrophobia	Wet flotation	Restricts	It might cause the client to have a panic attack if they are in an enclosed space.
Alcohol use within the last six hours	Sauna, steam room, hot tubs	Restricts	It might impair sweating and cause overheating of the body through dehydration.
High or low blood pressure	Sauna, steam room, hot tubs, cold treatments	Restricts	Can cause fainting and nausea. Client should seek medical advice before use.
Heart condition	Sauna, steam room, hot tubs, cold treatments	Restricts	Can cause fainting and nausea. Client should seek medical advice before use.
High fever	Sauna, steam room, hot tubs, cold treatments	Restricts	Might increase the client's already high temperature.

You should also not carry out spa treatments on a client:

- after they have had a heavy meal
- if they are under the influence of drugs
- during the first two days of their menstrual cycle (due to bleeding and tenderness in the abdominal area).

Activity

Design a consultation checklist for use during consultations for spa treatments. Be sure to include everything.

Temperatures, timings and frequency of spa treatments

Some suggested, timings, frequency and temperatures of treatments are suggested below.

Treatment	Temperature	Length of treatment	Frequency of treatment	Humidity levels
Heat treatments				
Finnish sauna	70–100°C	15–20 minutes	2–3 times a week	10–15%
Laconium	55–65°C	15–20 minutes	2–3 times a week	15–20%
Sauna pod	Depends on chosen setting	20–30 minutes	2–3 times a week	5%
Steam pod/cabinet	45–50°C	10–20 minutes	2–3 times a week	n/a
Steam room	40–43°C	15–20 minutes	2–3 times a week	n/a
Caldarium	40–45°C	15–20 minutes	2–3 times a week	n/a
Hydrotherapy treatments				
Spa pool	37–40°C	10–15 minutes	Daily	n/a
Hydrotherapy bath	37–40°C	15–20 minutes	2–3 times a week	n/a
Wet flotation	35°C	30–60 minutes	1–2 times a week	n/a
Dry flotation	35–40°C	30–40 minutes	1–2 times a week	n/a

The table above contains suggestions. You should always refer to the manufacturers' instructions for specific information.

Provide spa treatments

In this part of the chapter you will learn about:

- heat treatments
- hydrotherapy treatments
- exfoliation, body wraps, body masks, body brushing
- home-care advice and recommendations
- contra-actions to treatment.

There are a variety of treatments used within the spa environment. It is essential that you are aware of:

- how each treatment works
- the benefits/treatment objectives of each treatment
- how to use the equipment within a spa safely and correctly
- how to carry out safety checks/tests on each piece of equipment
- the guidance you need to provide clients on using the equipment.

Heat treatments

Sauna

A sauna is a room or pod that is heated to provide a dry heat with low **humidity**.

There are three main types of sauna:

- Finnish sauna (Tyrolean)
- laconium
- sauna pod.

Finnish sauna (or Tyrolean sauna)

This is a traditional wood-lined sauna cabin made from pine. It usually has two tiers of seating. An electric stove heats up specially made stones. Water is poured onto the stones and it evaporates quickly, with the heat rising to the top of the sauna. It is necessary for clients to shower before entering the sauna as this will start them sweating. As the heat rises, the upper tier of seating gets the hottest so advise new clients to sit on the lower level.

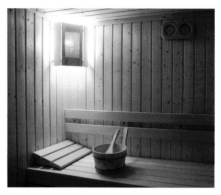

A sauna room

Humidity
The amount of water vapour in the air.

HANDY HINT
Humidity is low in saunas and high in steam rooms.

HANDY HINT
Traditionally in Scandinavian countries, sauna users would tap their skins with supple and flexible birch wood twigs to increase the blood circulation.

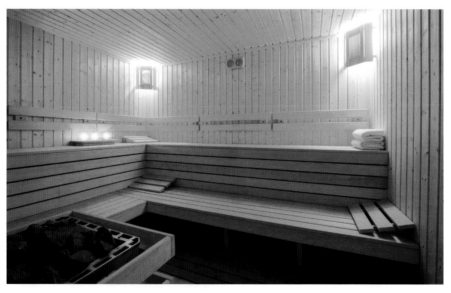

A Finnish sauna

Laconium

This type of sauna is based on a form of dry sauna used by the Romans. It has heated tiles on the floor, walls and seating. The heating usually comes from underfloor heating rather than a stove. **Aromatic essences** (eg lavender or eucalyptus), lighting and water features can be added to create a relaxing atmosphere. It gives a gentler heat than the traditional Finnish sauna. It allows the body to heat up gradually and is used for gentle cleansing and purifying of the skin because of the gentle heat. As the heat is not as intense, this type of sauna is quite sociable as most people can tolerate the heat.

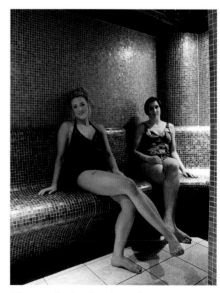

Clients relaxing in a laconium

Aromatic essences
Pleasant-smelling plant extracts used for scent.

INDUSTRY TIP

You can adjust the humidity in a sauna by ladling water onto the stones of the heater.

HEALTH & SAFETY

A thermal sensitivity test is when two test tubes are used, one filled with hot water and one with cold water. The client closes their eyes, and, at random, the therapist places the test tubes on the skin. The client has to distinguish which is hot and which is cold. If the client cannot tell the difference, then the treatment is contra-indicated.

Sauna pod

A sauna pod is used for an individual treatment. It is suitable for those clients who do not feel comfortable sharing a sauna with other people. The client's body is enclosed in the pod with a hole for the head. The pod is then heated up to a temperature that suits the client.

Health and safety checks on saunas

At the start of each day or 30–45 minutes before use, you need to switch on the sauna to allow it to heat up to the required temperature.

During this time, you will need to check the sauna to make sure that:

- there is no damage to seats/benches and walls
- the stove guard is in place and secure
- the sauna stones are in place
- the thermostat is in working order
- the door opens and closes properly
- all the lights are working correctly
- the emergency call button is working
- the directions for use, explanation of the benefits and list of precautions are on display
- there are no slip or trip hazards
- the water bucket is free from mould, has distilled water in it and that there is a ladle for pouring the water on the stones (Finnish sauna)
- the air vents are open and unobstructed.

Activity

Make a list of all the differences between a sauna and a steam treatment.

Client guidance on using a sauna

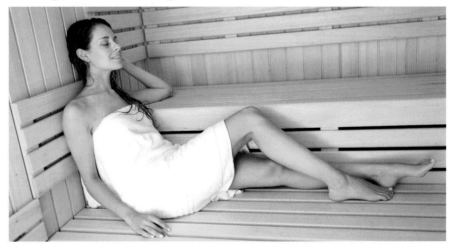

A client covering themselves with a towel in a sauna

Clients should:

- have had a thorough consultation to make sure that no contra-indications are present
- read the guidance notice on how to use the sauna safely
- remove all jewellery and metal piercings as the metal may heat up and cause a burn
- remove contact lenses and glasses
- remove all make-up
- sit on a towel if they are not wearing a bathing suit
- maintain modesty
- sit on the lower bench when they first enter and make a note of the time
- use the sauna for a maximum of 10 minutes
- take a shower after leaving the sauna to lower the body temperature (and if desired return to the sauna for a further 10 minutes)
- shower and relax for 20 minutes to allow the body temperature to return to normal
- drink plenty of water to rehydrate the body after use.

HANDY HINT

A dressing gown, slippers and disposable gown can be provided for clients using the sauna if needed (ie if they don't have a bathing costume).

Activity

Make a checklist of everything that the therapist needs to do when preparing the sauna and steam room area for use by a client.

Claustrophobic

Having a fear of enclosed spaces.

Steam room

Steam rooms originate from Turkish baths which have been in use for thousands of years. The inside of a steam room (including the seats) is completely tiled. Water is heated in a boiler and the steam is piped into the room. The whole room, and therefore the whole of the client's body (including their head), is covered in steam. Some people find steam rooms **claustrophobic**. There is a higher level of humidity so this is a wet heat treatment.

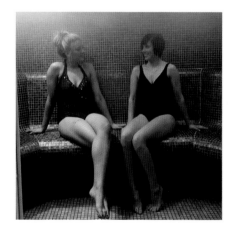

A steam room

Steam cabinet/bath

There are a number of different types of steam baths/cabinets available. They are often made of fibreglass, with a hinged door or a sealable plastic covering. The client sits on an adjustable seat inside and places their head through an opening at the top. You will need to place a towel around the neck area to help seal the unit and prevent steam from leaking out. Water is heated in a small tank inside the pod to create the steam. The steam reaches a temperature of between 45 and 50°C.

Caldarium

A caldarium is a steam room that has aromatherapy essential oils added to the steam. The heat does not become as intense as in an ordinary steam room. There may be a Kneipp hose within the caldarium that allows clients to apply cold water to their body to cool down during the treatment.

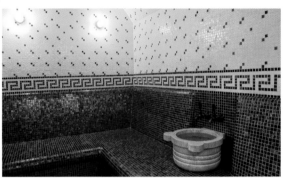

Caldarium

Hammam

This is another type of steam room that originates from Turkey/the Middle East. It is also found in North Africa. It is often decorated in mosaics with a blue, gold or brown colour scheme to reflect its eastern origins. It produces a hot, steamy aromatic effect. A traditional hammam would be made up of a series of rooms:

- the caldarium: the hot room
- a tepidarium: a relaxation room usually heated to body temperature
- a frigidarium: a cool room.

Traditionally the hammam treatment would involve going from the hottest room to the coolest room.

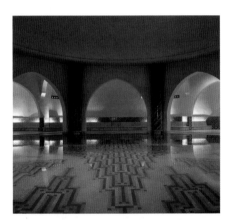

Hammam

Health and safety checks on steam rooms

At the start of each day, the steam room needs to be switched on to allow it to heat up to the required temperature. This time will vary according to the size of the room.

During this time you should check the steam room to make sure that:

- there is no damage to the seats and walls
- the ventilation is working and the warning notice on steam room usage is in place
- the thermostat is in working order
- the door opens and closes properly
- all lights are working correctly
- the emergency call button is working
- the directions for use, explanation of the benefits and list of precautions are on display
- there are no slip or trip hazards.

WHY DON'T YOU...
Have a look on the internet and research the types of products that can be used on the body in a hammam.

HANDY HINT
Chill treatments that reduce body temperature, such as plunge pools or ice rooms, will stimulate sensory nerve endings. As with heat treatments, this creates an analgesic effect which gives temporary pain relief.

Client guidance on using a steam room

Clients should:

- have had a thorough consultation to make sure that no contra-indications are present
- read the guidance notice on how to use the steam room safely
- remove all jewellery and metal piercings as the metal may heat up and cause a burn
- remove contact lenses and glasses
- remove all make-up
- sit on a towel if they are not wearing a bathing suit
- maintain modesty
- stay in the steam room for a maximum of 20 minutes
- shower and relax for 20 minutes after leaving the steam room to allow the body temperature to return to normal
- drink plenty of water to rehydrate the body.

Rasul

A rasul (also known as a serail) is a heated mud treatment that comes from the Middle East. Traditionally, it was performed within a ceremony based on social cleansing. The treatment takes place in a steam room (or a series of steam rooms) with a temperature of 42–60°C. The steam room may have two or more tiled seats which are often very decorative in their design. **Mood rocks** and twinkle lights are also commonly used to improve the experience.

Warm mud that is rich in minerals is applied all over the body by a therapist or the client. The client then relaxes in the warm, herbal-scented steam room or chamber. Sea salt may also be placed in the rasul chamber for the therapist or client to apply at the beginning of the treatment to provide additional exfoliation. After a short time, either the therapist showers the client with cool water or the client showers themselves with cool water to rinse away the mud.

> ### Activity
>
> Make a list of different spa treatments that could be combined with a sauna or steam room session to form a treatment package.

> **HANDY HINT**
>
> A dressing gown, slippers and disposable gown can be provided for clients using the sauna if needed (ie, if they don't have a bathing costume).

> **HEALTH & SAFETY**
>
> After a steam treatment the client's skin is sensitised and therefore they cannot have treatments such as waxing, etc.

> **HANDY HINT**
>
> The mud applied during the treatment has exfoliating and cleansing actions. The particular mud used may be local to the area or sourced for its health-promoting, medicinal and mineral properties.

> **Mood rocks**
>
> Glowing crystals.

> **HANDY HINT**
>
> In addition to the general benefits of heat treatments, rasul treatments help to exfoliate and cleanse the skin and improve skin texture.

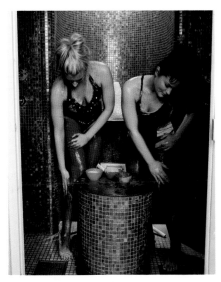

Clients applying mud during a rasul treatment

WHY DON'T YOU...
Do some research into the different kinds of mud that are used in a rasul treatment and find out the properties of each mud.

INDUSTRY TIP
When adding products to the rasul mud (eg grapeseed oil for ease of mud application), always make sure that the client does not have any allergies.

HANDY HINT
A rasul treatment can be used prior to a body massage to warm the muscles. It will make the massage more effective as it makes it easier for the therapist to get deep into the warmed muscles.

WHY DON'T YOU...
Work with a colleague to make a list of all the other spa treatments that would benefit a client after having a heat treatment.

Health and safety checks on a rasul chamber

You need to carry out health and safety checks on a daily basis. You need to check to make sure that:

- there is no damage to any surfaces
- all the lights are working correctly
- the emergency call button is working
- the directions for use, explanation of the benefits and list of precautions are on display
- there are no slip or trip hazards.

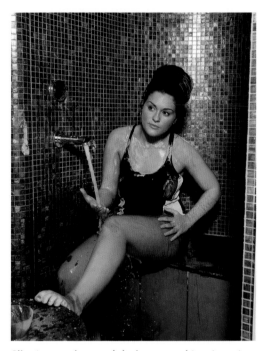
Client removing mud during a rasul treatment

Effects and benefits/treatment objectives of heat treatments

The benefits/treatment objectives of heat treatments include the following:

- They soothe aches and pains as muscles are warmed and relaxed.
- They create a sense of well-being.
- They improve skin tone and skin condition due to increased blood supply and oxygen and nutrients to the cells.
- They induce deep relaxation.
- They stimulate blood and lymph circulation.
- They increase body temperature – this stimulates the sudoriferous glands which results in increased perspiration; perspiration assists with deep cleansing and the removal of waste products.
- They help relieve stress.

Hydrotherapy treatments

Hydrotherapy is the use of water in the treatment of different conditions, including arthritis and related rheumatic complaints. Hydrotherapy differs from swimming because it involves special exercises that you do in a warm-water pool. It has greater benefit if hot and cold water are alternated during a treatment as this stimulates the circulation and leaves the client feeling **invigorated**.

The main types of hydrotherapy equipment are:

- spa pool/bath/Jacuzzi/whirlpool
- hydrotherapy baths
- blitz showers
- Swiss/Vichy shower.

Spa pool

Also known as a Jacuzzi or a whirlpool, a spa pool can seat up to ten people (depending on the size of the pool). Heated water is forced through jets. This causes the water to bubble and creates a gentle massaging effect on the body. The water from the spa bath is filtered and recirculated meaning that it is not changed after each client. Every week the spa attendant should carry out a full service on the spa pool equipment. The spa pool should be cleaned thoroughly every day to remove any residue.

You will need to carry out the following specific tests on the spa pool a couple of times a day to test the quality of the water and to make sure that it is safe:

- **pH balance** (acidity/alkalinity) – the pH needs to be balanced to make sure that the water is neither too acidic nor too alkaline. If it is too acidic, the water can become cloudy. If it is too alkaline, this may cause a build-up of limescale in the equipment.

- Water hardness (ie calcium content) – water contains calcium which may make it hard or soft. If there is too much calcium this may cause a build-up of limescale on the equipment.

- Water temperature – this needs to be tested to make sure that the spa pool isn't too cold or too hot.

HEALTH & SAFETY

Make sure that spa guests/clients always shower before any water treatment to prevent the spread of water-borne infections. Legionnaires' disease is caused by bacteria that grow in warm water that is recirculated (eg in a spa pool). Good hygiene in the spa wet areas is essential to prevent these bacteria from growing. Symptoms of the disease include tiredness, aching muscles, headaches, cough and fever.

Hydrotherapy

The therapeutic use of water in treatments.

Invigorated

Energised.

HANDY HINT

The nineteenth-century Bavarian monk Father Sebastian Kneipp reintroduced hydrotherapy as he believed that disease could be cured by using water to get rid of waste from the body.

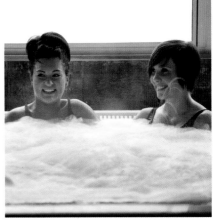

Spa pool

pH balance

A measure of the acidity or alkalinity of the water. If the water is acidic, the pH is less than 7 and if it is alkaline, the pH is greater than 7.

HANDY HINT

Chlorine is the most widely used disinfectant used in swimming pools. Bromine, like chlorine, can be used in the maintenance of swimming pools and also spa pools (hot tubs).

INDUSTRY TIP

The Langelier Saturation Index is a calculation that is used to show whether water is corrosive or likely to form limescale.

INDUSTRY TIP

As a guide, the pH of a spa pool should be between 7.2 and 7.6.

INDUSTRY TIP

As a guide, the water temperature in a:

- spa pool should be between 34 and 37°C
- swimming pool should be between 27 and 30°C.

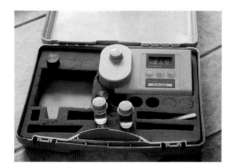

A Palintest® kit

DPD

Diethyl-p-phenylenediamine.

HANDY HINT

When placing the tablets in the water **reservoir** do not let them touch your skin because this will affect the pH reading, as the tablet will register the pH reading of your skin.

Reservoir

Part of a container that holds a liquid.

HANDY HINT

It is very important that the spa pool water and swimming pool water are tested regularly and that the levels are within those recommended by the manufacturer.

The results of the water quality tests need to be recorded for the **Environmental Health Officer** to review on their visit. By keeping records of these it shows that the spa is following health and safety requirements.

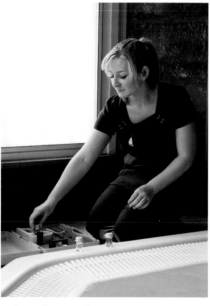
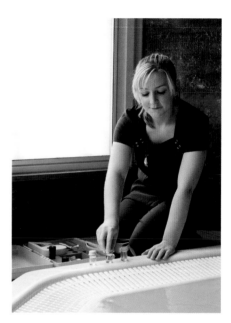

A therapist carrying out a pH test

pH testing

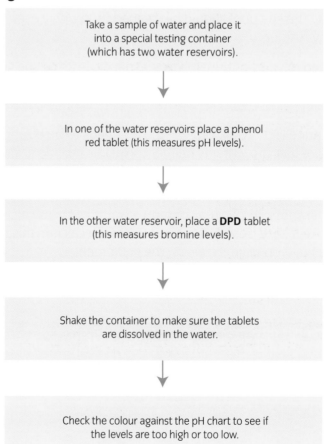

Take a sample of water and place it into a special testing container (which has two water reservoirs).

⬇

In one of the water reservoirs place a phenol red tablet (this measures pH levels).

⬇

In the other water reservoir, place a **DPD** tablet (this measures bromine levels).

⬇

Shake the container to make sure the tablets are dissolved in the water.

⬇

Check the colour against the pH chart to see if the levels are too high or too low.

Activity

Design a water treatment checklist for use in a spa.

WHY DON'T YOU...
Find out what corrosive water can do to a pool within a spa.

Client guidance on using a spa pool

Clients should:

- have had a thorough consultation to make sure that no contra-indications are present
- read the guidance notice on how to use the spa pool safely
- remove all jewellery and metal piercings
- shower and remove all make-up before entering the pool
- tie up long hair and use a shower/bathing cap if their hair has been coloured recently
- only enter the pool when it is not bubbling so the steps and floor of the pool are fully visible
- stay in the pool for a maximum of 20 minutes
- hold onto the rails for additional support when the water jets are massaging the skin
- take a shower and relax for 20 minutes after leaving the pool to allow the body temperature to return to normal
- drink plenty of water to rehydrate the body.

HANDY HINT

Watsu is a body treatment carried out in a warm pool with the emphasis on water shiatsu – the client is held by a practitioner moving the body through gentle stretches and rotations within the water to support the freeing of joints and muscles and promoting deep relaxation.

INDUSTRY TIP

A thermal suite within a spa has a range of hot and cold experiences to cleanse the body, relax the muscles and invigorate the client.

Health and safety checks on hydrotherapy equipment

You will need to carry out the following general health and safety checks on hydrotherapy equipment. You need to make sure:

- there is no damage to any surfaces
- the water is at the correct temperature
- there is a handrail in place and that it is secure
- all lights are working correctly
- the emergency call button is working
- the directions for use, explanation of the benefits and list of precautions are on display
- there are no slip or trip hazards
- the spa pool water is tested at the start of each day for temperature, water hardness and pH balance
- the spa pool water is monitored regularly throughout the day.

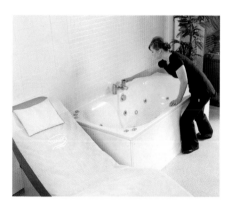

A therapist filling a hydrotherapy bath

 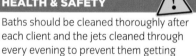
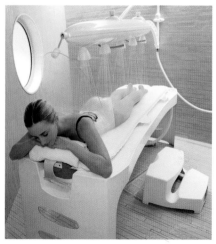

Vichy shower

Hydrotherapy bath

A hydrotherapy bath is designed for individual use. It has water jets positioned around the inside of the bath. These jets force water against the body, giving a gentle massage. Sometimes these baths have a water hose which can be used to direct water onto specific parts of the body. The water temperature in the hydrotherapy bath is usually pre-set to approximately 37–40°C. The bath may be used for relaxation or a pre-set programme can be used to target the jets at a specific part of the body.

Products may be added to the bath to further enhance the treatment.

Product	Example	Use/benefit
Algae	Marine minerals (eg seaweed)	Helps to stimulate the circulation. Helps to detoxify the body. Has a general toning effect.
Salt	Mineral salts (eg potassium, magnesium, calcium)	Helps to stimulate circulation. Helps to detoxify the body. Has a relaxing effect on tired and aching muscles.
Pre-blended aromatherapy oils	Essential oils – lemon and juniper or lavender and camomile	Depends on the blend used. The aroma will have an immediate effect on the senses. Relaxing and calming.
Milk		Ideal for mature or dehydrated skin. Very soothing and nourishing.

Blitz shower

A blitz shower uses powerful water jets to invigorate the circulation and revitalise tired muscles. The temperature can be varied from hot to cold for a more stimulating experience.

Swiss/Vichy shower

The client lies down on a cushioned treatment table. Above the table is a row of five to seven shower heads. While the client is lying down they are sprayed with water. It is used during spa treatments to remove products and as a form of hydro-massage.

Benefits/treatment objectives of hydrotherapy treatments

The benefits/treatment objectives of hydrotherapy treatments include the following:

- They increase joint flexibility by removing excess toxins and reducing swelling.
- They give a feeling of well-being.
- They stimulate the circulation.
- They bring relief from pain by soothing the nerve endings as the body relaxes.
- They stimulate the metabolism.
- They tone up the body.
- They build up the immune system by removing toxins and waste products.
- They increase lymph circulation which reduces fluid retention/ **oedema**.

Oedema

A condition where excess fluid collects in the tissues of the body.

Activity

Working in pairs, carry out a thermal sensitivity test on each other using hot and cold test tubes. Fill one test tube with cold water and one with warm water. Ask your partner to close their eyes and then place each of the test tubes onto their skin. Ask them to tell you which one is cold and which one is warm.

HANDY HINT

Kneipp therapy is the use of alternate hot and cold herbal baths to stimulate the circulation and create a feeling of well-being.

Other spa treatments

Flotation

There are two different types of flotation used in the spa:

- dry flotation
- wet flotation.

HANDY HINT

Dry flotation is often used alongside a body wrap treatment.

Dry flotation

As the name suggests, this is a dry treatment. Unlike wet flotation (where the client is placed into a tank of water), the client lies on a board on the surface of the water. This board is protected with a thick vinyl covering which also protects the client. The board is then lowered onto the water so that the client is floating on it. It is similar to lying on a water bed.

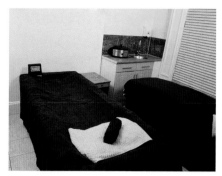
Dry flotation bed

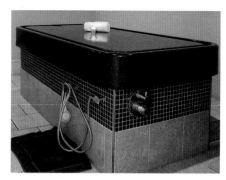
Heated hammam bed

Health and safety checks for dry flotation treatments

You need to carry out the following health and safety checks prior to treatments:

- Check the vinyl covering for any splits or tears.
- Make sure that the mechanism for raising/lowering the board is working.
- Check the temperature of the water in the bed (refer to manufacturer instructions).

Client guidance – dry flotation treatments

Clients should:

- have had a thorough consultation to make sure that no contra-indications are present
- shower and remove all make-up prior to treatment
- be aware that the bench will be lowered so that flotation can take place
- be comfortable and warm
- float for approximately 20 minutes
- shower after treatment and relax for 15 minutes to allow the body temperature to return to normal
- drink plenty of water to rehydrate the body.

HANDY HINT

During a dry flotation treatment, you could provide other spa treatments to clients (eg a body mask).

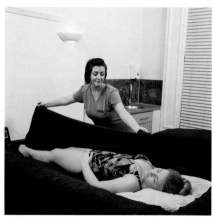
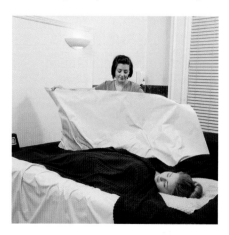
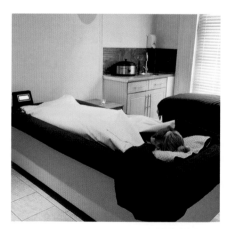

Dry flotation treatment

Wet flotation

A specially made bath or tank is filled with about 25cm of salt- and mineral-rich warm water (between 34°C and 36°C). The client floats in the water. As the water contains so much salt it is impossible to sink. This gives a feeling of weightlessness. This feeling of floating helps the muscles to relax and therefore reduces back pain and other muscular aches and pains. As the water won't allow the client to sink, they don't have to concentrate on supporting or moving the body, which allows their brain to relax.

Client preparation for wet flotation treatments

The flotation tank is soundproofed to help clients to relax. You should also provide clients with earplugs to make sure that they aren't disturbed by any noise. You need to make sure the room is in darkness as this slows the electrical activity of the brain. Darkness also helps balance the brain's activity so that the creative side of the brain becomes more dominant than the logical side of the brain.

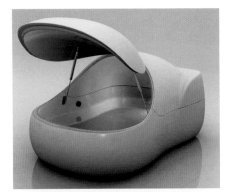
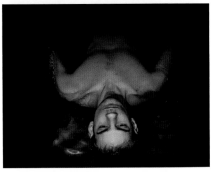

Wet flotation tanks

Health and safety checks for wet flotation treatments

You need to carry out health and safety checks twice a day. You need to check to make sure that:

- there is no damage to any surfaces
- the water is at the correct temperature (between 34°C and 36°C)
- the lights are working correctly
- the emergency call button is working
- the directions for use, explanation of the benefits and list of precautions are on display
- there are no slip or trip hazards.

In addition to the general checks, you should also check at the start of each day and during the day that:

- the water is at the correct temperature (approximately 34–36°C)
- the water is at the correct level and has no debris in it
- that the pH balance is 7.2–7.4
- the filters aren't blocked (and any other checks in line with the manufacturer's instructions)
- the intercom is working.

Client guidance – wet flotation treatments

Clients should:

- have had a thorough consultation to make sure that no contra-indications are present
- shower and remove all make-up before entering the flotation tank

- read the guidance notice on how to use the flotation tank safely
- have had a demonstration and explanation by the therapist on how the tank works (eg lighting, audio levels and opening and closing of the pod)
- wear ear plugs to prevent water getting into their ears
- relax
- be aware that the therapist will use the intercom to check the client is comfortable
- shower at the end of the treatment to remove salt and toxins from the skin
- relax for 20 minutes after the treatment
- drink plenty of water to rehydrate the body.

Benefits/treatment objectives of flotation treatments

The benefits/objectives of flotation treatments include the following:

- They help with jet lag.
- They can bring about pain relief.
- They help with insomnia.
- They induce relaxation of the mind, body and spirit to relieve stress.

Activity

Research two spas that include flotation as part of a pre- or post-treatment package.

Ice treatments

There are many different cold treatments available in a spa which will lower the body temperature and can be used as a pre- or post-body treatment.

A cold treatment can decrease blood pressure by lowering the body temperature, can relieve pain due to its analgesic effect on superficial nerve endings and can have a toning and tightening effect on the skin. It can bring about a general feeling of invigoration and energy.

There are a variety of ice treatments such as:

- Ice room – the client rubs crushed ice all over their body, cooling themselves down and stimulating the circulation.
- Cold plunge pool – usually a small deep pool near a sauna or steam bath. The client enters slowly and usually just 'plunges' their body and then gets out.
- Cold foot bath – the client can soak their feet in the bath for up to a minute. Can help circulation and tired feet.

HANDY HINT

Soundproofing and lighting are optional for a wet flotation. Some people may not like the feeling of darkness and silence. If a client doesn't like darkness or silence, then you should dim the lights and play some gentle music instead. Recommend total darkness as this helps the body and mind to switch off completely.

INDUSTRY TIP

Research has shown that flotation can help pain relief (eg pain caused by rheumatoid arthritis).

INDUSTRY TIP

Flotation can be used by clients who are pregnant.

HANDY HINT

Scandinavian countries for years have been combining the use of heat on the body from the sauna and then going out into the snow or cold water to clean the skin and encourage the feeling of well-being.

HANDY HINT

Spas with an ice room encourage clients to rub ice all over their bodies to cool down and get an invigorating sensation.

HEALTH & SAFETY

Check contra-indications thoroughly as ice treatments can be a shock to the system. Clients with heart (coronary) disease should not have cold treatments.

- Cold shower – the client showers under cool water for as long as they can tolerate. Alternating between warm and cold showers has a toning effect on the skin.
- Cold compress – this can be applied to a specific area of the body and is ideal for sprains or inflammation of a muscle.

HEALTH & SAFETY

After a cold treatment it is important that the client relaxes for 20 minutes, to allow the body temperature and blood pressure to return to normal.

Activity

Try having a cool shower next time you come out of the sauna/steam room to see how it makes you feel.

Body wrap treatments

Body wrapping is another popular treatment offered by many spas. Body wrap treatments help with detoxification, relaxation, improving the skin's appearance or can be used as part of a slimming programme. A mask or body wrap product is applied to the skin and the client is wrapped in plastic, foil or bandages (if it is a treatment to aid slimming).

Depending on the manufacturer's instructions the client may have a heated blanket applied or use the dry flotation bed. The wrap and heat from the blanket cause the body's temperature to increase. This then increases the circulation and encourages the body to sweat which gets rid of any impurities.

Body wrapping can also be used as part of a weight loss and toning programme. Body wrap treatments for this purpose often use bandages that are pre-soaked in a product that improves skin tone or a contour gel applied to the skin and then wrapped in dry bandages and then wrapped around the body to achieve weight loss. The objective of the wrap is to improve the skin tone and remove toxins which will help to give the skin a firmer and tighter appearance.

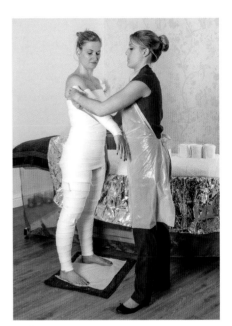

Body wrap treatment

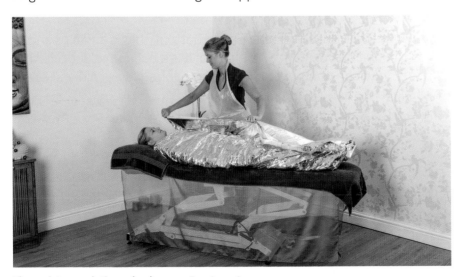

Therapist completing a body wrap treatment

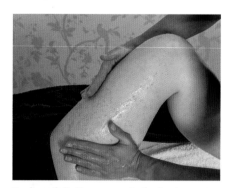

Body exfoliation as part of a body wrap treatment

Consultation for body wrap treatments

Before carrying out a body wrap treatment, you need to carry out a thorough consultation by:

- using open questions to establish the treatment objectives and identify any possible contra-indications
- referring to the client's record card to review previous treatments
- using visual aids to explain the treatment to the client.

You should also record the results of any patch/sensitivity tests that have been carried out. These tests will need to be carried out a minimum of 24 hours prior to treatment by applying a small amount of the product to the client's skin. Thermal testing can be carried out immediately before heat treatments to check the client's sensitivity to heat.

Treatment objectives – body wraps

As part of your consultation it is important to establish which treatment objective is most appropriate for your client:

- improve the appearance of underlying muscle tissue
- improve skin condition
- body contouring
- improve circulation
- improve the appearance of cellulite.

Body assessment

As part of the consultation for a body wrap treatment, you will need to carry out an assessment of the client's body. You will need to discuss with the client any specific conditions that they may want to try to improve with the treatment:

- Cellulite – this is usually found on the bottom, thighs and hips and has a dimpled appearance on the skin. It is a build-up of fat cells that slows down the removal of toxins. It quite often feels cold and can be the result of:
  - poor diet
  - lack of exercise
  - a slow metabolism
  - poor circulation.

- Fluid retention – this usually occurs around the ankles, in the lower limbs and in the abdominal area. It can be due to standing for long periods of time or hormonal changes, particularly around menstruation.

HANDY HINT

Anyone, male or female, whatever their shape or size, can suffer from cellulite.

INDUSTRY TIP

Dry skin brushing is excellent for the treatment of cellulite as it helps to stimulate the circulation. The client can continue the treatment at home every day before they have a shower.

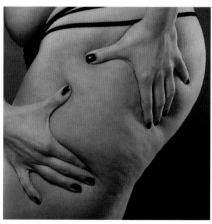

The thighs are a common site for cellulite

- Adipose tissue – commonly referred to as excess fat. It forms the subcutaneous layer below the skin and its main purpose is to store fat and release it as energy when needed by cells in the body. Women tend to store excess weight around the hips and thighs while men store it on the abdomen and waist.

- Postural problems – a client's posture can be affected by their occupation, muscle condition, lifestyle and general health. Postural faults that you should be aware of include lordosis, scoliosis and kyphosis. For further information on postural faults, see chapter 303.

Exfoliation

Exfoliation is the treatment to remove dead skin cells from the skin's surface. There are facial and body exfoliation treatments available to cleanse, brighten and stimulate the skin. In body treatments you can use cream scrubs, salt scrubs, peels or body brushing. It is an excellent pre-treatment to body massage, self-tanning application and body wrap treatments. Encouraging desquamation of the skin allows products to penetrate easily and more even absorption.

A full consultation should be carried out to make sure the treatment will be effective. Contra-indications to exfoliation include skin diseases, sensitive skin, eczema, psoriasis, bruising, recent scar tissue and sunburn.

Products, tools and equipment for body wrap treatments

Listed below are the products, tools and equipment that you will need to carry out body wrap treatments.

HANDY HINT

Body scrubs and body brushes are an ideal product to retail in the spa to encourage the client to continue their treatment benefits at home.

INDUSTRY TIP

Javanese Lulur and Balinese Boreh are two types of traditional exfoliation body treatments now incorporated into spa menus worldwide.

INDUSTRY TIP

Juniper essential oil is an excellent diuretic and is good in the treatment of cellulite and fluid retention.

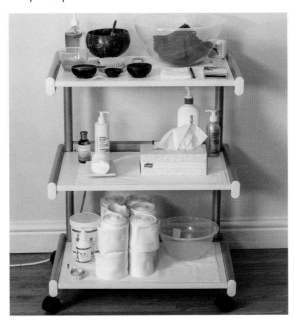

A range of products, tools and equipment used in a body wrap treatment

Product/tool/ equipment	Description	Use/benefit
Cleanser	Body cleanser – sprays	Removes surface debris, oils and barriers. Cleansing makes sure that the body wrap product/mask can penetrate into the skin.
Exfoliator	A cream/liquid containing small man-made abrasive beads or abrasive natural products (eg sea salt or fruit and nut kernels).	Gives a deeper cleanse.
Body wrap products	Body wrap products can be applied directly to the skin or via bandages applied to the limbs or body. Products can include seaweed, thermal products and cryo-based products.	Help to achieve the treatment objective such as detoxifying, inch loss, fluid reduction or skin conditioning.
Body masks	Mud-based, seaweed or milk-based products applied prior to wrapping the client.	Help to achieve the treatment objective. Improve the appearance of the skin. Improve skin tone. Detoxification.
Materials for wrapping the body (after applying mask or body wrap products)	Plastic wrap. Bandages. Linen strips. Foil blanket.	Used to help the product penetrate into the skin. Assist with body contouring.
Heated blanket/ wrap	Electric blanket that produces heat. Often broken down into zoned areas of heat so the client can choose which area to have heated. Manually controlled **thermostat**.	Helps to maintain body temperature throughout the treatment. Encourages body's temperature and therefore circulation to increase. Causes the body to sweat which gets rid of any impurities.
Couch	Adjustable therapy couch. Protected with couch roll.	For the client to lie on during the treatment.
Trolley	Clean trolley. Set up in an organised way for treatment. Trolley should have sufficient space for all your tools and equipment.	To hold the necessary equipment and products for the treatment.

Product/tool/ equipment	Description	Use/benefit
Bowls	For body wrap products. Flexible (ie bendy) bowls in varying sizes.	For **decanting** products. For mixing products. Need to be flexible and bend to break up mud that might have set in the bowl. Can be used to pour products directly onto the skin.
Spatulas	Usually made of wood. Can be plastic or metal.	For dispensing products to avoid cross-contamination. Used for mixing products.
Body brush	A natural bristle brush.	Used to brush the body when dry in long alternate strokes working in the direction of the lymphatic system. Aids desquamation of the skin. Helps with the removal of waste products. Increases circulation. Improves the appearance of cellulite. Improves skin colour and tone.
Sauna	Dry heat room.	Used before treatment. Increases body temperature to relax the client and allow for better penetration of the products.
Steam	Wet heat room.	Used before treatment. Increases body temperature to relax the client and allow for better penetration of the products.
Plastic wrap	Fine plastic disposable wrap.	To protect the therapy couch. To wrap the client in after they have had a body mask applied.

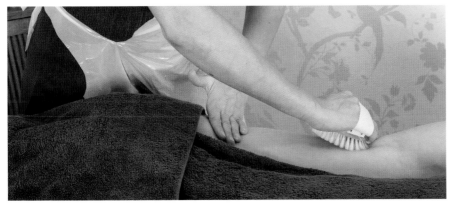

Body brushing is an ideal way to prepare the body for a body wrap

Thermostat

A device that controls temperature.

Decanting

Pouring from one container to another.

Watch the video of this body brush treatment on SmartScreen (unit 310).

INDUSTRY TIP

If you are using dry flotation as part of the treatment to help with relaxation and absorption of products, you will need to make sure that all the necessary equipment is set up – see page 509.

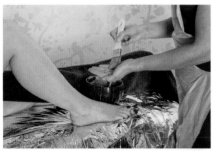

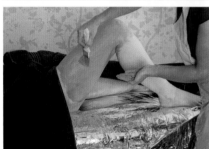

A client undergoing a body mask treatment

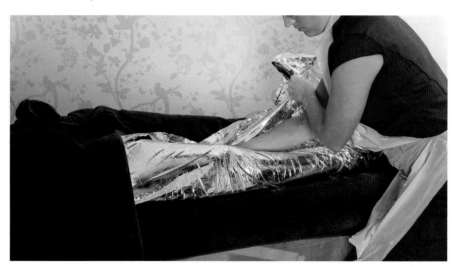

Watch the video of this body mask treatment on SmartScreen (unit 310).

HANDY HINT

There are over 20,000 different types of seaweed; most contain minerals, proteins and trace elements and are often used as nutritional supplements.

HANDY HINT

Laminara digitata is great for stimulating the lymphatic system and improving the appearance of cellulite because of its diuretic properties.

Other equipment that you may need:

- a tape measure – to measure improved skin tone on the client
- disposable paper underwear – for use by the client to avoid any damage to their own underwear
- couch roll – to protect the couch and for the client to stand on.

Body masks

During the consultation you will have agreed the client's treatment objectives. You will therefore need to select the right type of body mask to achieve these objectives.

Body masks are used to improve the appearance of the skin, improve tone and for detoxification. As with face masks, body masks can be setting or non-setting masks. You should be able to remove the mask from the client while they are on the therapy couch by using hot towels or mitts. However, it is better to have a shower cubicle so that the client can remove the product thoroughly. This method of removal is less messy and the shower cubicle can be cleaned easily to remove all traces of the product.

A client being covered in a foil blanket

The main types of body mask are:

- Mud masks – these are made of mud and clay from the sea bed. They are rich in active minerals and are used to detoxify, firm and cleanse the skin. Their smell is sometimes unpleasant so they may have essential oils added to make them smell better.
- Algae/seaweed masks – this type of mask contains a rich source of trace elements, minerals and salts. A variety of seaweeds are used:
  - fucus vesiculosus – detoxifies, firms, tones and hydrates
  - laminaria digitata – high in iodine with diuretic properties
  - ascophyllum nodosum – balancing and relaxing
  - spirulina – firms, antioxidant and anti-inflammatory.

■ Milk masks – these are rich in vitamins. Milk masks contain milk whey which contains calcium, magnesium, potassium and sodium. They are used to improve dry, sensitive skin and various skin conditions.

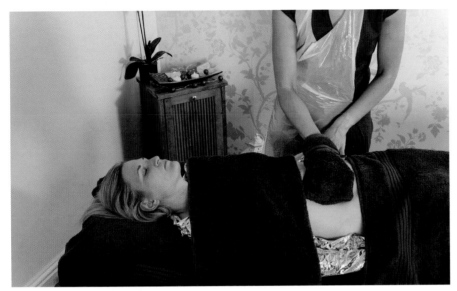

Using mitts to remove body products

Body contouring/slimming wraps

The aim of body contouring/slimming wraps is to help the client lose inches by improving muscle tone and aiding detoxification. These can be applied as a standalone treatment or can also be applied after the client has used the spa facilities. There are two main types of wrap:

■ Cryowraps – these are cold wraps. A cold wrap treatment reduces excess fluid in the hips, thighs and legs and improves the appearance of cellulite. The coldness of the wrap stimulates the circulation so this is an ideal treatment for someone who is just starting out on a weight-loss programme.

■ Thermal wraps – these are self-heating. The heat encourages perspiration which assists with the removal of waste products and toxins from the body.

Effects and benefits of a body wrap treatment

Specific benefits and effects of a body wrap will depend on the products that are used.

The effects and benefits of a body wrap treatment include:

■ removal of excess fluid

■ inch loss/improved skin/muscle tone

■ assists removal of waste toxins

■ fat dispersal

■ improved skin condition

■ improved circulation.

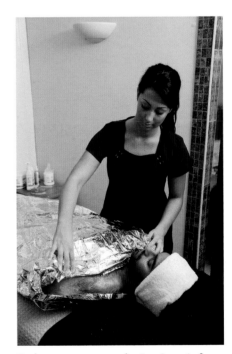

Body wraps are popular treatments for male clients

INDUSTRY TIP

Some spas use grape extract, coconut, herbs, flowers, hay and even peat in their body wrap treatments. Grape extract stimulates the circulation and improves the lymph system. Coconut is good for cleansing and moisturising. Flowers add a nice fragrance and hay and peat cleanse the skin and help to regenerate it.

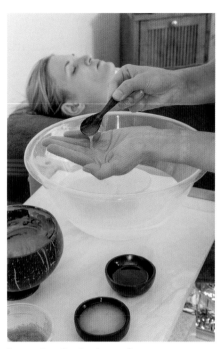

Preparing the body mask

Application of a body mask

- Carry out a consultation and agree the treatment objectives with the client.

- Prepare the treatment area. Make sure that a heated blanket and plastic or foil sheets are placed on the therapy couch and that all the necessary products are on the trolley.

- Mix the body mask in a bowl using warm water and a spatula. Make sure you follow the manufacturer's instructions.

- Ask the client to lie face up on the couch and cover them with blankets for warmth.

- If you are using an exfoliation or body brushing treatment, apply it at this point.

- Apply the mask using either a soft brush or your hands. Ask the client to lie on their side so you can apply it to their back. Then apply the mask to the front of the body.

- Work quickly to keep the product warm and avoid the client getting too cold.

- Wrap the plastic or foil blanket around the client and place a heated blanket placed over the top. This traps the heat next to the skin and improves the circulation. If you are using dry flotation, you do not need to place the heat blanket on the client as the warmth from the dry flotation will help to maintain the body temperature.

- Let the client relax for 15–20 minutes depending upon the manufacturer's instructions. Then either remove the product using hot towels/mitts or take the client to the shower to remove the body mask. Depending on the type of mask used, moisturiser or cream can be applied at this stage of the treatment.

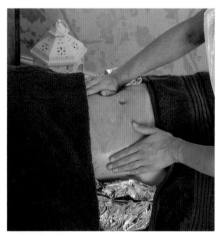

Applying the body mask

HANDY HINT

Increasing the body's temperature affects hydration levels. Make sure that the client has a good supply of water during the treatments.

INDUSTRY TIP

A head or foot massage can be given at this part of the treatment if appropriate.

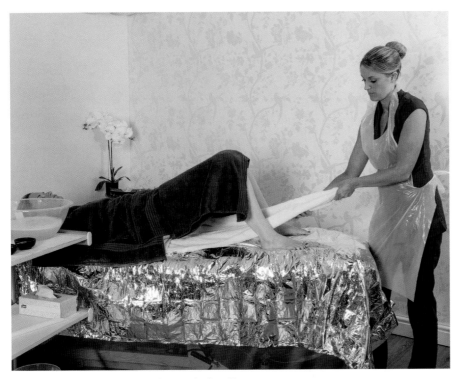

Removing the towel from underneath the client

- Remove the towels from underneath the client
- Once the client has removed the body mask, give them five minutes to relax before providing home-care advice and recommendations.
- Give the client a glass of water for rehydration and take them back to the reception area. Ask them if they would like to rebook and show them any retail products that you have recommended.

Application of slimming wraps

The following routine can be used when carrying out a slimming wrap treatment on a client.

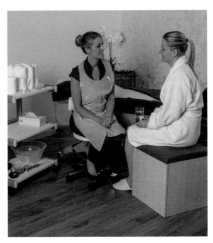

Client advice and recommendations

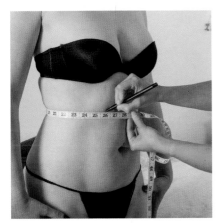

STEP 1 Measure the client before the treatment so you can give them details of its effects afterwards.

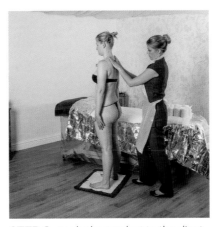

STEP 2 Apply the product to the client.

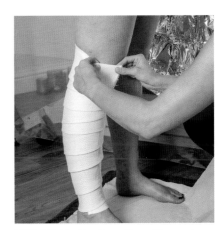

STEP 3 Starting from the ankle, apply the slimming wrap bandages to the client's leg making sure that they are snug but not too tight. Apply to both legs.

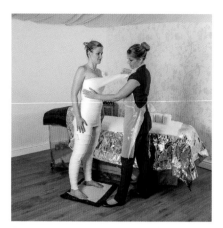

STEP 4 Apply the bandages to the client's waist. Make sure that you overlap the bandages so there are no gaps.

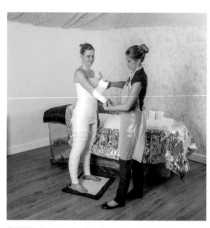

STEP 5 Apply the bandages to the client's abdomen.

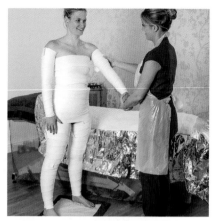

STEP 6 Starting at the wrist, apply the slimming wrap bandages to one arm and then apply the bandage to the other arm.

Watch the video of this body wrap treatment on SmartScreen (unit 310).

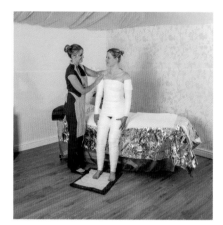

STEP 7 Apply the bandage to the client's bust area. You will have to ask the client to raise their arms.

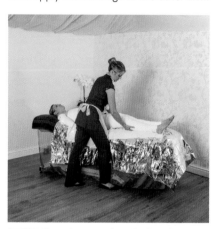

STEP 8 Make sure that the bandages are secure before you commence the treatment.

INDUSTRY TIP

Wraps may be combined with other treatments (eg a facial or a manicure). Remember to offer these additional treatments to the client.

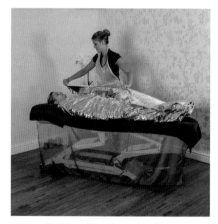

STEP 9 Allow the client to relax on the dry flotation bed or couch and apply the towels and foil blanket.

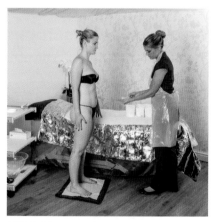

STEP 10 Once the treatment has finished, allow the client to shower if they are required to do so. Remember to measure them again and provide details of the inches they have lost on their body as a result of the treatment.

Activity

Make a list of everything you could do as a spa therapist to make sure a client's visit to the spa is a memorable treatment and experience.

Advice and recommendations

Following a spa treatment, you should give your client suitable advice to follow. This advice will help the client maximise the benefits of the treatment. Suggest that the client:

- drink plenty of water as this will help to flush out the toxins that have been released and rehydrate the body

- rest for at least 20 minutes following a heat treatment to allow their heart rate to return to normal

- avoid alcohol, caffeine, nicotine and drugs (unless prescribed) for 24 hours

- eat a light diet, avoiding processed foods and very spicy foods for 24 hours

- return for a programme of treatments (for all spa treatments) – a minimum of six should be recommended for them to see any real benefits

- look at their lifestyle to see if they can make any improvements

- use recommended home-care products to achieve the most effective results.

> **HANDY HINT**
>
> Make sure as a therapist you look after your own health and eat a well-balanced nutritious diet, and drink plenty of water throughout the working day to keep you hydrated.

> **HANDY HINT**
>
> Ensure you provide sufficient water, herbal teas and fruit in your spa, particularly if you offer many heat and water treatments, to keep your clients hydrated.

> **HANDY HINT**
>
> Make sure you maximise on retail opportunities by giving the client a prescription that gives details of the products that suit their individual home-care needs.

Client advice and recommendations

Watch a video of spa treatment advice and recommendations on SmartScreen (unit 310).

Contra-actions

A contra-action is an adverse reaction that can happen during after a treatment. The table below lists some contra-actions that might occur and the actions to take if any occur.

Contra-action	Cause	Action to be taken
Dehydration (causing fainting, sickness, dizziness and breathing difficulties)	Overheating causing excessive sweating and loss of body salts.	Client should rest and lie down. Drink plenty of water. Apply a cool compress to the forehead.
Cramps	Overheating causing excessive perspiration and loss of body salts.	Client should drink plenty of water. Stretch muscles.
Heat exhaustion (causing dizziness, sickness, headaches and fainting)	Loss of fluids. Loss of salts.	Client should rest and lie down. Drink plenty of water or fluids containing salts and minerals (eg sports drinks) to replace lost salts. Apply a cool compress to the forehead.
Severe erythema (including irritation and swelling)	Allergy to a product. Over-stimulation of the circulatory system due to heat.	Suggest that client takes a cool shower to remove products and lower the skin temperature. If irritation continues for more than 24 hours, client should seek medical advice.
Respiratory disorder (eg asthma attack)	Dry heat can affect the airways and cause an asthma attack.	Get the client to take their medication. If they are panicking, ask them to focus on controlling their breathing. If severe, seek medical advice.
Burning/scalding	Client didn't remove metal jewellery before treatment. Client has touched a heating source. Client has sat in front of the steam inlet in the steam room.	Apply cold water to burns. Cover burns with a dry dressing. If no dressing is immediately available, a sterile plastic wrap will protect the area from infection. If severe, seek medical help.

Answers at the back of the book.

1 A Palintest® is used to check:

  a For product allergies

  b The temperature of the spa pool

  c The pH balance of the spa water

  d The humidity of the steam room

2 What is a caldarium?

  a Sauna

  b Spa pool

  c Body wrap

  d Steam room

3 Why is milk added to a hydrotherapy bath?

  a To detoxify

  b To soothe and nourish

  c To stimulate the circulation

  d To stimulate lymphatic drainage

4 What is erythema?

  a Redness of the skin

  b Severe swelling

  c A severe headache

  d Sweating/perspiration

5 Which one of the following is a contra-action to spa treatments?

  a Increased pulse rate

  b Increased perspiration

  c Fainting

  d Ingrown hairs

6 What was the name of the monk who believed that disease could be cured by using water to get rid of waste from the body?

  a Kneipp

  b Algae

  c Hammam

  d Galen

7 What does 'hydro' mean?

  a Hot

  b Cold

  c Water

  d Temperature

8 Which one of the following is a specific effect of a seaweed body wrap?

  a Detoxifying

  b Moisturising

  c Desquamation

  d Nourishment

9 What should the temperature of a Finnish sauna be?

  a 70–100°C

  b 60–80°C

  c 45–60°C

  d 40–45°C

10 Which one of the following treatments can a client have if they are pregnant?

  a Sauna

  b Rasul

  c Flotation

  d Seaweed wrap

11 What does PPE stand for?

  a Protective personal equipment

  b Positive personal energy

  c Personal protective equipment

  d Personal publication equipment

12 A dry flotation treatment should last:

  a 10–15 minutes

  b 15–20 minutes

  c 10–20 minutes

  d 30–40 minutes

13 What is a laconium?

a Sauna

b Spa pool

c Body wrap

d Steam room

14 If you are claustrophobic, you have a fear of:

a Heights

b Other people

c Enclosed spaces

d Spiders

15 Cold treatments can:

a Increase blood pressure

b Soothe sensory nerve endings

c Decrease blood supply

d Lower blood pressure

16 Bromine is a chemical used to:

a Sterilise equipment

b Disinfect pools

c Measure the pH balance

d Reduce limescale on equipment

17 Oedema is a condition where:

a The immune system is boosted

b Metabolism is stimulated

c Excess fluid collects in tissues of the body

d Lymph circulation is increased

18 The water temperature in a wet flotation tank should be:

a 34–36°C

b 60–80°C

c 45–60°C

d 40–45°C

19 Adipose tissue is commonly referred to as:

a Fluid retention

b Excess fat

c Cellulite

d Poor posture

20 Spirulina is a form of:

a Salt

b Mud

c Milk

d Seaweed

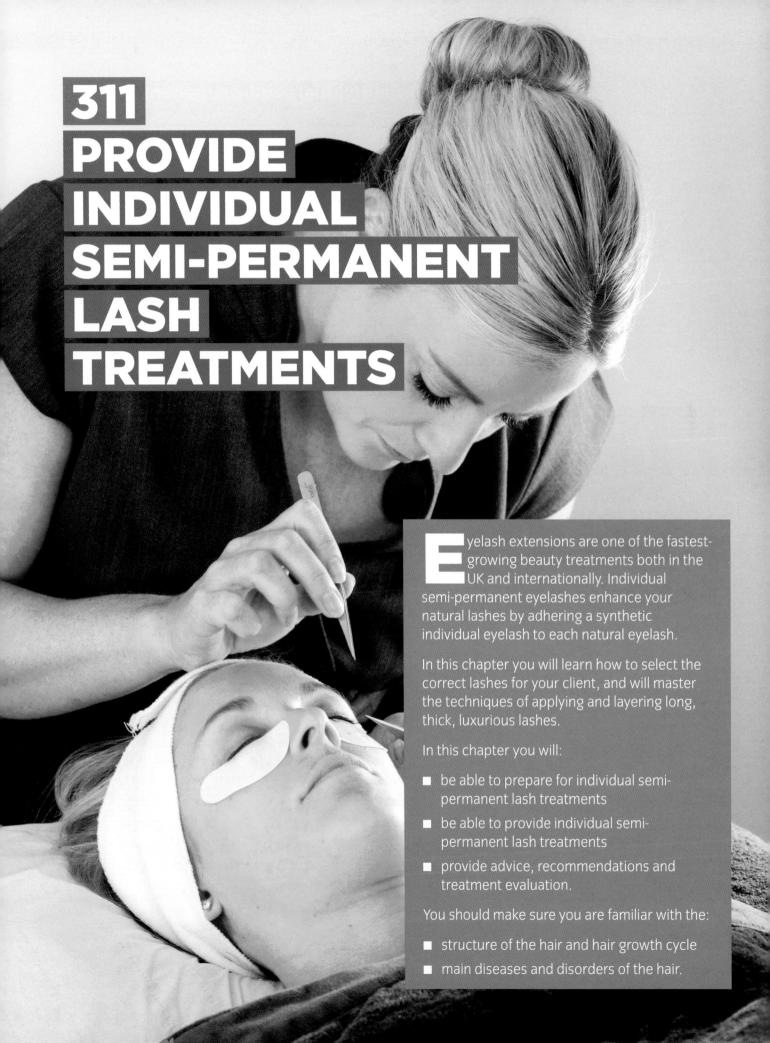

311 PROVIDE INDIVIDUAL SEMI-PERMANENT LASH TREATMENTS

Eyelash extensions are one of the fastest-growing beauty treatments both in the UK and internationally. Individual semi-permanent eyelashes enhance your natural lashes by adhering a synthetic individual eyelash to each natural eyelash.

In this chapter you will learn how to select the correct lashes for your client, and will master the techniques of applying and layering long, thick, luxurious lashes.

In this chapter you will:

■ be able to prepare for individual semi-permanent lash treatments

■ be able to provide individual semi-permanent lash treatments

■ provide advice, recommendations and treatment evaluation.

You should make sure you are familiar with the:

■ structure of the hair and hair growth cycle

■ main diseases and disorders of the hair.

Prepare for individual semi-permanent lash treatment

Semi-permanent lashes, also known as eyelash extensions, are lashes applied with a strong **adhesive** to bond the lash to the natural lash to give a long-lasting effect. The bond is designed to last until the lash cycle naturally sheds the lashes, and are then infilled with new lashes after a couple of weeks.

Adhesive

A sticky substance, eg glue.

Semi-permanent lashes are available in various lengths, colours and thicknesses so they can be tailored to the client's preference.

Factors that will affect the eyelash treatment

The following should be considered when completing your consultation, as these could alter the treatment.

Client's age

Most people opt for individual lashes to produce a bold and dramatic effect. As you get older the thickness and quantity of lashes change. This must be taken into account when choosing lashes. Use lashes to enhance the client's appearance.

Client's natural lash

When consulting with your client, you need to look at the length, thickness and curvature of their natural lashes. When choosing to apply the single lash you should select one that will complement their natural lash – if you do not, the appearance and **durability** may suffer.

Durability

How long-lasting something is.

Eyelash colour

Choose a lash that will complement the client's hair colour. You may recommend an eyelash tint on the natural lash prior to wearing single lashes to give them more definition. As the lashes are only applied to the top lashes, the tint will enhance the bottom lashes.

Skin colour

Select lashes that will complement the skin tone and be sure to question your client during the consultation on what colour foundation and also mascara they normally wear.

Natural eye shape

This must be considered when selecting the lashes and also for applying lashes, as you could use corrective techniques for various eye shapes.

Eye shape	Correction technique
Small eyes	Use longer lashes in the middle and medium towards the outside of the eye.
Close-set eyes	Use shorter lashes on the inside of the eye and a variety of medium and longer lashes in the middle and towards the outside
Wide-set eyes	Use longer lashes in the centre and medium towards the inner eye and a mixture of short and medium towards the outer corners

Preparation of the therapist

For this treatment you will be working in close proximity to the client, so personal hygiene is very important. You must make sure that your uniform is clean, your breath is fresh, any long hair is secured away from the face and your nails and hands are clean. For more about your own presentation, see the Values and behaviours chapter.

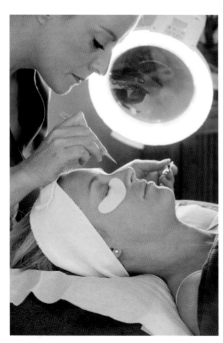 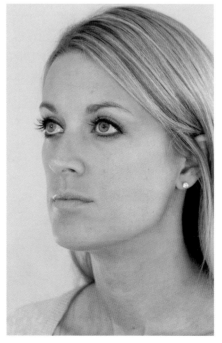

A client before and after an individual semi-permanent lash treatment

Preparation of the client

The application of semi-permanent lashes can take up to two hours and the client will be in a semi-reclined position during the treatment. It is very important to make sure the client is comfortable at all times and that they are positioned at the correct height for you to work on them without straining your back. Apply a hairband to your client to ensure that their hair is away from their face so you can clearly see their eyes.

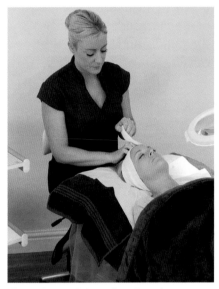

Therapist applying a headband

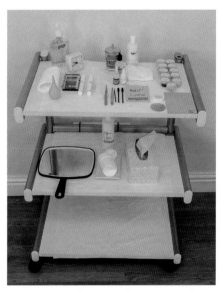

Trolley layout for a semi-permanent lash treatment

Preparation of the treatment area

■ Suitable lighting is very important while performing lash treatments. A clear view is required throughout to ensure that the chosen product is applied in a correct, safe and effective manner. You can wear a magnifying head lamp or use a free-standing magnifying lamp if you would like to.

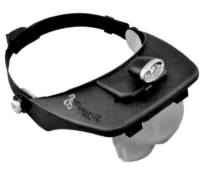

Head magnifying lamp

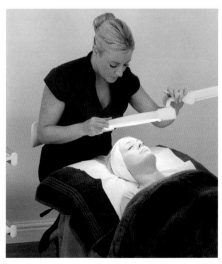

Therapist using a magnifying lamp

THE CITY & GUILDS TEXTBOOK

- The treatment room needs to be at an appropriate temperature, so that both you and the client are comfortable.

- The room needs to be warm enough for the client to feel comfortable throughout their treatment, but if it is too hot this may cause them to perspire and could affect the consistency of the products.

- If music is playing it should be at a noise level acceptable to all and appropriate for both young and mature clients.

- Privacy is a very important aspect of ensuring that the client feels comfortable throughout their treatment. Make sure that the treatment room door is closed and remember never to leave your client on their own in the treatment room.

- All tools should be sterilised using the most suitable means. Use an autoclave for small metal tools such as tweezers.

- The therapy couch or chair must be disinfected before and after use, and can be protected for the duration of the treatment by placing disposable couch roll on it.

- Use a tiered trolley to place products and tools on. It needs to have wheels so that you can move it around and position it next to you to allow for easy access to the products/tools you will need during the treatment. It should be made of a material which is easily cleaned.

- You may need to place a bolster under your client's knees as they will be lying down for some time and provide a blanket to keep them warm.

> **INDUSTRY TIP**
>
> As you lie down the blood pressure drops, causing the body to cool down, so make sure you have a blanket to cover your client, should they feel cold.

The consultation

The consultation is very important, as it is necessary to find out what type of look the client wishes to have before the application, whether they want to appear natural, somewhat enhanced or achieve a dramatic effect. A portfolio of before and after pictures is an ideal way to show the client the effects they could achieve. Allow the client plenty of opportunity to ask questions and be confident with your answers. The desired length of the lashes should be discussed, but do explain that it is not possible to select the exact length of lashes until after the consultation and you have looked at the natural lashes.

During the consultation you should also check that the client has had a patch test to ensure that they are not allergic to any of the products used during eye treatments. The patch test should include testing for adhesive, micropore tape, eye patches and solvent. Each test must be carried out in accordance with the manufacturer's instructions for the product, including the procedure and timings, eg 24 hours prior to the treatment. Record the results of the patch test on the client record card. Interpreting the results is important; they will be either a positive or a negative reaction to the products.

 Watch a video of a lash treatment consultation on SmartScreen (unit 311).

✔ Positive test result – the skin will appear irritated and inflamed, and swelling may occur. Ask your client to seek medical advice and do not continue with the treatment.

✗ Negative test result – the skin will appear normal with no reaction. If this is the case you can continue with the treatment.

Information to record before, during and after the treatment:

- the client's name, contact details and date of birth
- the date of the treatment
- the occasion (eg wedding)
- type of lashes required (eg natural, enhanced or dramatic)
- type of adhesive used
- lash length and thickness used
- lash colour used
- approximate quantity used
- any reactions (eg nervous client, client kept opening their eyes)
- contra-indications or contra-actions
- the cost of the treatment
- advice and recommendations, detailing when the client needs to return for maintenance/infills
- the client's signature and yours – before the lash treatment.

> **Activity**
>
> Create a list of frequently asked questions and answers. Ask friends, family and colleagues what they would like to know before and after having the treatment to get ideas.

If during the consultation you find that the client cannot wear semi-permanent lashes, you can offer one of the alternative treatments below.

- Perming – this treatment takes about an hour to carry out and gives a curl to the natural lash. Unlike when using lash curlers, the curl is permanent until the lashes finish the growth cycle and are lost.
- Eyelash and eyebrow tinting – this is the application of a dye to the natural lashes and eyebrows in order to add definition. Changing their colour gives the illusion of thicker, fuller lashes.
- False flare lash extensions – these are a small cluster of around five synthetic lashes, which can be applied to the client's natural lash. They are heavier and less natural looking than semi-permanent lashes, and do not require a medical-grade glue, resulting in a much shorter duration of wear.

INDUSTRY TIP

Ask the client's permission to take before and after photos of the treatment, and use them to build a portfolio. This will be helpful to show other clients your standard of work and the variety of lashes that they can choose from.

INDUSTRY TIP

Very fair-haired clients will benefit from a lash tint in advance of the individual lash application.

HEALTH & SAFETY

Always ensure you get a signature from the client before commencing a treatment. This signature represents the client's agreement to the procedures you have discussed with them. Should there be any legal dispute as a result of the treatment, the client's signature provides evidence of their **compliance**.

Compliance

Willingness to go along with a set plan.

■ Strip lashes – these come in pairs and are applied to the edge of the eyelid. They are available in a variety of lengths, styles and thicknesses, and give a dramatic effect. They should be removed each night with care, and can be reused.

Contra-indications

During the consultation, you need to establish whether there are any contra-indications which will prevent or restrict treatment. It is important to remember that only a medical professional can give a diagnosis. You should advise the client to get anything that appears to be a contra-indication checked by their GP.

As this treatment concerns the eye area, most contra-indications will relate to the eyes.

Contra-indication – preventing treatment	Description
Conjunctivitis 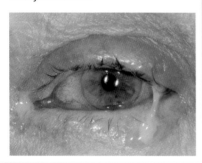	An inflammation of the membrane covering the eye. The eyes may be itchy and red, and pus may be present.
Dry-eye syndrome 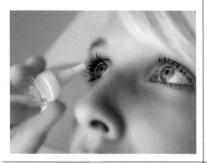	The eyes feel dry and the client will need to apply eye drops every hour or so. Lashes may irritate and the eye drops may dissolve the adhesive bond on the artificial lashes.
Eye infections 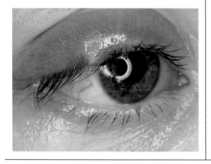	The eyes feel dry and the client will need to apply eye drops every hour or so. Lashes may irritate and the eye drops may dissolve the adhesive bond on the artificial lashes.

Contra-indication – preventing treatment	Description
Alopecia 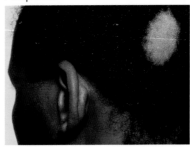	This is hair loss which can be triggered at any time, so each semi-permanent application must be assessed separately. It may be that there are no hairs present to attach lashes to, or the application may trigger alopecia, resulting in the lashes (natural and artificial) falling out.
Severe skin disease/disorders 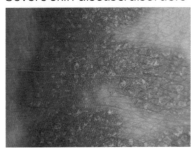	These include psoriasis, eczema and dermatitis. Depending on their severity, the treatment may cause further irritation to occur.
Trichotillomania 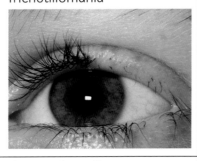	This is a condition where a client pulls their own hair out, from the head, eyebrows and/or lashes. The client may cause further damage by pulling the lash extensions out.
Skin/product allergies 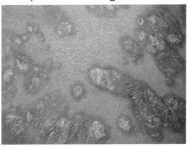	The client should not react to the adhesive, as it does not come into contact with their skin; however the gel pads, micropore tape or the gloves the therapist is wearing may cause an allergic reaction. Check for allergies during the consultation.
During chemotherapy 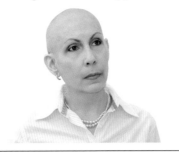	This may result in hair loss including the lashes. Even when lashes remain, application should be avoided as the extensions will put further pressure on the already weakened roots.

The following contra-indications should also be taken into consideration, with the treatment either not being carried out, or restricted and modified as necessary:

- fungal, bacterial and viral infections
- during radiotherapy
- cuts and abrasions in the area
- infestations
- epilepsy
- diabetes
- high/low blood pressure
- undiagnosed lumps and swellings.

Products and equipment

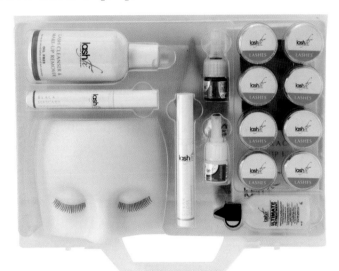

A professional semi-permanent lash kit

Products

A selection of products is required to carry out this treatment to a professional standard.

Product	Use
Non-oily eye make-up remover	To cleanse the eye area without leaving an oily barrier.

Product	Use
Adhesive	A professional adhesive which is suitable for use around the eyes. It is incredibly strong, so care must be taken during application. Do not apply too much, otherwise the client's eyes may stick together.
Anti-wrinkle gel patches	Placed over the lower lashes during treatment to protect the under-eye area and also to prevent the upper and lower lashes sticking together during the treatment.
Adhesive remover	Used for the removal of excess adhesive or for lashes that have been positioned incorrectly and need to be removed and reapplied.
Sterile eye wash	To flush out the eye if anything enters it.
Professional sealer	Helps to seal the lashes and prolong their life.

Lashes	Effects
J curl	Natural lash curl
C curl	Enhanced curve
D curl	Dramatic curl
Rainbow lashes Designed lashes	Lashes come in a variety of colours and effects to create a fun look, give instant glamour or add impact for a special occasion. Gem lashes and feather lashes are other varieties that can be used.
Y-type lashes	These offer a speedier application time and fewer are needed – however, they do not always look quite as natural, and are really only suitable for naturally thick lashes due to their weight.
Different diameters This is a W-lash which comes in sizes of 10, 11 and 12mm	Most lash companies will supply lashes of all lengths in different **diameters**. The diameter will affect the end result – the thickest lashes should be reserved for the most dramatic effect on naturally strong lashes.

Diameter

The distance across the lashes.

Activity

Practise separating lashes on a strip lash using tweezers and a magnifier so you feel confident when working with the natural lash and can improve your technique. This is quite tricky and needs lots of practice.

HANDY HINT

Many people confuse 'practice' and 'practise'. 'Practice' is a noun while 'practise' is a verb. Here are some examples:

I practise my spellings

My spellings have improved with practice.

Equipment

You will need the following general equipment for this treatment:

- cotton wool
- pillow
- magnifying lamp
- mirror
- headband
- scissors.

The specialist equipment needed to perform the treatment is detailed in the following table.

Equipment	Use
Adhesive cup 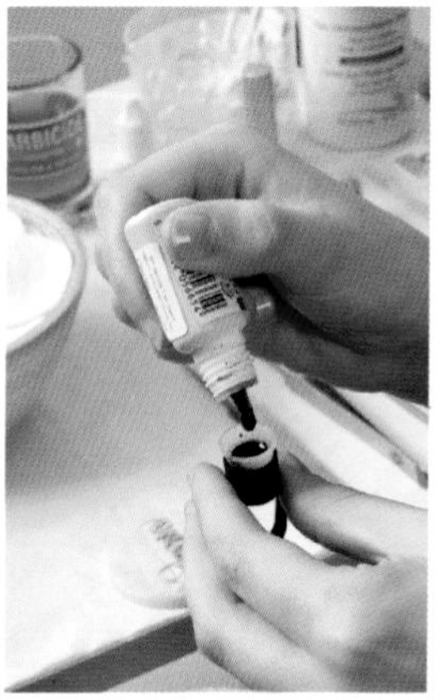	A small cup that holds a small amount of adhesive to prevent it drying out before it can be used.
Cup ring 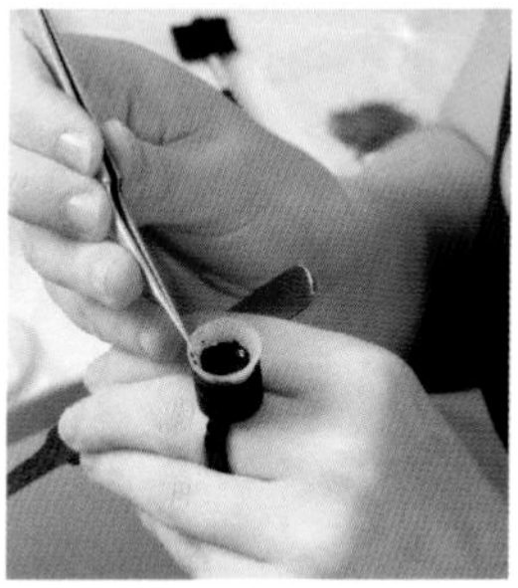	A small ring which is placed on the fingers or thumb – the adhesive cup sits in it.
Adhesive stone	A flat, smooth stone on which the adhesive can be placed as an alternative to an adhesive cup and ring. Usually made of jade, it helps to keep the adhesive cool during application of lashes.

Equipment	Use
Disposable eyelash combs	Used to comb through the lashes before, during and after the treatment.
Micropore tape	If the lashes are not already on pre-taped strips, they will need to be taken out of their container and placed on the micropore tape to enable the correct lash to be chosen for quick application. Micropore tape can also be used to hold back the upper layers of lashes to enable a layering effect.
Eyelash blower	A small rubber blower which is squeezed over the eyelashes to help the adhesive dry.
Tweezers	Needlepoint tweezers are required to separate the lashes, and for the application of the lash.
Barbicide	Barbicide is a translucent blue disinfectant solution used to clean metal tools.

Provide individual semi-permanent lash treatments

Apply lashes

Watch the video of this lash application treatment on SmartScreen (unit 311).

Once the consultation has taken place and you, the treatment area and the client are prepared, lash application can begin. You will be applying approximately 50 lashes per eye so it is important to allow plenty of time for the application. Each brand of lashes will have its own routine for you to follow, which will help you to apply the lashes safely and achieve a great look for your client. However, here is a general description of the techniques required for applying lashes.

Position the client comfortably with support cushions where necessary (bear in mind the two-hour treatment time) and sanitise your hands.

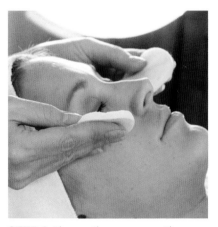

STEP 1 Cleanse the eye area with a recommended eye make-up remover.

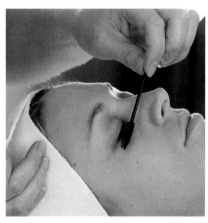

STEP 2 Comb through the lashes and separate using a disposable brush/comb.

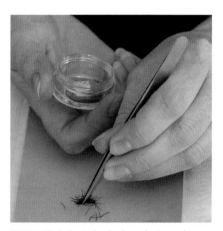

STEP 3 Select the lashes that you have discussed from the consultation.

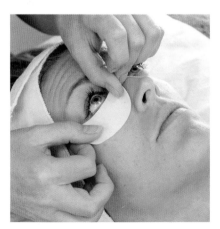

STEP 4 Apply a gel pad or micropore tape to hold the bottom lashes down.

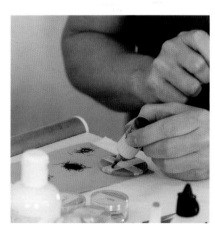

STEP 5 Apply micropore tape to the jade stone and place a pea-sized amount of glue onto the tape.

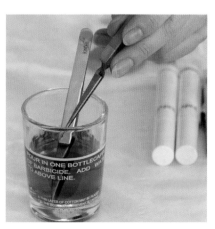

STEP 6 Remove the tweezers from the Barbicide.

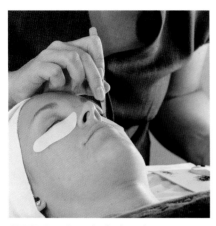

STEP 7 Select the lashes that you are going to use.

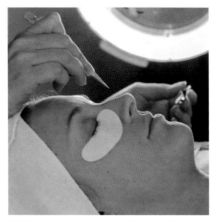

STEP 8 Commence application by isolating a natural lash, holding the tweezers at a 45° angle in your non-working hand.

INDUSTRY TIP

As a guide, the semi-permanent lashes should be no less than one-third longer than and no more than half as long again as the length of the natural lash. If the lash is too long, it will put too much weight on the natural lash, which may cause it to fall out or drop the lashes down.

HANDY HINT

Cover the surface of the isolated hair with adhesive by stroking the glue from the single lash extension along it (avoid contact with the skin of the eyelid).

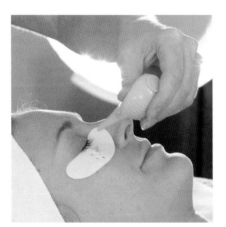

STEP 9 Use a blower to dry the glue.

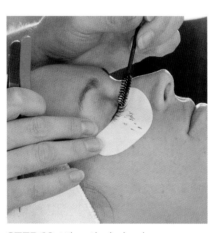

STEP 10 When the lashes have bonded, comb the lashes through to separate, avoiding the root.

HANDY HINT

Work from eye to eye to allow the adhesive to dry; this also allows you to position the lashes in the same places on both eyes.

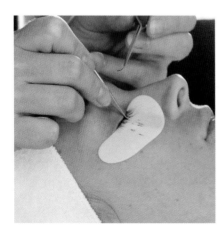

STEP 11 Continue applying lashes across both eyes until they are full. Lashes should be positioned at spaced intervals along the lash line in order to achieve a balanced look and avoid adjacent lashes sticking together during application.

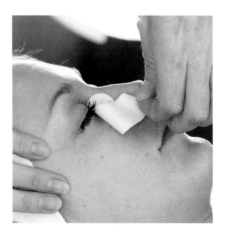

STEP 12 Remove the gel pad/micropore tape.

INDUSTRY TIP

Once you've applied a lash, and before the adhesive is fully set, check the positioning to make sure the lash is pointing in the same direction as the natural lash. If there is any excess adhesive it can be removed at this stage using a disposable micro-brush. Do not brush along the lash, as this may remove it if the adhesive is not dry.

INDUSTRY TIP

If you are right-handed, apply the lashes to the back of your left hand, position the adhesive pot on your left thumb and also use this hand with the tweezers to isolate the natural lash. Use your right hand to dip the lash into the adhesive and then apply it. If you are left-handed, reverse the method.

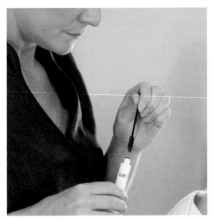

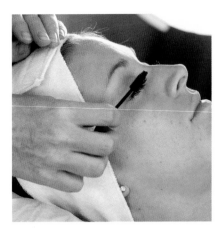

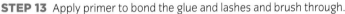

STEP 13 Apply primer to bond the glue and lashes and brush through.

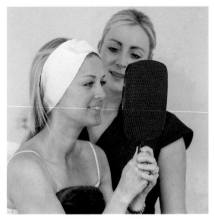

STEP 14 Show your client the end result with a mirror.

Lashes can be layered to create a fuller effect. Use micropore tape to hold back the uppermost lashes. This is then repeated with the next layer of lashes. The individual lashes are then applied to those natural lashes closest to the inner upper lid. The layers of micropore tape are removed in reverse order, and extensions applied to the released lashes. When isolating lashes, they are selected from the different natural layers.

Adapting the lashes to suit the client's facial characteristics

Looking at the different types of natural lashes below will help you decide what type of lash to apply.

Naturally curly lashes

These will require a shorter lash extension, as a maximum bonding area is recommended. Use 'C' lashes.

Strong, healthy lashes

These can take extra-thick lash extensions if desired, which should only be applied to strong, healthy lashes that are naturally thick, so that they can carry the weight.

Deep-set eyes

Use slightly longer lashes so the extra length makes the eyes more noticeable. However, they should not be so long that they irritate the upper eye area if the eyes are very deep-set. Choosing the straightest lashes available will help you avoid this.

Round eyes

Lashes used on round eyes should be shorter at the inner corner and gradually extend in length toward the outer eye.

Maintenance and removal of semi-permanent lashes

To keep the lashes looking their best, the client should return every two to three weeks to have loose lashes removed and new lashes applied. You should advise the client of this during the initial consultation.

In rare cases the client may not like the feel of semi-permanent lashes, or they may simply decide they no longer wish to wear them; in this case you need to be able to remove them. It is extremely important that you tell the client not to try to remove the lashes themselves, as this may lead to the natural lashes being pulled out.

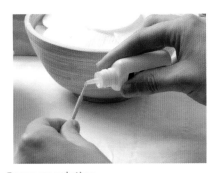

Remover solution

Removal of individual lashes

- Position the client comfortably with support cushions where necessary and sanitise your hands.
- Cleanse the eye area with a recommended eye make-up remover.
- Put a small amount of adhesive remover into an adhesive cup, then dip a micro-brush into the remover.
- Apply a gel pad or micropore tape to hold the bottom lashes down.
- Using two micro-brushes – a dry one underneath the lash and one dampened in adhesive remover on the top – stroke along the lash to be removed. This dissolves the adhesive and helps with the removal of the lash.
- When all the lashes have been removed, wipe the eye area with damp cotton wool to remove any remaining adhesive or adhesive remover. If the adhesive remover enters the eye it will become sore and the eye will need flushing out.
- Advise the client that the eye area may feel tender for a couple of hours. If any tenderness persists they should seek medical attention or return for their eyes to be flushed through with saline solution.

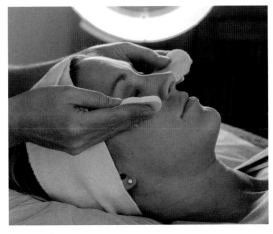

Wiping the eye

Advice and recommendations

Once the lashes have been applied, the client needs to know how to look after them to prolong their life. The client should be advised to:

- avoid getting the lashes wet for at least two hours after application
- avoid heat treatments including hot water in the area for 48 hours
- avoid oil-based products, as these may break down the adhesive bond
- avoid waterproof mascara, as it requires removal with an oil-based product
- avoid using an eyelash curler as it will loosen the lashes
- always pat the eye area dry; do not rub as this will loosen the adhesive bond
- return for maintenance appointments every two to three weeks
- not remove the lashes themselves – a special adhesive remover needs to be applied to avoid breakage of the natural lash
- seek medical attention in the event of an allergic reaction.

Watch a video of lash treatment advice and recommendations on SmartScreen (unit 311).

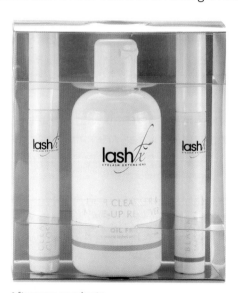

Aftercare products

You can use an oil-free make-up remover and mascara which the client will be able to purchase after the treatment. See chapter 301, Promote and sell products and services to clients, for advice on how to initiate a sale.

Contra-actions

A contra-action to this treatment will usually be a result of an allergic reaction. If this happens during the treatment, stop it immediately. The cause of the allergy needs to be found – you cannot assume that it is the lashes, as it may be the gel pads or the cleansing products used during the process. The reaction may be made worse if you try to remove the lashes. Advise the client to seek medical attention and, if possible, give them a list of ingredients and some remover to supply to the medical practitioner.

Stinging or watery eyes

These may be just natural reactions, or they may be caused by sensitivity to the adhesive. Gently blot the eyes frequently, as the tears will affect how well the lashes adhere. Adhesive for sensitive eyes is available, but usually has a weaker set. If the watering is excessive, the treatment may have to be stopped, with a careful explanation to the client. You will then need to wash out the eye using a specialised eye wash and remove the lashes if it is too severe.

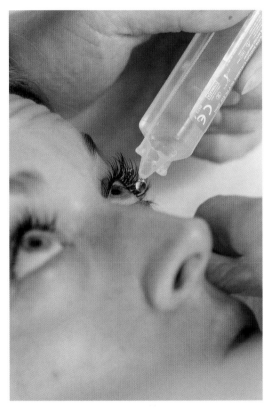

Applying an eye wash to the eye

Client feedback

When the treatment is finished it is important to gain feedback from the client to make sure they are happy with the treatment and the finished results. This can be achieved by asking the client to complete a written questionnaire, or verbally, by asking them open questions. Peer evaluation by a more senior member of staff will ensure that you gain useful feedback, including tips on what you did well and how you can improve in the future.

Answers at the back of the book.

1 What is the maximum length a semi-permanent lash can be when applied to natural lashes?

a ¼ longer

b ⅔ longer

c ½ longer

d ¾ longer

2 Following a treatment, how often should a client return to the salon for maintenance to their individual permanent lashes?

a Every two to three weeks

b Weekly

c Monthly

d Never

3 Eyelash extensions are suitable for all clients. True or false?

a True

b False

4 The J-curl permanent lash is described by which of the following?

a Dramatic

b Natural-looking

c Enhanced

d Colour coded

5 What is the approximate number of permanent lashes that are applied per eye?

a 30

b 40

c 50

d 60

6 Which one of the following would prevent a permanent eyelash treatment?

a The client wearing glasses

b Contact lenses

c Trichotillomania

d Tinted lashes

7 Before application or removal of permanent lashes, which one of the following should the lower lashes be covered with?

a Wet cotton wool

b Oil

c Micropore tape

d Dry cotton wool

8 Which one of the following is the best method of sterilising tweezers?

a An autoclave

b A UV cabinet

c Alcohol-based sanitiser

d Soap and water

9 What type of tweezers are used for the application and removal of permanent lashes?

a Automatic

b Slant-edge

c Needlepoint

d Round-tip

10 Which glue should be used to apply semi-permanent lashes?

a Flare lashes glue

b Latex glue

c Semi-permanent lash glue

d Hair extension glue

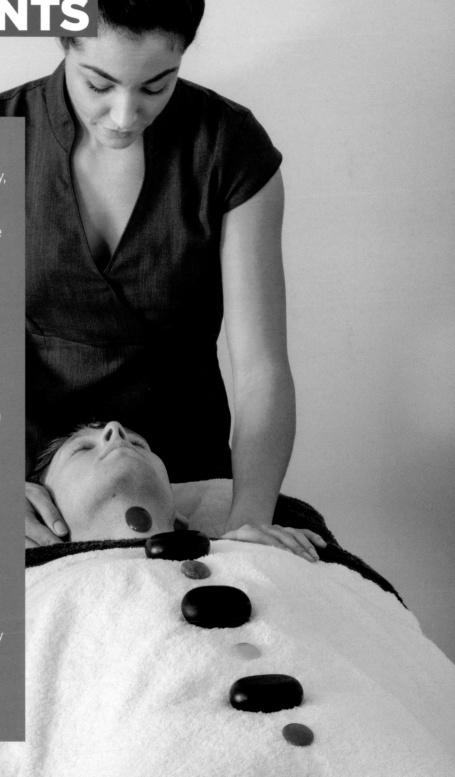

320
PROVIDE BODY STONE THERAPY TREATMENTS

The technical name for using heated or chilled stones in therapy is geothermotherapy, with 'geo' meaning from the earth and 'thermo' meaning heat. Heated and chilled stones are applied to the body (often alternately) for the purpose of healing by changing the body's physiological responses.

In this chapter you will:

■ prepare for stone therapy treatment

■ provide stone therapy treatment

■ provide advice, recommendation and treatment evaluation.

You should make sure you are familiar with:

■ the structure and function of the skin

■ the structure, function, position and action of the muscles of the body

■ the location, function and structure of the bones of the body

■ the location, function and structure of the circulatory and lymphatic systems

■ the function of the renal system.

The philosophy of stone therapy

Stone therapy has been around in one form or another for more than 2000 years: in saunas, for warming baths, for relieving pain and even for warming beds before hot water bottles and electric blankets were invented. At one time, fasting Japanese priests would place hot stones along their abdomens to slow down digestion. Warm stones have also been used during labour to give comfort and relieve pain. Acupuncturists in ancient Japan and China used pointed stones to stimulate meridians before the advent of needles. Even the ancient Egyptians used stones for healing.

We tend to associate modern geothermotherapy with Native American healing rituals. American Mary Nelson is credited with the modern development of this popular treatment, called LaStone. Pat Mayrhofer, an American massage therapist, has, along with Mary Nelson, also been prominent in teaching the natural therapeutic value of stone therapy. Using hot and cold stones, she demonstrated the benefit to the circulation and increased speed of recovery from injury.

The popularity of stone therapy initially grew in the UK largely due to the work of Jane Scriven. Jane trained with Mary Nelson and brought LaStone and its unique philosophy to the UK market.

Stone therapy has since been simplified from the original LaStone therapy that Mary developed, and many brands now have their own version of a geothermotherapy treatment, which goes to show just how flexible it is.

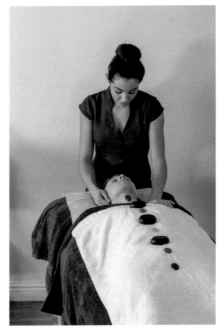

A relaxed client with stone placement

Prepare for stone therapy treatment

Preparation of the therapist

As a therapist you will be working in close proximity to your client throughout this treatment. It is very important that you are dressed and presented in a professional manner. See chapter 301, Promote and sell products and services to clients, for more information.

Before you start any treatment you should make sure you are fully prepared physically by doing the hand exercises in chapter 303, and that you are mentally focused. The client is paying for your time and attention and you should avoid any distractions.

Preparation of the treatment area

The treatment area should be fully prepared before the client arrives. You should make sure that all work surfaces have been cleaned and are tidy and organised. Any equipment that needs to be cleaned and sanitised, such as the heater and the stones, needs to be ready before you begin. Make sure that any equipment or products that you need are ready and easily accessible before you start, so that you do not have to interrupt the flow of your treatment to go and get anything.

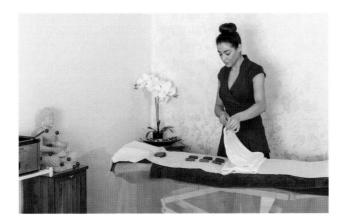

A prepared treatment area

Preparation of the treatment environment

The client needs to be comfortable during the treatment. Check and adjust the following so that the client can relax and enjoy their treatment:

- Aim for subtle lighting, with no glare in the client's eyes.
- Ask the client if they mind if you put on soft, gentle, relaxing music. Some clients may prefer to have their treatment in silence.
- Make sure the room is warm, cosy and free from draughts.

VALUES & BEHAVIOURS

Personal hygiene and protection requirements.

INDUSTRY TIP

If you are aiming to entice the male market you should make sure that the reception area is neutral and has non-gender-specific advertising. Include current magazines for your male clients as well as ladies' magazines.

VALUES & BEHAVIOURS

Effective, hygienic and safe working methods.

HANDY HINT

When choosing footwear, remember that flip-flops can be noisy, and should also be avoided for safety reasons. Work shoes should be fully enclosed and secure on the feet.

- Make sure the room has a pleasing aroma – avoid the build-up of stale odours, pay attention to personal hygiene and use of fragranced products.
- Remember to take into account the client's need for privacy.
- Avoid any unnecessary noise during your treatment – for example, when you remove the stones from the heater, do so with care.
- Make a quick check of the working area for hazards, and remove them or take steps to reduce any risks.

You also need to make sure you are working in such a way to maintain environmental and sustainable working practices.

Preparation of the client

For full details on preparing a client for a massage treatment, see chapter 303.

Consultation

A detailed consultation to establish the client's priorities and needs must take place before every treatment using appropriate professional communication techniques. Further information on the consultation process can be found in the Values and behaviours chapter. A stone therapy treatment uses both hot and cold stones, and therefore an important part of the consultation is to carry out a thermal test (see chapter 303 for information on thermal testing). You can use a hot stone and a cold stone for thermal testing. Ask the client to look away while applying the hot and cold randomly to a treatment area and then ask them to state which is hot or cold.

Contra-indications

You will need to make sure you are familiar with each of the disorders and diseases listed below. Guidance can be found in chapter 302, Anatomy and physiology, in the relevant systems of the body. The following are contra-indications that you will need to be particularly aware of when offering stone therapy treatment. You will then be able to take the necessary actions to protect the client, whether this is to refer them for further advice or restrict or adapt your treatment.

Treatment should be avoided completely in the case of the following:

- contagious skin diseases (fungal, bacterial, viral, infestations)
- severe eczema
- severe psoriasis
- severe skin conditions
- deep vein thrombosis

 Watch a video of a stone therapy consultation on SmartScreen (unit 320).

- during active cancer treatment
- during chemotherapy
- during radiotherapy
- obesity.

Treatment should be restricted in the case of the following:

- broken bones
- recent fractures and sprains
- cuts and abrasions
- recent scar tissue
- skin disorders
- skin allergies
- product allergies
- epilepsy
- uncontrolled diabetes
- high/low blood pressure
- metal pins or plates
- piercings
- pregnancy
- medications
- varicose veins
- undiagnosed lumps and swellings.

Equipment

You will need a treatment couch (with a pillow to support the client's neck), a trolley and a bin to dispose of waste. For more information on equipment, refer to chapter 303.

The heater and stones should be prepared ahead of your client's arrival. The top shelf of the trolley should be cleansed and covered with a towel to absorb any water and also to give a quiet surface to place the stones on. The trolley can then be moved as you need to gain access to the stones. Avoid moving a heavy heater on a trolley.

HEALTH & SAFETY

A contradictory reaction to the application of heat is when erythema does not colour. The body reacts as if it is chilled and the skin has a blue-white appearance. This may be a sign of arteriosclerosis (remember, you cannot offer a diagnosis) and the treatment should be stopped immediately. Advise the client to consult their GP.

HEALTH & SAFETY

If you are in doubt about carrying out the treatment, ask the client if they have been advised by their doctor to avoid hot baths, saunas or steam treatments. This will include clients with heart, lymphatic conditions and diabetes.

HANDY HINT

If there is a sink next to the work area, place a towel in it to give yourself somewhere quiet to place used stones.

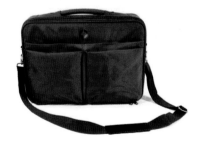

Stone heating bag

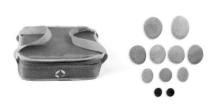

Stone cooling bag

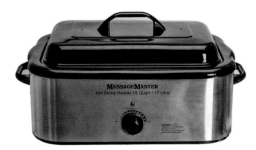

A stone heater

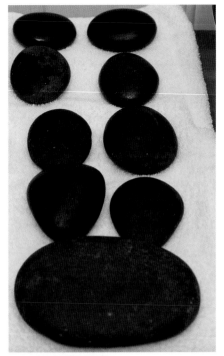

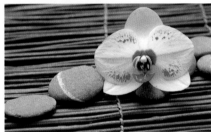

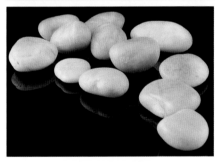

A selection of treatment stones

The stones

To perform a stone therapy treatment it is necessary to have a selection of stones. These vary in size, shape, colour and temperature.

Massage stones vary in shape – they may be round, oblong or half-moon. They also come in various sizes, from large stones which are placed on the sacrum to more delicate stones which can be placed between the fingers and toes or over the eyes. A full body treatment can use up to 55 different stones.

It is important to check stones before the treatment to see that they have no cracks or chips in them. Damaged stones can be felt by the client and may cause stretching of the skin or injury.

Hot stones

■ Basalt – these stones are made of fine-grained volcanic rock, created when the molten lava from a volcano is compressed. They are rich in iron and magnesium. Water from the sea or a river wears away the sharp edges, leaving a smooth, naturally shaped stone. Basalt stones appear darker once oil has been applied to them. They remain hot up to four times longer than other natural stones and release this heat slowly, making them ideal for hot massage. There are several different varieties of basalt stone.

Cool stones

■ Marine – as the name suggests, these stones are found in water, specifically around volcanic islands. They are rich in minerals, as they are formed from the sediment on the ocean floor. They are patterned, and are usually a grey-green colour. Marine stones are cool to touch and are therefore used for cooling an area, reducing inflammation and promoting vasoconstriction.

■ Marble – marble is an organic rock, which means it comes from living organisms. It contains calcite and limestone (forms of calcium carbonate). In its original state, marble can feel rough to touch. It is a heavy stone which is also very cool. Marble stones are expensive as they are handcrafted to make them smooth enough for massage, and to fit small contours of the face. They are used to reduce inflammation and to cool areas of the body when the skin becomes overheated. Marble can be easily scratched and needs to be looked after carefully to prevent damage.

■ Semi-precious – these are crystals or gemstones which vary in colour. They are said to have properties which enable them to open the chakras and therefore help with rebalancing the mind, body and spirit. A set of seven different stones is used for stone therapy, with each relating to one of the colours of the chakras; the correct stone is placed on the corresponding chakra point during treatment.

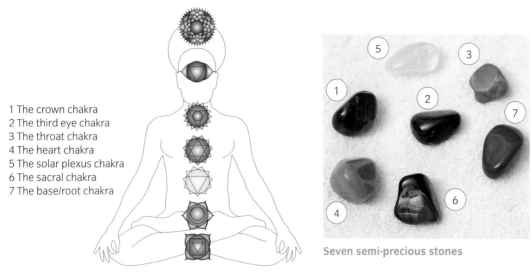

1 The crown chakra
2 The third eye chakra
3 The throat chakra
4 The heart chakra
5 The solar plexus chakra
6 The sacral chakra
7 The base/root chakra

Chakras

Seven semi-precious stones

Thermotherapy (hot stones)

Hot stones can be used for placement. If the client is lying on the stones these must always be covered with a pillow case, sheet or towel. When they are applied as part of treatment they should be subtly introduced to the body with a flowing action. Effleurage with the hands first: hold the stone, effleurage with the side of the hand and then slide in the stone.

<table>
<tr><td colspan="2">**HANDY HINT**</td></tr>
<tr><td colspan="2">Stones with high iron and magnesium content tend to stay hotter for longer.</td></tr>
</table>

Stone shape/size	Image	Hot stone uses	Cold stone uses
Toe/finger stones, small and flat in appearance, approximately the size of a 10p		Between fingers and toes.	Between fingers and toes. Can be placed over the eyes to reduce puffiness and inflammation.
Small and round, 15–50mm in size		Placement stones on face. For massaging the body, by using the full surface area or the edge.	Placement stones. Effleurage.

Stone shape/size	Image	Hot stone uses	Cold stone uses
Medium round, 60–75mm in size (palm size)		Placement stones. For massaging the hands, arms and deltoids.	Placement stones. Effleurage.
Large, thick and round, 75–100mm in size		For spinal layout. Placement stones. For massaging the larger muscle groups using the full surface area, or for deeper work using the edge only.	Placement stones. For working large muscle groups.
Oblong, pointed or trigger stone, 60–90mm in length		For deep tissue work – to apply pressure to areas of tension the pointed ends can be used, in the same way as thumbs.	Oblong: pillow stone placed behind neck. Pointed: deep tissue work.
Contour stones (pillow and hand stones), 90–130mm in size		Placement stones. For use on the soles of the feet, held in the hands or behind the neck.	
Extra-large stones (mother and father stones), too large to handle for massage, 110–130mm in size		Placement stones used on the sacrum or abdomen.	Placement stones used on the sacrum or abdomen.

Cryotherapy (cold stones)

When applying cold stones, hover the stone over the area first, then effleurage with the back of the hand before sliding or positioning the stone into place. If using a cold stone for deeper work, ask the client to take a breath in and place the stone onto the body as the client breathes out.

Activity

Activity

Find a partner and blindfold them. Carefully practise placing different hot and cold stones on them. Ask your partner to give you feedback. If you apply the stones well, it should be hard for them to tell which is hot and which is cold.

Activity

Get to know your stones. Take a set of stones and put them into groups according to their use. You will need to know exactly what they all do, and in which area of the body. Check the results with your tutor to see if you are correct.

Preparation and cleansing of the stones

After each use, the stones should be washed in hot soapy water, then placed on a clean surface or towel to air dry. Once dry they should be sprayed with a sanitising spray such as isopropyl alcohol. In the training environment the stones should be packed away to avoid damage. However the stones are stored, they need to be positioned somewhere they are not going to be moved to avoid cracks and chips.

Cleanse and re-energise the treatment stones

According to the theory behind stone therapy, stones absorb energy. They will fail to heat through and hold their heat when they have absorbed too much negative energy, and this is why it is necessary to energise them. This should be done on a regular basis depending on how often the stones are used. It is recommended that the stones are re-energised at least once a month. This does not include precious stones.

1. Wash and scrub the stones in hot soapy water.

2. Leave the treatment stones outside somewhere safe for a day in the sunlight, or for example on a sunny windowsill, to absorb the sun's energy. (Do not leave precious stones in direct sunlight, as it can make the colours fade.)

3. Place the stones outside at new moon to absorb the moon's energies; this is safe to do with all stones, including crystals.

In between treatments

- Store stones on a bed of natural sea salt, as this will draw out any impurities (with the exception of marble, as the salt may soften and split these stones).

- Hot stones can be recharged with a crystal called labradorite. Place it in the storage box with them or on top of the stones where they are on display.

- Cold stones can be recharged with moonstone.

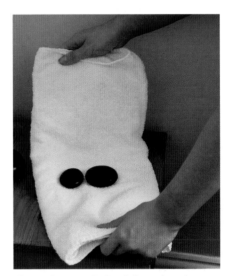

Cleaned stones being left to dry after use

HANDY HINT

When the stones are not holding their heat, it is a sign that they need energising.

INDUSTRY TIP

Thunderstorms re-energise stones, so if possible place them outside during a storm. While not very practical, returning the stones to the earth and covering them with soil is another way to re-energise them.

The heater and cooler

The heater

The water heater must be designed for the purpose of heating stones – no other device should be used, as you will not be covered by your insurance. The heater must be large enough to either hold a full set of stones for a full body treatment, or a set of back stones if carrying out a shorter treatment. You should also make sure you read the manufacturer's instructions on how to operate the heater safely. The heater should have a thermostatic control, so that the temperature of the water can be easily set, monitored and maintained. Before you turn the heater on, check for any damage to the equipment, flex or plug. Make sure the heater is placed on a stable work surface and can be accessed easily. Hot stone heaters can take up to 45 minutes to heat a full set of stones from cold.

Thermal bags are also available. These heat the stones by dry heat and are designed with the mobile therapist in mind. The bag has a washable insulated lining, which is heated through a power supply. They are considered more economical and environmentally friendly than heating a tank of water.

There are a couple of simple steps you need to take to maintain the heater ready for use.

- With the heater unplugged, wash it with hot soapy water, paying particular attention to the water-line as this is where any residue will collect.
- Place a rubber mat at the bottom of the heater to prevent any noise the stones might make by knocking together.

The cooler

This is used to store marine and marble stones to ensure that they remain cool. There are two options for cooling stones:

- They can be placed in a freezer bag and stored in the top of a fridge.
- They can be placed in a cooling container – an insulated container or a bowl or bucket filled with iced water. Alternatively, place them on freezer blocks, as these are less messy and can be reused.

Accessories

Other things you will need are:

- thermal gloves, for removing the stones from the heater – this will reduce the risk of burning or contact dermatitis
- a wooden ladle to help you lift the stones out of the heater
- net bags to place the stones in, to keep them organised in the tank

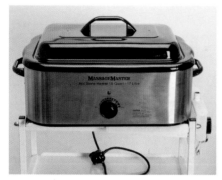

Stone heater

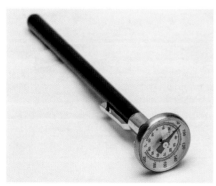

Thermostat to show temperature

- thermometer – if the heater does not have a built-in thermostat, use a waterproof thermometer to check the water temperature, which should be 47–50°C

- props (rolled towels, cushions or pillows) to support the client's limbs during treatment.

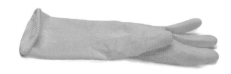
Thermal gloves

Activity

The amount of oil you use will depend on several factors including the client's skin type (texture and condition) and the size of the client. Some oils are viscous and absorb less easily, while others are less viscous and absorb more easily than others.

A typical full body massage will use about between 20–40ml of oil (as a rough guide, 10ml for the back, 5ml for the scalp and 5ml for the face).

If a bottle has 473ml, how many treatments will you get out of the bottle:

- for a back massage (using 10ml each)?

- for a body massage (using 20ml and 40 ml each)?

What percentage of the bottle will you use per treatment?

You are left with 10ml of oil at the end of your treatment, which you have to dispose of. How much profit have you just lost?

> **INDUSTRY TIP**
>
> Stones should be completely air dried before putting away in a closed storage box or bag. This is to maintain hygiene. Damp stones and a dark storage bag will harbour bacteria and odours.

Massage mediums

An oil is used during treatment to enable the stones and hands to glide across the skin. This makes the treatment more comfortable and prevents dragging of the skin and excessive friction. The medium also leaves the skin feeling soft and supple. The oil used will also help to transfer the heat across the surface of the skin by **conduction** and **convection**. Any product used should be one that is easy to clean from the stones following treatment as some oils are more water-soluble than others and to prevent a residue build up in the heater. The oil is always applied to the client rather than the stones during treatment. See chapter 303 for more about massage mediums. Essential oil blends should be avoided, as the heat will affect the blend and may also increase absorption, creating adverse contra-actions.

> **Conduction**
>
> When heat is transmitted through a material because there are differences in temperature.

> **Convection**
>
> When heat is transmitted through hotter materials rising and colder materials sinking.

Activity

Ask your tutor if you can have a selection of different oils. Use the ones you covered in your massage unit– try at least four and compare their texture and feel on the skin. Which oils did you prefer the feel of? Write down your reasons and discuss your findings with your colleagues.

> **INDUSTRY TIP**
>
> Always use a light oil – a great oil to try is jojoba. This is good for all skin types and is more water-soluble than some other oils, making it easy to remove from the stones. Avoid heavy or rich oils, as these can be difficult to remove from the stones and are more likely to stain towels and sheets.

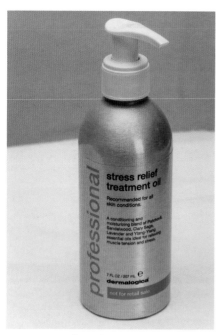

Massage medium for stone therapy

Skincare products

If the client is having their face treated, you will need cleansing products. Each company will have its own product range and training to support its use. You will find a simple cleansing routine in chapter 304.

Consumables

You will also require some consumables:

- damp cotton wool to remove cleanser and toner if required
- tissues
- couch roll to protect towels and maintain hygiene
- spatulas, to decant products hygienically.

Provide stone therapy treatment

Sensitivity testing

Before providing a stone therapy treatment, the client should have a sensitivity test. This is a safety procedure to ensure that the client is able to distinguish between different temperatures. You can use your stones to carry out this test with one small cold stone and one hot stone. Ask the client to look away and randomly introduce the stones on an area while asking the client to tell you whether the stone is hot or cold.

Physiological effects and benefits of stone therapy treatment

The physiological effects of stone therapy treatment are the same as those described in chapter 303. Stone massage is much more effective than manual massage which is why is has becomes such a popular treatment. It is stated that each massage stroke with a stone is equivalent to five to ten strokes with the hands. The stones apply pressure and compress the tissues in a different way from massage, while the heat increases and relaxes the muscles so that they can be stretched and relaxed to a much greater degree.

Using stones gives the following enhanced benefits:

Hot stones provide:

- vasodilation
- decreased blood pressure
- stimulation of digestion
- increased cellular metabolism
- relaxation of muscle spasms

- increased muscle flexibility
- softening of muscle tissue
- increased range of joint mobility
- increased activity of the parasympathetic nervous system; being more relaxed will also help to improve sleep patterns.

Cold stones provide:

- vasoconstriction
- increased blood pressure
- increased activity of the sympathetic nervous system
- reduced pain
- decreased digestive function
- reduced inflammation
- reduced cellular activity
- reduced swelling and lymph congestion
- enhance mental stimulation.

Cold stones are excellent for any type of inflammatory condition due to their vasoconstrictive effect. This in turn reduces cellular activity in the area. The cold has a numbing effect on nerve endings, reducing pain perception.

The best effects are achieved when cold stones are applied with hot stones as the two have opposite physiological effects. They create a pumping effect within the tissues as the vasoconstriction is alternated with vasodilation. This has a fantastic effect on reducing congestion, and generally stimulating the circulation.

> **INDUSTRY TIP**
>
> Make sure your hands are warm, as this will be more comfortable for the client. Warm muscles and tendons are more flexible and so this will also help to protect your hands from strain. A simple way to achieve this is to place your hands in warm water before starting.

Psychological effects and benefits of stone therapy treatment

Stone therapy has many psychological effects, similar to the physiological effects. It is fantastic for stress relief and is very relaxing. The treatment helps to calm the mind and create a sense of well-being.

Depending on the techniques used, the psychological effects of stone therapy include:

- induced state of relaxation
- reduced stress levels
- feeling of well-being
- uplifting effects.

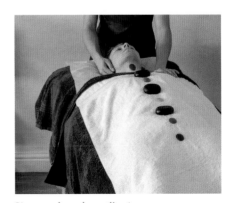

Stones placed on client

Activity

18 basalt stones cost £48.75. How much does this work out per stone?

64 basalt stones cost £79.99. How much does this cost per stone?

Assume that these prices are inclusive of VAT and you are VAT registered. As you can claim this back, you need to deduct 17.5% from these figures before your next calculation.

How many additional treatments will you need to carry out in your salon to cover the cost of a new set of stones? Each treatment has a net profit of £22.50 per hour and a stone therapy takes 75 minutes.

How much profit will you make in 15 minutes?

How much profit in 75 minutes?

You add a set of 14 marble stones at £35.99. How much do these work out per stone and how many additional treatments will you need to do to cover this cost?

Which is the most cost-effective type of stone?

Activity

You over-measure your oil by 15ml. The bottle contains 130ml and costs £4.39. What percentage have you just wasted and how much have you lost in profit?

Calculate how much you would lose if you over-measured for 12 treatments.

Massage techniques

The techniques you use to apply the stones and your choice of hot or cold stones will enable you to achieve your client's treatment objectives. Most treatments combine hot and cold stones, and with correct technique and placement the client should not easily be able to tell the difference between the two.

The use of stones is not only beneficial to the client, but also to the therapist. You do not need to apply as much pressure as in a conventional massage, thereby preventing wear and tear to the joints and reducing the risk of repetitive strain injury. The philosophy of less is more is very true in this case: one stroke with a stone is equal to five to ten strokes with a hand.

In chapter 303 you were introduced to the main massage techniques. You should familiarise yourself with these before studying the new techniques you will also use for stone therapy.

Piezoelectric

Rhythmic tapping of two stones to create a sound wave of vibration both across the skin and deep into the muscle tissues.

Technique	Use with hot stones?	Use with cold stones?	Application
Effleurage	Yes	Yes	Apply the massage medium with your hands to the client using slow effleurage. This will allow the client to become accustomed to your touch. Never just place the stones onto the body and start to massage with them. The stones should be introduced to the body in a subtle way. Hold the stone in your hand with the palm upwards. Slide the back of the hand onto the body and start to stroke, then slowly turn the hand over to introduce the edge of the stone. Check the heat before applying the flat surface onto the skin, and keep the stone moving.
Petrissage	Yes	Yes	The stones are introduced to the body with an effleurage. Once contact is established, a range of petrissage movements can be carried out.
Frictions	Yes	Yes	Using the edge of the stone, rub it back and forth to create friction. Work across the fibres of the muscles.
Tapping (**piezoelectric**)	Yes	No	The effects created by this movement are similar to the vibrations used in Swedish massage, but they are much more profound and create an excellent rippling effect out across the muscle fibres. One stone is held and stays in contact with the body and the second stone is tapped on top of it. This technique is noisy but very therapeutic, creating vibrations deep into the muscle, and is ideal for tension nodules. It is also excellent for stimulating the lymphatic system.

Technique	Use with hot stones?	Use with cold stones?	Application
Tucking	Yes	No	Once the stones have been used and have started to cool, they are tucked under the client's body to deliver warmth to an area. This prevents them losing too much contact with the body by being removed and placed on another surface. Tucking should be a smooth action, sliding the stone into place under the body once it is no longer required.
Placement	Yes	Yes	This can be used as a method of relaxation at the start of the treatment. This is a technique used to warm the muscles before the treatment begins. The stones are placed directly onto the client. The client may lie on the stones – with their skin protected by a sheet or pillowcase placed on the body.
	Yes	No	When using hot stones, they may be placed directly in contact with the skin, such as in between the fingers and toes, or in the hands.
Trigger points	Yes	Yes	By using the rounded point of a hot stone and pressing into an area of tension or a nodule within muscles, tension can be alleviated. The client should take a breath in, then the stone is pressed into the area of tension while they breathe out and held there for 30–90 seconds.

Adapt massage technique

The treatment objectives of stone therapy are:

- relaxation and a sense of well-being
- reduction of joint and muscle pain
- invigoration and uplifting
- improvement of skin and body condition
- anti-cellulite.

It is important that massage movements are adapted to suit the client's treatment objectives, unless it is a signature treatment following a set routine. The selection and use of stones will depend on the client's requirements. Some general guidance is given below.

Treatment objective	Adaptation of treatment
Relaxation and sense of well-being	Use long slow effleurage strokes, slow petrissage. Use more hot stones. Emphasise placement of stones to calm and relax. More time can be spent on the face and head or feet during placement to enhance relaxation depending on the client's preference.
Reduction of joint and muscle pain	Placement of cold stones will reduce inflammation and desensitise the nerve endings, reducing pain. Work around the joint with alternating hot and cold stones using slow draining movements. You could also incorporate joint mobility around the wrist and ankle to help. Muscular pain responds well to placement on trigger points.
Invigoration and uplifting	Keep strokes brisk but still continuous. Use more cold stones, particularly around the face and scalp. Increase frictions and tapping to invigorate.
Improvement of skin and body conditions	Choose an appropriate oil specific to the client's needs so that they feel their skin and body are benefiting from their treatment. Frictions and petrissage will help to exfoliate the skin even with the oil.
Anti-cellulite	Alternating hot and cold stones to stimulate the circulation and lymph. Deep massage over the cellulite – be cautious as hard fat/cellulite can be quite painful to massage deeply. Frictions will help to increase the circulation.

VALUES & BEHAVIOURS

Flexible working attitudes

INDUSTRY TIP

Remember that the heat from the stones will increase the absorption of any product that they are used with. Caution should be taken with oils that have ingredients that may aggravate the skin. Most clients will benefit purely from a base oil and the thermal and **cryo** effects.

Cryo

Icy cold.

HANDY HINT

Is it affect or effect?

Affect – verb, to influence or make a difference or make a change.

 The client was *affected* by the poor treatment.

Effect – noun and verb. The noun means a change that is a result or consequence of something. The verb means to bring about a change.

 The client was really pleased with the *effect* of her treatment.

 You must *effect* these changes at once.

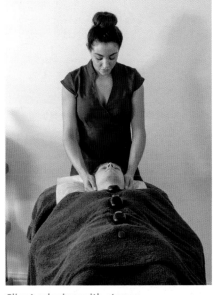

Client relaxing with stones

Client group	Suggested adaptations/modifications to treatment
Elderly	The client may have impaired senses and possibly poor circulation, so monitor the temperature of the stones carefully. Skin may be thin with a lack of subcutaneous tissue, so avoid deeper movements, and always use light pressure. Avoid tapping due to possible changes in the bone structure (joint stiffness, arthritis, osteoporosis).
Overweight	Use deeper pressure, more vigorous movements, petrissage and tapping. If the client is obese they should be advised against treatment, as the body may not be able to cope with the heat effectively. There may also be difficulty in locating trigger points.
Underweight	Use lighter pressure over bony areas. Avoid tapping and be cautious with trigger points; there may not be adequate muscle tissue to use this technique comfortably. Techniques will need to be fine-tuned and kept delicate due to lack of adipose tissue. Use extra covers to keep the client warm.
Good muscle tone	There will be firm, well-toned muscles and skin and the client will be within a normal weight range. All massage techniques can be used, in particular friction and trigger points. Use firm, deep movements. Alternating hot and cold stones will be very beneficial.
Poor muscle tone	Both muscles and skin tissue may be of poor tone. Try to gradually lead in to a state of relaxation, gently stretching the muscles with the stones. Avoid any wringing if there is loose skin. Use deeper movements over large areas and incorporate tapotement and petrissage. Gentle tapping will help to stimulate the muscles.

Activity

Imagine that a muscular male athlete, an elderly woman and an overweight client all wish to have a stone therapy massage. Think about how you would adapt your massage in order to meet the clients' needs and make sure that they remain comfortable throughout the treatment.

Stone placement

Stone placement is a popular way to relax the client. Seven stones are placed at the chakra points of the body, and semi-precious stones are placed in between them. As well as relaxing them, this also helps to rebalance the client.

Chakra name	Location	Colour
1 Crown	Top of the head	Purple
2 Third eye/Ajna	Middle of the forehead centred above the eyebrows	Indigo
3 Throat	Middle of the throat at the neck, above the collar bone	Blue/ turquoise
4 Heart	Centre of the chest, by the heart	Green
5 Solar plexus	Below the sternum	Yellow
6 Sacral	Below the navel	Orange
7 Root/base	Base of spine/lower pelvic area	Red

Spinal layout

Ask the client to lie on the couch in a supine position. Wrap the client in a sheet and cover them with an additional towel or cover if required.

Tell the client that they must tell you during treatment if any of the stones you are using are too hot or uncomfortable in their placement or application. Collect the spinal layout stones from the heater and place on a towel.

Place the 16 spinal layout stones in position, tucking the butterfly stones that will sit under the sacrum into the pillowcase.

The spinal stones consist of:

■ four narrow stones which sit in a butterfly shape under the sacral lower back area

■ four round, thick stones which sit under the lumbar region (latissimus dorsi muscle) of the back

■ four smaller, round stones that are a bit flatter in shape and sit under the ribs (top of the latissimus dorsi)

■ four narrow, oblong-shaped stones which sit under the upper back (under the rhomboid muscles)

■ one oblong stone which can be placed behind the neck, inside a sock for comfort if desired.

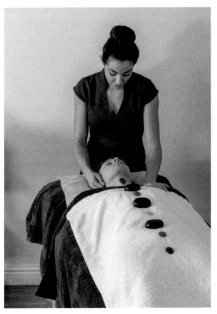

A client with chakra stones positioned on them

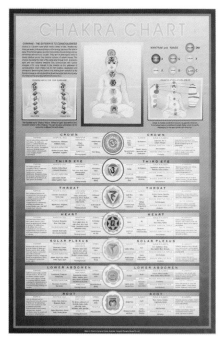

An example of a chakra chart

Help the client to lie down onto their back and onto the stones, which should be carefully positioned for comfort. They should lie on the stones for between 10 and 30 minutes. Reassure the client that this should be a pleasant sensation. Adjust any stones as required so that the client is lying comfortably.

Offer the client the hand stones to hold – you may also like to place stones between the toes and fingers.

You can now either place chakra stones, or treat an area on the front of the body. For a back treatment the client may be left to relax on the stones and benefit from the deep tissue warmth before turning them over to massage the back.

Chakra placement

Stand on the left-hand side of the couch. You can use either precious stones for the placement, or hot and cold stones. It is recommended that cold stones are not used on their own for this treatment, but are mixed with hot stones.

- Start with the first chakra and work in a clockwise direction, creating a semicircle in between each chakra point and the next.
- Think of each chakra flower opening and envisage the correct chakra colour (see page 565), then slowly slide the stone into place.
- Lift the hand with a semicircular movement in a clockwise direction to the next chakra point.
- Continue until all the chakra stones are in position.

You can leave your client to relax for a few minutes if you are doing a relaxation treatment. If you are doing a back treatment you can begin to massage around the neck and décolletage.

If you are doing a full-body stone therapy treatment, you will start the treatment on the client's right leg (the one on your left as you stand at the foot of the couch). Once the spinal placement treatment and/or treatment of the front of the body is complete, you should always remember to close the chakras to keep the energy in. This is done by simply reversing the sequence you performed to open the chakras. Start with the crown chakras and take your hand in an anticlockwise direction, while picturing the chakra flow closing. As you work down the rest of the chakras, place your hand on top for a moment and then slide and slowly lift the stone from the body. You should finish with the heart chakra.

On completion of the treatment, gather up any tucked stones and remove them to the trolley. Remove any placement stones. Let the client know that the treatment is complete.

Stone therapy treatment routine

Below is a suggested stone therapy routine. There are many different versions and you may be taught something different – this is only for guidance.

A stone therapy treatment will be flowing and will use a range of techniques. You should maintain contact between stone and skin as much as possible. Your treatment should be seamless while you adjust or arrange stones. Be aware of noise and keep movement of the stones to a minimum.

Treatment timing

A full stone therapy treatment will take between 75 and 90 minutes to carry out. A back treatment on its own will take 45 minutes.

Suggested sequence

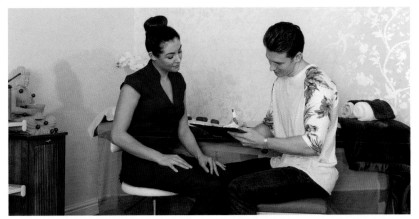

Carry out a full consultation and fully explain the treatment process to the client. Agree the treatment objectives and plan and gain the client's consent.

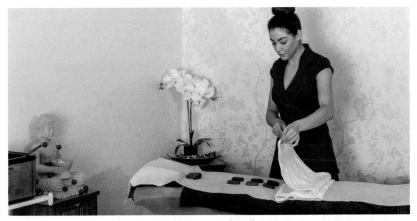

Carefully position your spinal layout on the couch. Cover the stones with a towel or sheet as they should not be in direct contact with the client's skin. This is to prevent any risk of skin burning as the heat can sometimes build up when left in a static position.

Routine for *supine* position

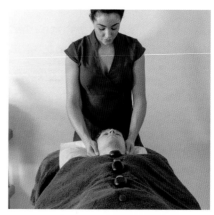

STEP 1 Assist the client onto the couch in a sitting position, then guide the client onto the spinal layout. Make sure the stones are positioned correctly and are comfortable. Tuck a flat stone behind the neck. Give the client the hand stones to hold. Place a bolster under the knees to help support the client's lower back.

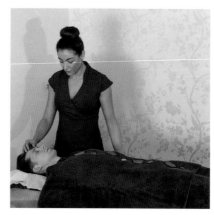

STEP 2 Position the chakra layout first, then place the hot stones between each chakra.

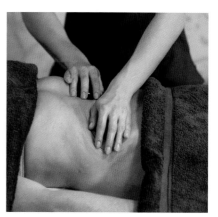

STEP 3 While the client is relaxing on the spinal layout, begin the massage working around the décolleté, shoulders and upper arms. Massage each arm, applying oil with effleurage and then working the area with the stones.

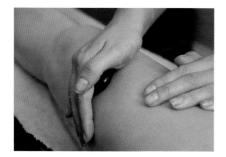

STEP 4 Leaving the chakra stones in place, massage the leg. Effleurage to start and to apply oil. Work in a logical sequence starting at the top of the thigh, around the knee, lower leg and then foot.

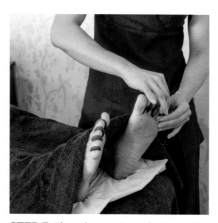

STEP 5 Place the toe stones between the toes. If only performing a back treatment, leave the client to relax for 10–20 minutes before turning the client over.

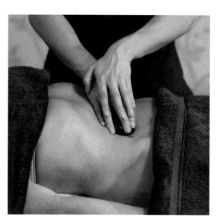

STEP 6 If treating the abdomen, apply oil with effleurage. Work gently to avoid discomfort.

INDUSTRY TIP

Always introduce your oils after effleuraging with the back or side of the hand, then slide with the stone so that the client becomes accustomed to the application. Never just place a hot stone on the skin. Hot stones should never be applied in a static position unless they have a towel or sheet between them and the client's skin; the exception is when you tuck stones which have been used during treatment and have cooled slightly as a result.

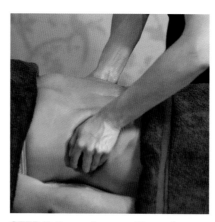

STEP 7 Remember, as with regular massage, to work across the abdomen.

STEP 8 Or massage in a clockwise direction (to assist digestion).

Routine for *prone* position

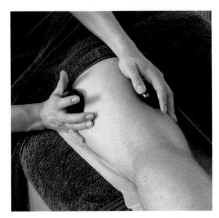

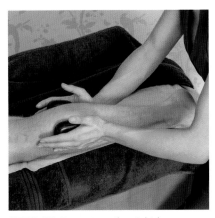

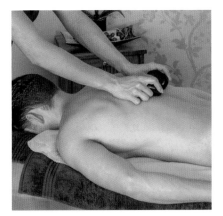

STEP 9 Start with the left leg. Follow a similar sequence to the front of the leg. Apply oil with effleurage and then work from the upper leg to the lower leg using a range of appropriate techniques.

STEP 10 Repeat on the right leg.

STEP 11 Apply a liberal amount of oil with effleurage to the back. This will give you a large area to work on and you will be able to apply a range of techniques to suit the client's needs. Be cautious around the spinal column and avoid working too deeply around the kidney area.

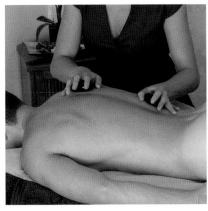

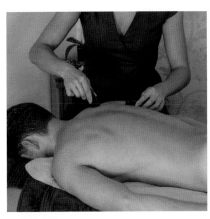

Watch the video of this stone therapy treatment on SmartScreen (unit 320).

STEP 12a

STEP 12b

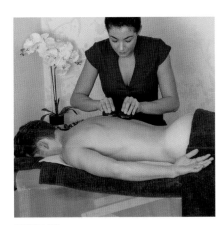

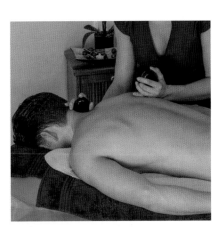

STEP 12c

STEP 12d

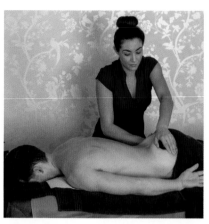

STEP 13 Make sure you include the top of the gluteals as this can be beneficial for relaxing the back; these muscles often get very tight. You may also like to include a scalp treatment to finish.

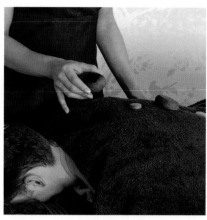

STEP 14 Finally apply your chakra closing balancing technique. You should allow the client to relax for one minute to allow the energy to be centered and balanced. After this time carefully remove hot stones gently tapping each stone upon removal. Then remove the chakra layout starting from the base chakra.

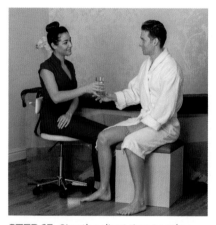

STEP 15 Give the client time to relax before helping them to sit up. Give them a glass of water and go through advice and recommendations.

Provide advice, recommendations and evaluate the treatment

Following the treatment you should give the client suitable personalised advice to follow. Think about the treatment you have just given and the effects that the client will experience. This will help to maximise the benefits the client gets from the treatment.

Remember to follow up with any recommendations you can give the client on lifestyle changes, postural awareness, skin care, products and further treatment.

In addition to the advice you will find in the massage chapter, clients should be advised to avoid UV after treatment. As the skin will be preheated, it will increase the risk of sunburn.

> **Activity**
>
> Review any lifestyle changes that you might discuss with the client as part of advice and recommendations. This might include a change in dietary habits or increasing activity levels. Make sure the client is aware of the benefits of any advice you give to encourage them to take up your recommendations.

Contra-actions

For detailed information about contra-actions, refer to chapter 303.

Burns

Burns are a particular consideration when offering stone therapy. They should never occur, but can happen if you:

✗ fail to check and monitor the temperature of the heater or do not use one with a thermostat

✗ apply placement stones directly to the skin without protection

✗ don't check the temperature of the stones before application.

Make sure to consider all of the above when offering a professional treatment to avoid injury to your client.

For information on client feedback and evaluation, see the Values and behaviours chapter.

Answers at the back of the book.

1 Marble stones are made of which of the following?
   a Calcium carbonate
   b Calcium silicate
   c Calcium phosphate
   d Calcium nitrate

2 Which of the following is not a benefit of cold stones?
   a Stimulation of digestion
   b Reduced pain
   c Reduced inflammation
   d Enhanced mental stimulation

3 A cool box is used for which of the following stones?
   a Basalt and marble
   b Semi-precious and basalt
   c Marine and basalt
   d Marine and marble

4 Which one of the following describes a trigger point?
   a An area of tension knots
   b The crown chakra
   c The largest stone
   d The heater on/off switch

5 What is the maximum temperature a stone heater should reach?
   a 25°C
   b 37°C
   c 50°C
   d 60°C

6 Which of the following can be used to carry out a thermal sensitivity test?
   a Hot and cold stones
   b Cotton bud and cold stone
   c Orange stick and cotton bud
   d Orange stick and hot stone

7 Where is the third eye located?
   a The feet
   b The chest
   c The stomach
   d The head

8 Which one of the following stones will remain cold the longest?
   a Basalt
   b Marble
   c Jade
   d Slate

9 How long does a full stone therapy treatment take?
   a 60 minutes
   b 75 minutes
   c 30 minutes
   d 95 minutes

10 Which one of the following stones holds heat the longest?
   a Basalt
   b Marble
   c Jade
   d Marine

TEST YOUR KNOWLEDGE ANSWERS

Values and behaviours

1 a,	2 d,	3 a,	4 b,	5 b,
6 c,	7 d,	8 a,	9 b,	10 b

Health and safety legislation

1 d,	2 b,	3 d,	4 c,	5 a,
6 d,	7 a,	8 c,	9 b,	10 d

301 Promote and sell products and services to clients

1 b,	2 d,	3 c,	4 c,	5 b,
6 d,	7 c,	8 c,	9 b,	10 a

302 Anatomy and physiology

1 a,	2 a,	3 b,	4 c,	5 d,
6 a,	7 c,	8 d,	9 d,	10 d,
11 a,	12 d,	13 a,	14 d,	15 a,
16 c,	17 a,	18 a,	19 b,	20 c,
21 d,	22 c,	23 c,	24 c,	25 c

303 Provide body massage

1 c,	2 b,	3 b,	4 d,	5 c,
6 d,	7 b,	8 c,	9 a,	10 d

304 Provide facial electrotherapy treatments

1 c,	2 a,	3 b,	4 d,	5 d,
6 a,	7 d,	8 c,	9 a,	10 b

305 Provide body electrotherapy treatments

1 b,	2 c,	3 c,	4 a,	5 c,
6 c,	7 b,	8 b,	9 a,	10 b

307 Provide electrical epilation

1 a,	2 d,	3 a,	4 a,	5 c,
6 b,	7 c,	8 d,	9 a,	10 c

308 Provide Indian head massage

1 d,	2 c,	3 d,	4 d,	5 c,
6 a,	7 c,	8 a,	9 c,	10 d

309 Tanning treatments

1 c,	2 d,	3 b,	4 b,	5 c,
6 d,	7 c,	8 b,	9 c,	10 b

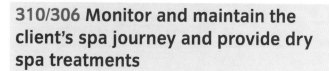

310/306 Monitor and maintain the client's spa journey and provide dry spa treatments

1 c,	2 d,	3 b,	4 a,	5 c,
6 a,	7 c,	8 a,	9 a,	10 c,
11 c,	12 d,	13 a,	14 c,	15 d,
16 b,	17 c,	18 a,	19 b,	20 d

311 Provide individual semi-permanent lash treatments

1 c,	2 a,	3 b,	4 b,	5 c,
6 c,	7 c,	8 a,	9 c,	10 c

320 Provide body stone therapy treatments

1 a,	2 a,	3 d,	4 a,	5 c,
6 a,	7 d,	8 b,	9 b,	10 a

INDEX

NOTES

THE CITY & GUILDS TEXTBOOK